Textbook of
Orthopaedic Nursing

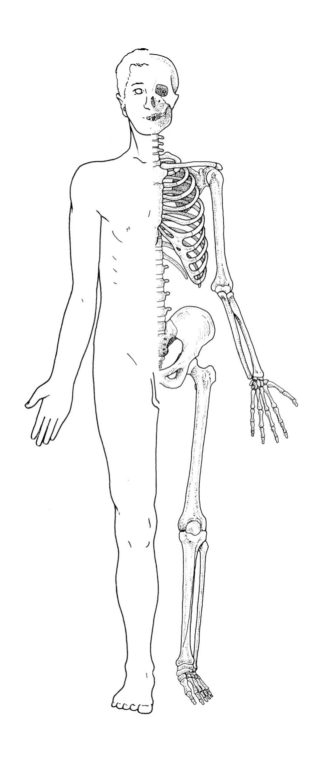

Textbook of
Orthopaedic Nursing

by

ROBERT ROAF

M.A., B.Ch., M.Ch.Orth., F.R.C.S., F.R.C.S.E., L.R.C.P., D.Obstet., R.C.O.G.
Emeritus Professor of Orthopaedic Surgery, University of Liverpool; Consultant
Orthopaedic Surgeon to the United Liverpool Hospitals and The Robert Jones
and Agnes Hunt Orthopaedic Hospital, Oswestry, Shropshire

and

LEONARD J. HODKINSON

S.R.N., R.N.T, O.N.C., F.R.S.H.
Regional Nurse (Professional Education and Development)
Northern Regional Health Authority
Formerly Principal Tutor at The Robert Jones and Agnes Hunt Orthopaedic
Hospital, Oswestry, Shropshire

THIRD EDITION

BLACKWELL SCIENTIFIC PUBLICATIONS
OXFORD LONDON EDINBURGH
MELBOURNE

© 1980 by
Blackwell Scientific Publications
Editorial offices:
Osney Mead, Oxford, OX2 OEL
8 John Street, London, WC1N 2ES
9 Forrest Road, Edinburgh, EH1 2QH
214 Berkeley Street, Carlton
    Victoria 3053, Australia

First published 1971
Second edition 1975
Third edition 1980

Printed and bound in
Great Britain by
William Clowes (Beccles) Ltd
Beccles and London

DISTRIBUTORS

USA
    Blackwell Mosby Book Distributors
    11830 Westline Industrial Drive
    St Louis, Missouri 63141

Canada
    Blackwell Mosby Book Distributors
    86 Northline Road, Toronto
    Ontario, M4B 3E5

Australia
    Blackwell Scientific Book Distributors
    214 Berkeley Street, Carlton
    Victoria 3053

British Library
Cataloguing in Publication Data

Roaf, Robert
    Textbook of orthopaedic nursing.
        3rd ed.
    1. Orthopedic nursing
    I. Title II. Hodkinson, Leonard John
    610.73'677   RD753
    ISBN 0-632-00473-8

Contents

SECTION D Practical Management of the Orthopaedic Patient

Section A

Science of Orthopaedics

1

Scope of Modern Orthopaedics

Introduction

The word *orthopaedic* was devised by a French surgeon, Nicolas Andry in 1743. It has two roots derived from the Greek words: *Orthos* = straight, and *Paedios* = of a child. Thus the term 'orthopaedic' implies 'to straighten a child'.

History and orthopaedics

To examine the background to the coining of such a word. During the eighteenth and nineteenth centuries standards of living for many people throughout Europe were very low. Poverty coupled with malnutrition, bad communal hygiene and drunkenness made our cities, as well as the urban and rural areas, breeding grounds for the diseases associated with malnutrition and low standards of hygiene.

Tuberculosis was prevalent; it was spread either by inhalation in the over-crowded ill-ventilated slum dwellings, or by ingestion, being swallowed in polluted milk. Tubercular infection commonly resulted in the destruction of bones and joints.

Infections of all varieties spread easily through a vulnerable people. They commonly caused osteomyelitis and suppurative arthritis with resultant severe crippling deformities.

Avitaminosis D due to ignorance and related poverty with malnutrition caused bending and bowing of bones, particularly in infancy; the deformed infant eventually became the crippled adult.

Poliomyelitis, or rather its childhood form (that is, infantile paralysis), was endemic. Most town-dwelling children were infected early in life and would either recover and gain resistance to it, die from it, or survive with varying degrees of paralysis from mild weakness of a muscle or muscle groups, to complete paraplegia or tetraplegia.

There were many other diseases which were always present in a latent form but would periodically flair up as epidemics in the population, affecting and destroying large numbers of people. The four diseases, avitaminosis D, osteomyelitis, poliomyelitis and tuberculosis were, however, the main cause of the conditions which produced orthopaedic problems. All left severe deformities which remained for the rest of the victim's life. Thus the cities were filled with children and adults who were crippled and deformed; because they were handicapped and limited in their function they were unable to work and earn; because they were unable to earn they had to beg. Thus the vicious circle of begging related to disease continued.

To add to the miseries of the sick-poor there was a lack of welfare facilities and adequate treatment. Such treatment existing was empirical and often based on false assumption rather than scientific facts. There were no such things as antibiotics, chemotherapy, blood transfusion or even efficient surgical technique. The work of Lister and Pasteur had not begun, knowledge of the basis of inflammation, of sepsis, and the relationship between micro-organisms and diseases was unknown.

Although there were many charitable organizations at work attempting to help the beggars and the cripples, their work represented only a small fraction of the effort needed to overcome the plight of the disabled-poor. It was not until the later years of the nineteenth century that any adequate action was taken in the treatment of these diseases.

Towards the end of the nineteenth century there was initiated a strong altruistic movement to care for and treat the handicapped and the disabled. It was from this movement that the present welfare facilities originated. This was a time when many surgical homes and orthopaedic hospitals were founded. They removed the slum child with disability or disease from a city environment to an atmosphere of fresh air, sunlight, good feeding, and freedom from worry about money and finding food. They also provided rest, prolonged, enforced and uninterrupted, under medical and nursing supervision.

Orthopaedic pioneers

There were many pioneers of this movement to help the orthopaedic disabled; so many that it is probably unfair to refer to those who have gained most notice through their biographers. The two who are still considered the founders of the modern practice of orthopaedics and orthopaedic surgery, however, deserve special mention. They were Hugh Owen Thomas and his wife's nephew, Robert Jones.

Hugh Owen Thomas (1843–1891). Hugh Owen Thomas was the last of a line of bone-setters from the island of Anglesey in North Wales. His forebears had practised a form of folk medicine, the experience of which was passed on from father to son through many generations. They treated both men and animals and were renowned for their ability to set broken bones and reduce dislocated joints. In doing this they developed many practical procedures and forms of splinting which were efficient and effective. Hugh Owen Thomas was not only experienced in these arts, he was also a qualified

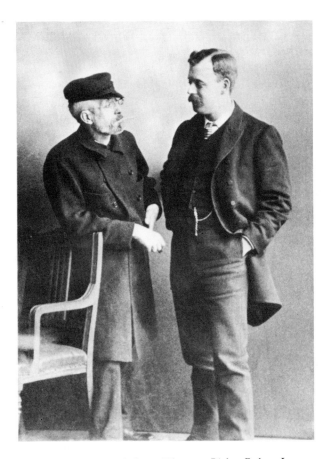

Fig. 1.1   *Left*—Hugh Owen Thomas; *Right*—Robert Jones.
(By permission of the President and Council of Liverpool Medical Institute.)

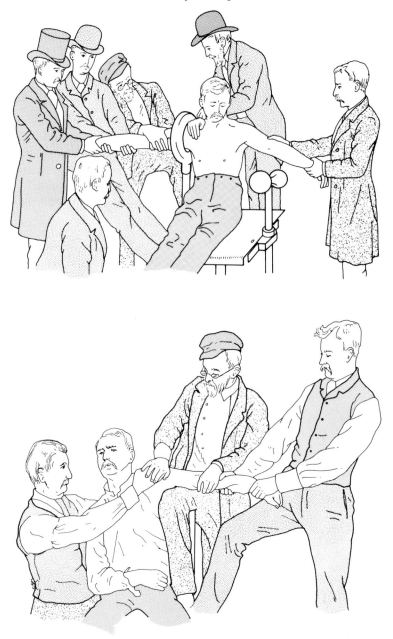

Fig. 1.2   Line drawings of activities at 11 Nelson Street, Liverpool, in the last century, showing reduction of late dislocations of the shoulder. Both Hugh Owen Thomas and Robert Jones are represented.

doctor with a medical degree from Edinburgh University. He was thus able to bring the abilities of the bone-setters into his medical practice; with his medical qualification his teachings and principles were acceptable to other members of the medical profession.

He practised at 11 Nelson Street, Liverpool. He was a busy general practitioner who was not restricted only to the care of orthopaedic patients. Probably the best known feature of his way of life was the free Sunday morning clinic. This was for the poor of the city of Liverpool. Most of the patients who attended were sufferers from skeletal tuberculosis, rickets and other chronic bone diseases, malunited fractures and other results of accidents which were common in the seaport of Liverpool.

Sir Robert Jones (1857–1933). Robert Jones came to live at the home of his uncle and aunt at 11 Nelson Street, Liverpool in 1873 at the age of sixteen years. From then on he was imbued with the principles and ideals of Hugh Owen Thomas. When qualified as a surgeon, he was able to advance still further the practices and principles of Hugh Owen Thomas, particularly when he served as a consultant to the accident service of the Manchester Ship Canal when it was under construction. Later he was Inspector of Military Orthopaedics to the British and Commonwealth armies of the 1914–18 War.

He was endowed with a warm personality which enabled him to establish good relationships with everyone whom he met. He was thus a major factor in gaining acceptance of 'orthopaedics' as an important branch of medicine when previously it had been a minor neglected part of the profession.

These two men were the true founders of the practice of orthopaedics.

Orthopaedics today

The days of empirical treatment and bone-setting with treatment in open air long-stay hospitals have now passed. Today the treatment of affections of the bones, joints, muscles and nerves is based on knowledge gained by research and has advanced alongside all the other branches of medicine and surgery. No longer can the practice of orthopaedics be considered the 'empire' of one individual surgeon. Today the team in the treatment of skeletal conditions includes members of other branches of medicine and science all pooling their knowledge for the general welfare of the patient. The team will include:

1 *The orthopaedic surgeon.* He is the specialist in disorders affecting the

locomotor system. Usually he will be entirely responsible for the patient's treatment: at other times he will call for help from others with special knowledge. He is the leader of the team.

2   *The anaesthetist*. Orthopaedic treatment has moved steadily towards surgical intervention in more cases than ever before. Such an approach leads to more rapid recovery than was possible in the early days of orthopaedic care. In addition to giving the highly technical anaesthetics required at operation, the anaesthetist plays his part in the management of patients with multiple injuries, particularly with crush injuries of the thorax when special ventilation equipment is required for the survival of the patient.

3   *The traumatologist*. This is usually an orthopaedic surgeon with a keen interest in the management of severely injured people. Multiple injuries are caused by the fast transport accidents that are the hazards of modern living. He makes the many rapid decisions which are necessary for the survival of the patient before the arrival of specialists in particular facets of patient care, e.g. the *neurological surgeon* for head injuries; the *thoracic surgeon* for chest injuries; the *ophthalmologist* for injuries to the eye; the *otolaryngologist* for injuries to the throat, nose and ear; the *gynaecologist* for injuries to the female genital organs; the *abdominal surgeon* for injuries to the abdominal organs.

4   *The nurse*. Good management of orthopaedic patients calls for dedicated nursing care. The nurse is the person who spends most time with the patient. She is the one who can give the most efficient report on changes in his condition and is his mainstay during the worst phases of his illness. Without good nursing, no surgical care is possible.

5   *The physiotherapist*. In all aspects of patient care physiotherapy is required; more than in any other branch of medicine the orthopaedic patient requires the full attention of a physiotherapist. She is mainly responsible for full restoration of function of muscles, joints and nerves in the rehabilitation period. She can also do a great deal for the patient at all stages of his illness.

6   *The occupational therapist*. She is a specialist in enabling the patient to gain full recovery of function through active use of mechanical equipment such as fret-saws, printing presses and other machinery. She does more than this however. The occupational therapist can do much to enable the patient to adapt to living with a disability by the development of new skills and the assistance of various aids to daily routines.

7   *The radiologist and radiographer*. Without these valuable members of the team, diagnosis and many forms of surgical and other treatment would not be possible.

8   *The pathologist*. Blood chemistry, blood transfusion, accurate histological and bacteriological diagnoses and the resulting specific treatment depend upon this member of the team and his staff.

9   *The physician*. It is realized more and more that conditions such as rheumatoid arthritis are the responsibility of both physician and orthopaedic surgeon.

10   *The pharmacist* and with him the many pharmaceutical firms who provide research into drug therapy. The use of antibiotics, chemotherapeutic drugs, analgesics and the many other medications in the armamentarium of the pharmaceutical department play a major part in the treatment of the orthopaedic patient.

This list could continue but the process would be tedious for the reader. The social worker, the dietician, the chaplain, the splint maker and other engineering staff are all worthy of mention, as all contribute to the treatment of the patient.

The practice of orthopaedics has moved far away from the days when patients were fixed to a spinal frame or plaster bed for an indefinite period of years. Hospitalization and nursing care is a costly process; patients cannot afford to be away from their place of work, nor can the State afford the large sums which are needed if patients are away from work for a long time. A prolonged stay in an institution is detrimental psychologically as well as demoralizing.

The treatment of the patient must therefore be a specific regime which will return him to his normal environment in the shortest possible time. This means the full use of all the facilities provided by surgical and scientific progress. It may mean gaining advice and help from engineering consultants, chemists and biologists in order to supply efficient metal joints to replace worn out natural joints; it is necessary to ensure that the metal joint will not be rejected by the body and will be of the best design for its prolonged function. Orthopaedic surgeons now use devices which will hold the cut surfaces of a bone in close apposition while they heal; this can avoid the necessity of embedding the patient in a heavy lump of plaster for months.

The work of the metabolic physician has also affected the outlook of the orthopaedic consultant. If a fracture will not heal or a bone is osteoporotic, he wants to know the dietary or chemical means of overcoming this problem and sends the patient to a metabolic unit where his biochemical disorder can be investigated. There are many other aspects of modern orthopaedic practice which will be discovered by the nurse as she works in this field. She must always be aware, however, of the need to blend the traditional principles of the past with modern advances in techniques which are occurring daily in our hospitals, and be sure that technique does not conquer reason and compassion.

2

Bone Growth and Repair

The nature of bone

Although bone is one of the hardest tissues in the body, the dead, boiled bones of the classroom skeleton give a wrong impression of the true nature of living bones. Bone is a living tissue with all the needs of any living material, these are: respiration; assimilation; excretion; reproduction; response to stimulation.

Respiration. The cells of bone require oxygen for metabolism and give off carbon dioxide which must be removed from their environment. If either process ceases the cells of the bone tissue will die in the same way as any other living tissue.

Assimilation. Nutrition is necessary for growth, replacement of worn cells, and other activities, therefore protein, fat, carbohydrate, water, mineral salts and vitamins must reach the cells of bone in a steady consistent supply.

Excretion. Products of metabolism are being made continually and must be taken away from bone cells and tissues. These include such products as excess water, lactic acid and urea.

Reproduction. During the growth phase, up to the age of sixteen to eighteen years in most people, the bones are increasing both in length and diameter. After growth has ceased new cells must still be produced to replace worn out old ones. This requires a steady process of cell division and the production of new, fresh cells.

Response to stimulation. All tissue reacts to chemical, mechanical, or nervous irritation and bone is no exception. It must repair itself when broken or damaged, respond to increased stresses by improving its strength in given areas, provide protrusions to which muscles are attached, and react in general to the need for increased size and length.

Classification of bone tissue

Bone tissue may be classified as compact or cancellous.

Compact bone tissue. This is the main supporting tissue in every bone. It is greatest in quantity in the shafts of long bones.

It has the important function of providing a strong supporting tissue where it is needed, in the cylindrical shafts of the long bones, for example. Elsewhere it forms the shell of bones which are mainly composed of cancellous bone tissue.

On naked eye inspection it looks dense and devoid of spaces with only entry holes for blood vessels and nerves. Under a microscope however it can be seen to be penetrated by many canals travelling parallel to each other with profuse numbers of communicating branches passing from one canal to another. These canals are for the transmission of blood to and from every cell of the bone and for the passage of nerves to all parts of the bone which make bones sensitive to pain (Fig. 2.1).

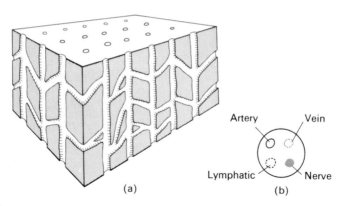

Fig. 2.1   (a) Section of compact bone showing canals carrying blood vessels, nerves and lymphatic vessels. (b) The contents of a haversian canal.

Cancellous bone tissue. In contrast to compact bone, cancellous bone has a great number of spaces in it. When these spaces are empty, for example in deproteinised dead bone, the appearance of the tissue is similar to the filigree work of the jeweller with a great number of spaces between the fine threads of bone.

Functionally it reduces the weight of every bone by replacing the density of compact bone. Cancellous bone however, also has strength. The fine threads are arranged in lines called trabeculae which follow the directions most likely to receive stress in the bone when force is applied (Fig. 2.2).

Throughout the cancellous bone, red bone marrow is found in the space. This is the material from which the erythrocytes of blood are produced.

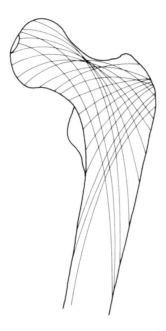

Fig. 2.2   Trabeculae and stress lines.

The formation, ossification and composition of bone

In the fetus and infant, bones ossify, or harden, in one of three ways, depending upon their structure and shape.

1   *Intramembranous ossification*. This occurs in the formation of flat bones such as those of the cranium and scapulae. The bones are first represented in the fetus as two layers of membrane. Between those two layers bone mineral is laid down.

2   *Intracartilaginous ossification*. This type of ossification is seen in the formation of long bones such as those of the limbs. The bones are first represented, in the fetus, by bars of soft cartilage. Within this cartilage bone mineral is laid down.

3   *Sesamoid ossification*. Small bones are formed in muscle tendons.

The unique properties and functions of bones can be most easily understood

*if we first consider the development of a typical long bone as found in the arms
or legs. This will clarify the mechanisms by which bones grow, repair themselves,
alter in shape and adjust to changing circumstances.*

The formation of a typical long bone

The fetus takes 280 days to form; in the earliest days it consists only of a
sphere of cells, called a morulla. These cells increase in number by division
into new cells. At this stage there is no sign of the formation of particular
types of tissues, and clearly there is no bone.

By the end of sixty days, however, the skeleton is formed in cartilage which
has similarities in structure to the hyaline cartilage found on the ends of
mature long bones. From this point ossification begins.

In a typical long bone, which is represented as a bar of soft cartilage at
this stage, a centre of ossification forms in the central point of the bone
shaft. At this centre the cartilage cells enlarge and form up into rows. Lime
salts are then arranged around the line of cells, increasing in quantity until
each cell is entirely surrounded; these cartilage cells then atrophy and are
destroyed. The destroyed cartilage cells are then replaced by bone cells
around which hard ossified matrix impregnated with mineral salts forms.
From this centre the hardening process spreads throughout the bar of
cartilage until most of the cartilage is replaced by bone. Long bones have at
least three such centres of ossification; some have many more (Fig. 2.3).

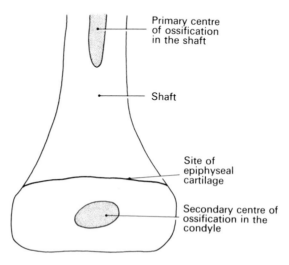

Primary centre
of ossification
in the shaft

Shaft

Site of
epiphyseal
cartilage

Secondary centre of
ossification in the
condyle

Fig. 2.3   Fetal cartilage showing centres of ossification and growth of bone.

So the complicated process of destruction of cartilage and its replacement by bone continues. Within these centres of ossification specialized large bone cells, *osteoblasts*, which build bone, and *osteoclasts* which destroy bone, are active. Enzymes also contribute to this activity. Between them they increase the size of the bone; shape it; make openings for arteries, veins and nerves; carve out the medullary canal and make the spaces in cancellous bone for marrow.

A long bone has three distinct parts during this growing phase—the shaft, or diaphysis, and the two ends, or epiphyses, placed at each end of the shaft (Fig. 2.3). Each of these three parts is separated from the other by a layer of cartilage; this epiphyseal cartilage is essential for the growth, in length, of the bone; it persists until complete growth in height has been achieved by the individual. At the epiphyseal cartilages the growth is active and new layers of bone are deposited at first on either surface of this cartilage, but later on only on the shaft side.

The diameter of the shaft of the bone increases by the presence of osteo-blasts and osteoclasts under the membrane surrounding the bone which is known as the *periosteum*. Here bone is deposited to make the bone thicker and stronger as greater weight must be carried by it.

Down the centre of the shaft, bone is eroded away to make the medullary canal. This passes down the whole length of the bone. It serves to reduce the weight of the bone and convert the shaft into a strong cylinder. This is filled with yellow marrow.

At the ends of the bone, on the surfaces that form synovial joints, a smooth glossy cartilage is laid down.

Classification of types of bones

Bones may be classified as: long; short; irregular; flat; sesamoid.

Long bones
Examples: Humerus, radius, ulna, femur, tibia and fibula.

These are bones with a structure as shown in Fig. 2.4. They form the longest bones of the arms and legs; they must therefore be strong supporting structures. Each bone has a shaft, composed of a cylindrical rod of compact bone (the diaphysis), with a projection at each end of the shaft (the epiphysis), composed mainly of cancellous bone with a thin outer casing of compact bone.

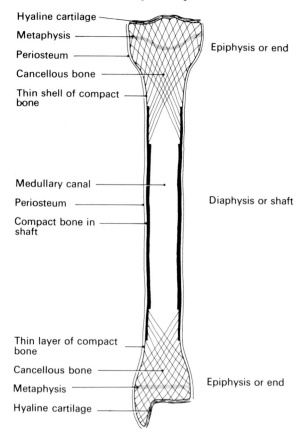

Hyaline cartilage

Metaphysis

Periosteum

Cancellous bone

Thin shell of compact bone

Epiphysis or end

Medullary canal

Periosteum

Compact bone in shaft

Diaphysis or shaft

Thin layer of compact bone

Cancellous bone

Metaphysis

Hyaline cartilage

Epiphysis or end

Fig. 2.4   Longitudinal section through a long bone.

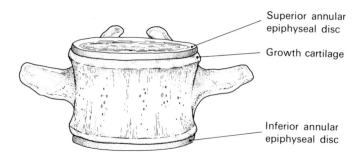

Superior annular epiphyseal disc

Growth cartilage

Inferior annular epiphyseal disc

Fig. 2.5   An anterior view of a vertebra showing the annular epiphyseal discs on the superior and inferior surfaces of the vertebral body.

Short bones and irregular bones

Examples. Short bones—metacarpals, metatarsals and phalanges.

Irregular bones—Vertebrae (Fig. 2.5) and innominate bones.

These are composed mainly of cancellous bone with a thin covering of compact bone.

Flat bones

Examples. Scapula and cranial bones.

These can be so thin that they are translucent. They form between membranes in the fetus and serve to give attachment to muscle groups (the scapula) or to form a protective box for the brain (the cranium).

Sesamoid bones

Example. The patellae.

These are bones which grow in tendons at points where the tendon is subjected to friction as it passes over a bony projection.

Periosteum

Surrounding every bone (except in joints) is a membrane, the periosteum. This is a fibrous covering which has important functions to perform:

(a) It is the means of attachment of muscles, ligaments and joint capsules.

(b) It holds blood vessels onto the surface of the bone to maintain a blood supply and venous return to and from the bone surface.

(c) In the growing phase the special growth cells, osteoblasts, which form new and absorb old bone, are active under the periosteum. They serve to increase the size of the bone on its surface.

Growth of bones

As the child increases in height and weight so must the skeleton. The long bones increase in length and diameter, and other bones grow larger to meet the need for development of all the tissues of the body.

This process of growth commences at birth and continues steadily until the body is completely grown. It is most obviously active however in the early months of life and at puberty when a growth 'spurt' occurs.

Growth occurs in bone:

(a) underneath the periosteum,

(b) at cartilage situated at the junction of the shaft and end of long bones (Fig. 2.3),

(c) in centres of ossification at various sites in all bones (Figs. 2.3 and 2.5),

(d) at special growth plates at the top and bottom of vertebral bodies (Fig. 2.5).

In all these areas of growth in bone, specialized cells, larger and different in microscopic appearance to other bone cells, are situated. They are *osteocytes* and are divided into two classes:

Osteoblasts. These are cells which lay down mineral salts in cartilage in the formation of bone. They increase the bone in diameter and length and form tuberosities on bone.

Osteoclasts. The function of these is to alter the shape of bones by removing redundant bone which is no longer needed.

Conditions affecting bone growth

There are various factors which may adversely affect the activity of the osteocytes. These are infection, excessive radiation (as in radiography or radiotherapy), reduced blood supply, trauma, malnutrition and some diseases of bone such as achondroplasia.

Blood supply to bone

Every bone must have a blood supply; thus, large bones have many nutrient arteries, whilst smaller bones have only one or two (Fig. 2.6a and b).

The nutrient arteries and veins are distributed to a bone:

(a) under the periosteum,

(b) into the centre and bone marrow,

(c) into the ends and protruberances on the bone.

The blood supply to the bone or any part of the bone may be impaired:

(a) if the nutrient artery is blocked or cut,

(b) if the periosteum is damaged,

(c) if a bone is broken or if a fragment is separated from the main body of the bone.

If the blood supply to a bone is interrupted and the bone or a part of it dies, it is called *avascular necrosis*. When seen on radiographs, avascular necrosis usually shows as increased density of the bone.

A poor blood supply is not conducive to healing when a bone has been broken; non-union may be the result.

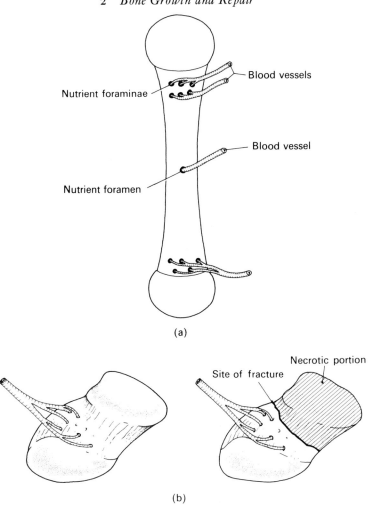

(a)

(b)

Fig. 2.6   (a) Blood supply to long bone. (b) Blood supply to scaphoid bone. *Left*—dorsal aspect showing blood and vessels entering the bone as nutrient arteries. *Right*—the same bone showing how a fracture can cause avascular necrosis.

The nerve supply to bone

An important aspect of our physiology is the awareness that something is damaged or diseased. This is part of the nervous mechanism which reports back to the brain every alteration in pressure or position in our bodies. The bones of the body are involved in this mechanism and every bone is traversed by a network of sensory nerves which are connected to the central nervous system. Thus, damage to a bone by trauma, infection or any other lesion results in pain.

The pain in a bony lesion can be intense. When a bone is broken the disconnected ends tend to grate against each other, causing intense pain (crepitus) until the site of the break is fixed and immobilized. The pain is accompanied by spasm of the muscles related to the bone; this is a form of physiological splinting.

Repair of bone

'Rest, prolonged, enforced and uninterrupted'—this was the maxim of Hugh Owen Thomas who initiated many of the basic orthopaedic principles practised today.

When a bone is broken, some form of immobilization is necessary for the bone to unite effectively. This may take the form of:

(a) *Physiological splintage.* Even in a wild or primitive state animal bones will unite. The beast will slink off to its lair to rest until the repair is advanced. Pain at the site of the fracture will result in:

  (i)   guarding of the limb,
  (ii) avoiding the use of the limb,
  (iii) muscle spasm in the limb,
  (iv) the desire to rest the whole body until some repair has occurred.

Such a process is not conducive to a good repair and the animal will often be left with a deformed and shortened limb. It also occurs in the human body when a fracture goes untreated.

(b) *External orthopaedic splintage.* There are many devices available for the immobilization of a limb (see Chapter 29) which can be applied on the surfaces of the limb.

(c) *Internal fixation of fractures.* The idea that compression stimulates osteogenesis is an old one and it has been employed in joint fixation and arthritis for many years (Key, Charnley). More recently the principle has been employed in the fixation of fractures. It is, however, comparatively difficult to differentiate the effects of compression from the associated effect of firm fixation. Firm fixation is clearly desirable with any operation on a fracture and if the fracture is a transverse one, pressure which ensures that the bone ends are in close contact clearly helps mechanical fixation and ensures there is a smaller gap across which new bone must grow. But whether compression has a further specific osteogenic biological effect is uncertain. Compression devices for fractures (Fig. 2.7) have some disadvantages. In the first place they are relatively bulky, and this may lead to problems of skin closure especially in the tibia. Secondly, the compression force is distributed unequally across the bone, and while one side may be compressed firmly together the opposite side may actually open up (Fig. 2.8). If the compression is too great bone necrosis may occur at the site of compression. One further disadvantage is that there may be interference with the local blood supply in the presence of a strong compression plate. These plates do appear to produce osteoporosis and though the fracture unites it does not fully consolidate and if and when the plate is removed violent use may cause a re-fracture. The same phenomenon is seen if a bone is fixed with two plates.

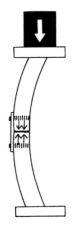

Fig. 2.7 Compression plate on tension side (correct).

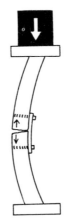

Fig. 2.8 Compression plate on concave surface (incorrect).

There is a considerable amount which is unknown about the ideal biological conditions for rapid union of fractures. Strong rigid plates are certainly invaluable in many conditions, but it is important to remember that final restoration of function ultimately depends on biological factors.

Callus formation

The natural repair of bone is by the formation of new bone around the site of the break in the bone. This new growth of bone is called a *callus*. Callus formation occurs in stages (Fig. 2.9a–d):

1 *Haematoma*. The bone bleeds at its broken ends. The blood collects together in the periosteal sheath or adjacent tissues and serves to fasten the broken ends together. Blood so shed forms into a firm clot.

2 *Fibrous union*. Clotted fibrinated blood results in the connection of the fragments by fibrous soft tissue.

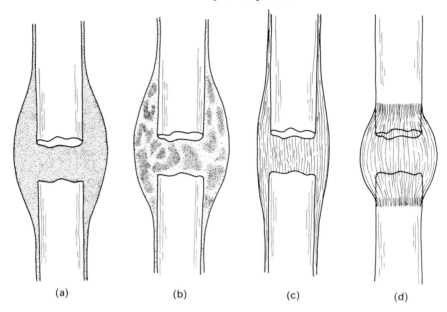

(a)   (b)   (c)   (d)

Fig. 2.9   Series showing callus formation in bone repair. (a) Bleeding from the bone ends into the periosteum. (b) Clotting of the blood and union by congealed blood. (c) Fibrous union by soft fibrous tissue. (d) Formation of hard bony callus.

3   *Bony union.* The fibrous union is invaded by osteocytes which convert the soft tissue into hard bone by depositing mineral salts in it and shaping it. The eventual repair is often stronger than the original bone.

There are factors conducive to good callus formation:

(i)   Efficient immobilization.

(ii)   Freedom from infection at the site of injury.

(iii) Absence of anaemia or other generalized conditions.

(iv) A normal endocrine balance.

(v)   A good dietary intake of all the factors required which make up a balanced diet.

Complications of repair

Callus formation does not always proceed efficiently because:

1   Sometimes nerves are involved in the callus, resulting in paralysis of the muscles distal to the fracture.

2   The callus may be prominent subcutaneously, as in a fracture of the clavicle, giving a poor cosmetic result.

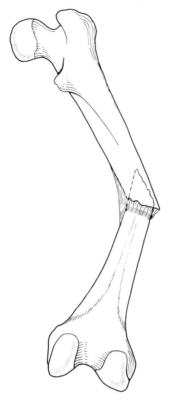

Fig. 2.10   Malunion of bone.

3   The callus may extend to other bones and cause unwanted union with adjacent bones (in fractures of the radius and ulna, for example).

4   The osteocytes may extend their activities beyond the formation of the callus to invade soft tissue, such as the capsule of a joint or adjacent muscle—*myositis ossificans.*

5   Union may not proceed beyond the fibrous stage so that the patient has a soft inefficient fibrous repair.

6   The end result may be a shortened or deformed bone if good alignment of the fragments is not achieved after a fracture (Fig. 2.10).

3

General Considerations of Disease and Deformity

Causes of disease

Ever since mankind started keeping records, there is evidence that people have held theories about the causes of diseases; treatment has often been based on such theories, e.g. if a certain disease was considered to be due to witchcraft, appropriate measures were taken. The ancient Greeks codified such theories into two main groups:

1 That disease, like other human ills, was due to implacable fate. Nowadays 'fate' would be recognized as a super-mathematician who invented the 'laws of probability'.

2 That diseases and ills were due to the malevolent influence of capricious gods and goddesses who could be persuaded to modify their actions by sacrifices, bribes and promises.

Interestingly enough, injuries were not included in this theoretical system, and from early times have been treated on common sense, pragmatic and empirical lines. For this reason the treatment of injuries has usually been of a higher standard than the treatment of diseases, concerning the origin of which erroneous and fallacious theories have so often been held.

In the last hundred years there have been considerable advances in our knowledge of the causes of disease and, in general, most doctors nowadays believe that a diseased condition arises from a multitude of factors acting together—for instance, tuberculous infection may be due to a combination of a congenital abnormality, faulty diet, unhealthy environment, a weak constitution, further weakened perhaps by another infection such as influenza or typhoid, and, at the same time, the patient must have been subjected to close contact with a source of the micro-organism of tuberculosis—e.g. another person or infected milk.

It is, however, traditional to divide causes of disease into *congenital* and *acquired*, and provided one understands that these are not alternatives but often act in combination, it is useful to retain this classification.

Congenital conditions. Congenital causes of disease may be divided into three types:

1   Those due to hereditary factors.
2   Those due to abnormalities of the chromosomes arising either at the time of formation of the gametes, or at the early stages of cell division after fertilization.
3   Abnormalities due to adverse influences acting on the developing fetus, e.g. toxic drugs such as Thalidomide, German measles virus, impairment of the blood supply of the placenta.

The word *congenital* literally means anything with which a child is born and which can be demonstrated at birth; it is not the same as a hereditary state. A hereditary condition may not reveal itself until the patient is middle-aged in some instances.

Acquired conditions. It is customary to divide acquired causes of disease into traumatic, infectious, toxic, dietetic, endocrine, degenerative, metabolic and neoplastic. Again, these sub-divisions are not exclusive and indeed, the development of a neoplasm, for instance, may be due to a combination of genetic, endocrine, toxic and infectious factors. Perhaps the most helpful way to look at the causation of disease is to realize that many factors may be involved which may be added together and, acting in combination, produce the diseased state.

Deformities

Deformities may be due to misshapen bones, distortion of joints, or a combination of the two. Bones may be misshapen due to derangement of growth, or to injuries or to destruction, e.g. by infections or tumours. Joints may be distorted either due to softening of the joint capsule, unequal muscle pull, fibrosis and scarring of adjacent tissues, including muscles, skin and joint capsule, or due to injuries. If the joint is so distorted that the articular surfaces are no longer in contact, it is said to be *dislocated*; if the relationship of the articular surfaces is abnormal but they are still in contact with each other, the joint is said to be subluxated.

Repair of bone

After a fracture, the gap between the bone ends and the surrounding tissue is filled with a blood clot or haematoma, into which primitive connective tissue cells and blood vessels grow (Fig. 2.9, page 22). These primitive connective tissue cells turn into bone-forming cells (osteoblasts) and, at the same time, a network of collagen fibres is laid down by fibroblasts. Bone salts are deposited in and around the collagen fibres by the osteoblasts and this leads to the replacement of the blood clot first by immature fibrous tissue and then by true bone. At the same time a certain amount of cartilage is formed; this normally becomes replaced by bone (Fig. 2.9). Under adverse conditions, e.g. poor blood supply, infection, excessive movement, the normal process of bone repair may be disturbed, leading either to the formation of mature fibrous tissue (fibrous union) or of cartilaginous tissue (pseudarthrosis).

Once the fracture has been united by bone, reshaping and remodelling of the new bone (callus) occurs in accordance with the mechanical stresses to which the bone is subjected. In general, strong bone is produced where a bone is subjected to considerable force, and bone which is not subjected to mechanical stress becomes porotic or is removed. Remodelling of bone in accordance with mechanical forces in particular increases where it is subjected to greater pressure and this is known as Wolf's law.

The normal locomotor system

Movement of the human body is carried out by muscles controlled by the nervous system, causing the bony skeleton to move at its many joints (Fig. 3.1). In good health this process is free from pain and extreme effort and

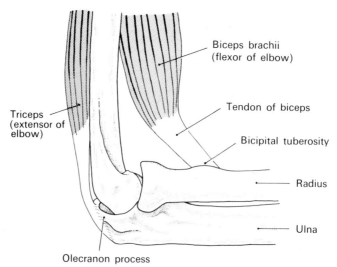

Biceps brachii
(flexor of elbow)

Tendon of biceps

Triceps
(extensor of
elbow)

Bicipital tuberosity

Radius

Ulna

Olecranon process

Fig. 3.1   Muscles controlling the elbow joint.

the normal body is capable of moving over great distances without distress or severe fatigue.

In those fortunate people who have no physical problems the bones are strong and able to bear weight—the structures of the skeleton grow in proportion to each other; there is no pain in any bone or joint; there is a full range of movement at every joint; muscles pull and relax in co-ordination and there is no paralysis.

The problem of deformity

We tend to think that the normal body is that which we see in a long mirror; normality is, in fact, a matter of comparison with others. A mother may consider her child's body to be perfectly normal until she sees him standing alongside another child; or we may consider our sight or hearing to be normal until they are tested. Most people have some minor defect in their body which they have never noticed or which troubles them so little that they take no action. Even when there is an obvious minor deformity most people live a reasonable life and remain independent of extensive help from others or of aid from appliances such as crutches or wheelchairs.

When a deformity is severely disabling, however, modification to living is necessary. Thus the person with a stiff hip or knee must learn a new way to sit down, or climb stairs, or enter a car or bus. The painful or stiff spine means that lying down in bed can be difficult and any attempt to reach the legs or feet calls for extreme effort. A person with a stiff elbow is unable to attend to the hair, face or reach the mouth to take food or drink with that limb. Paralysis of either upper or lower limbs can create immense problems.

Note that so far there has been no reference to 'patients'. A patient is one who is sick in hospital and under the direct care of a doctor. Many people live, work and earn their living with deformities; they do not go to the doctor with their disability because they have learned to live with it.

Normal posture

Another problem of the disabled person may be that of reaching a state of exhaustion long before a person with no disability. The reason for this is as follows: the upright position of a healthy individual with good posture requires the minimum of muscular effort to support him. The body is supplied with many muscles which work to support an upright structure.

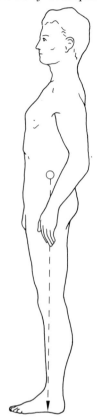

Fig. 3.2   When posture is normal the centre of gravity (represented by the circle on the abdomen of this figure) is centred over the base. If a plumb-line is dropped from the centre of gravity (if this were possible) it would end at a point exactly between the feet.

    Minimum muscular effort is needed to support this posture.

If all the structures are correctly positioned over the base (Fig. 3.2) then no group of muscles must work harder than another in order to keep the body upright. An analogy to explain this is shown in the supporting ropes needed to hold up a radio mast (Fig. 3.3). The four supports are pulling in four different directions; as long as the mast is exactly vertical the ropes are strong enough to hold it. Should (a) the wind pressures in one direction be too great and/or (b) one rope break, the mask will topple over. The muscular arrangement of the body in the upright position is similar—as long as all groups of muscles are balanced and pull together, the posture is good and the body can remain comfortably standing, walking or sitting for a long time.

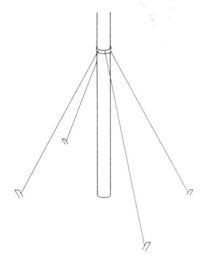

Fig. 3.3   Guy ropes holding mast in position.

Abnormal posture

Abnormal posture may take many forms; one leg may be shorter than the other; one leg may be bent in one direction or another; the spine may have abnormal curves which distort the shape of the trunk, or the spine may be stiff.

The abnormal curves of the spine may be:

(a) *Kyphosis:* This word is derived from the Greek word which means a hill or mountain. This implies therefore that the person has a protrusion on the back (Fig. 3.4). The hump may be of many different sizes or shapes. Such a deformity often reduces the height of the individual and may reduce the size of the thorax or abdomen, causing respiratory or digestive problems for him. He is often cyanosed and has anoxia.

(b) *Lordosis:* This term refers to the stature of the body as the person leans backward in a 'lordly' fashion (Fig. 3.5). Often this individual has a rigid spine which causes him many difficulties.

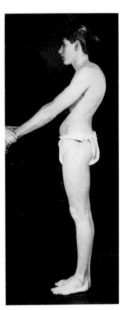

Fig. 3.4   Kyphosis.

(c) *Scoliosis:* This term is derived from the Greek and means 'worm-like'. The spine is bent in one or more curves from side to side (Fig. 3.6, and also 18.3, p. 276). As with the person who has a kyphos of his spine, the volume of thorax and abdomen is often reduced, causing respiratory and digestive problems. The bends in the spine also tend to reduce the height.

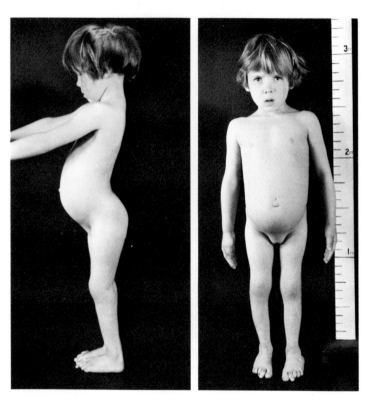

Fig. 3.5   Lordosis.

When the spine is curved abnormally, the trunk is also deformed and muscle balance is disturbed. One group of muscles must pull that much harder than the others and thus becomes fatigued first. This fatigue may take the form of local pain, or exhaustion of the whole body. Distances which can be covered, or work performance may therefore be limited.

Fractures and dislocations

The usual cause of a fracture is, of course, an injury, but if a bone is weakened by disease, a trivial injury may cause it to break—this is known as a patho-

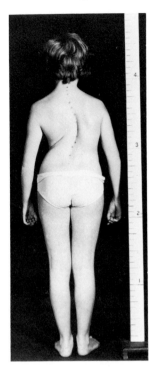

Fig. 3.6   Scoliosis.

logical fracture. Such pathological weakening may be local, e.g. due to infection, or tumour, or generalized as in senile osteoporosis and in the congenital abnormality of fragilitus ossium.

Fractures may be classified in a number of ways, e.g. by the type of injury:

(a) Direct, due to a blow or direct pressure as in a fracture of the os calcis due to a fall from a height.

(b) Indirect, due to strong muscle pull, e.g. a transverse fracture of the patella with separation due to a sudden strong contraction of the quadriceps muscle.

Or fractures may be classified by the shape of the bone fragments, i.e. transverse, oblique, spiral, butterfly, comminuted.

Further, it is important to differentiate between open and closed fractures. In open fractures there is communication between the fracture site and in the surrounding environment. This means that there is a considerable risk of infection being introduced with the likelihood of osteomyelitis and non-union or delayed union.

If there is no wound or no communication between the fracture site and the surrounding environment, the fracture is a closed one; such fractures are often termed 'simple'.

Open fractures are often called 'compound'; unfortunately closed fractures, though often called 'simple' are frequently very complicated. It should be noted that a fracture with a skin laceration which does not communicate with the fracture site is *not* a compound fracture.

4

Endocrine Disorders

There are a group of important organs which are characterized by the fact that they form chemical compounds which are discharged directly into the blood stream. These are sometimes known as ductless glands, as the product of the gland is not discharged along a duct, as for instance, with the salivary glands or pancreas, but is discharged directly into the blood stream. The substances they discharge are known as *hormones*; hormone is the Greek for a messenger, as the hormones take messages to other parts of the body. The glands are sometimes known as endocrine glands. There are six major endocrine glands (Fig. 4.1).

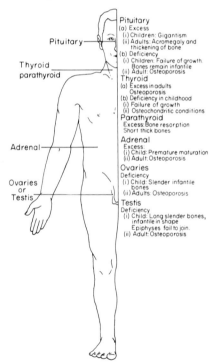

Pituitary
(a) Excess
   (i) Children: Gigantism
   (ii) Adults: Acromegaly and
        thickening of bone
(b) Deficiency
   (i) Children: Failure of growth.
       Bones remain infantile
   (ii) Adult: Osteoporosis
Thyroid
(a) Excess in adults
   Osteoporosis
(b) Deficiency in childhood
   (i) Failure of growth
   (ii) Osteochondritic conditions
Parathyroid
   Excess: Bone resorption
   Short thick bones
Adrenal
   Excess:
   (i) Child: Premature maturation
   (ii) Adult: Osteoporosis
Ovaries
   Deficiency
   (i) Child: Slender infantile
       bones
   (ii) Adults: Osteoporosis
Testis
   Deficiency
   (i) Child: Long slender bones,
       infantile in shape
       Epiphyses fail to join.
   (ii) Adult: Osteoporosis

Pituitary

Thyroid
parathyroid

Adrenal

Ovaries
or
Testis

Fig. 4.1   Situation of endocrine glands with indication of the influence of their hormones on bone growth.

The gonads

Firstly there are the sex glands which are responsible for the characteristic changes which occur in children towards puberty. The growth of hair on the male face, the development of muscle bulk and the characteristic male form, the breaking of the voice, the development of the penis and pubic hair are all dependent on an adequate secretion of the hormone produced by the testis known as *testosterone*. In girls, the secretion of the ovary—namely, *oestrin*, is responsible for the characteristic changes, the growth of the pelvis and breasts, the characteristic female form with an increase of subcutaneous fat and ultimately for the phenomenon of menstruation which is dependent on hormones secreted by the ovary. Lack of sex hormones is one cause of osteoporosis.

Pituitary gland

The most important gland is the pituitary gland which is situated at the base of the brain. This consists of two parts; an anterior lobe which is responsible for the regulation of most of the other endocrine glands—for instance, secretions from the anterior lobe of the pituitary control the sex glands, the adrenals, the pancreas and the thyroid. In addition, the pituitary secretes a hormone which is responsible for growth in length of bones; this is often known as the growth hormone. If there is a deficiency of growth hormone the patient is stunted and the bony epiphyses do not join with the shafts. If, on the contrary, there is excessive secretion of growth hormone in the growing period, the patient becomes abnormally tall, and this is one cause of gigantism. In the mature patient where the epiphyses have already united to the shaft, it is not possible for there to be further growth in length of the bones, but the bones become thickened and in particular the jaw and skull become thickened and enlarged, giving rise to a characteristic appearance. This is called acromegaly.

Pituitary disorders are often due to a tumour of the pituitary gland and this may have other effects, leading to pressure on the optic chiasma and blindness and headaches and, in severe cases, to increased intracranial pressure and disturbance of brain function.

The posterior lobe of the pituitary gland is responsible for the control of renal function through a hormone known as pituitrin, which also causes constriction of blood vessels and contraction of plain muscle, especially the uterine muscle, in addition to inhibition of the formation of urine by the kidneys.

In addition, tumours of the pituitary are often associated with disturbances of the adjacent part of the brain or hypothalamus, and a typical picture of a sub-pituitary child is the fat, slow, rather backward child who tends to sleep a great deal and whose intelligence is below the average; the development of the sex glands is inhibited or delayed.

Thyroid gland

Another very important endocrine gland is the thyroid. The thyroid hormone is known as *thyroxine*. The thyroid gland controls the rate of the body's metabolism, for instance, if there is a deficiency of thyroid, the patient is slow and lethargic; the pulse is slow; the skin is dry and coarse; intelligence is usually below average, the patient feels the cold very severely and tends in general to be slow. In addition, there is a loss of hair and the outer halves of the eyebrows. There may be characteristic changes in the voice which becomes hoarse, and in the vertebral column it is common to find wedge-shaped vertebra in the thoraco-lumbar region. If this condition is severe in childhood it will lead to cretinism, characterized by dwarfing and mental retardation, and in adults will lead to myxoedema with a characteristic facies and appearance.

The opposite condition of excessive thyroid function leads to a rapid pulse, flushing, dilated blood vessels and a rather nervous active temperament which tends to be very emotional. If mild, the condition can be treated medically, but if severe, it is usual to treat the condition surgically by excising the greater part of the thyroid gland.

Parathyroid glands

The parathyroid glands are, from the orthopaedic point of view, probably the most important ductless glands. Their secretion is known as *parathormone*. These are responsible for the rate at which calcium is removed from the blood by bone and *vice versa*. For instance, if there is excess of parathyroid secretion, calcium is mobilised from the bones, the bones become soft and there is a high blood calcium. This will lead to pains in the bones, the bones become fragile and are easily fractured. In the early stages this condition is hard to diagnose as the symptoms are vague, the patient complains of generalized pain and depression and may often be diagnosed as suffering from a psychoneurosis. X-rays of the fingers and gums often show characteristic areas of bone absorption. In classical cases, there is a raised blood calcium and this may lead to complications such as renal calculi, but where the diagnosis is in doubt elaborate calcium balance tests must be performed, and in any patient with a negative calcium balance,

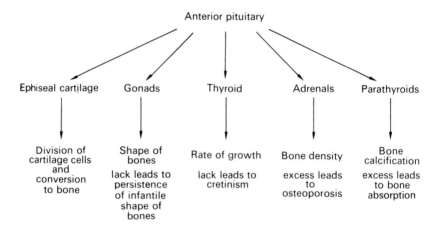

Fig. 4.2   The relationship of endocrines and their target organs.

hyperparathyroidism must be suspected. Hyperparathyroidism may be primary—for example, due to a tumour or adenoma of the parathyroid glands; or it may be secondary, in particular if there is chronic renal disease with renal rickets. This has the effect of stimulating the parathyroid glands, leading to secondary hyperparathyroidism.

The opposite condition of diminished hyperparathyroid secretion used to occur when the parathyroid glands had been inadvertently removed in the course of a thyroidectomy. This leads to a low blood calcium and a condition of tetany. The treatment is to give adequate amounts of calcium.

Adrenal glands

These consist of two parts: cortex and medulla. Disorders of the adrenal cortex are important as they give rise to osteoporosis, among other things. Patients with hypersecretion of the renal cortex characteristically have a moon-shaped face; they have striae; osteoporosis, and may develop other disorders such as diabetes. Hyperadrenalism may occur due either to disorders of the adrenal glands, or to the therapeutic administration of cortisone or other steroids. The opposite condition of diminished secretion of adrenal cortical hormone gives rise to the condition known as Addison's disease, in which there is muscular weakness, bronzing of the skin, low blood pressure and, if untreated, this condition ultimately results in death.

The adrenal medulla secretes adrenalin. The injection, or discharge of adrenalin causes tachycardia; vasoconstriction; bronchodilation and raised blood pressure.

Pancreas

The pancreas has two functions: firstly, to secrete digestive enzymes along the pancreatic duct into the gastro-intestinal tract; secondly, there are certain interstitial cells known as the islets of Langerhans which secrete a hormone known as *insulin*, this controls glucose and carbohydrate metabolism. If there is a shortage of insulin the patient will develop a condition known as *diabetes*, in which there is a failure of glucose metabolism, the blood sugar is raised and acetone bodies are usually found in the blood and urine, giving rise to the condition of ketosis with air hunger. There are many complications of diabetes which are of importance to the orthopaedic surgeon, in particular, diseases of the blood vessels, peripheral nerves and spinal cord. Also, diabetes is a common condition and patients with diabetes frequently suffer from orthopaedic disorders, e.g., fractures or torn cartilages. It is therefore important to exclude the possibility of diabetes before performing any orthopaedic operation, or to consider diabetes in any severe pain in the limbs, particularly if it is associated with obvious signs either of ischaemia or muscle weakness.

The metabolic unit

Patients with disorders of the endocrine system or with nutritional diseases may be investigated and diagnosed in a metabolic unit. This consists of a small clinical unit in a hospital with a team consisting of medical, biochemical, nursing, dietetic and medico-social staff.

In this unit the patient's intake of food and output is carefully analysed so as to estimate accurately the quantity and composition of all that the patient is both ingesting and excreting. This means that the dietician supplies a weighed diet containing a known quantity of all the constituents of the diet the patient says he was consuming prior to his admission to hospital. Under this regime the Basal Metabolic Rate of the patient is estimated and his total output of faeces and urine is measured and analysed. This is the first stage of his management and is useful for diagnostic purposes. If, for example, his output of an essential chemical element such as calcium exceeds his total intake of that element, then this indicates a deficiency of this factor in that he is in negative calcium balance. A day-to-day chart shows whether or not the intake and output are fluctuating or steady.

After the condition is diagnosed, a regime of treatment is established using the same methods but modifying the intake of food, vitamins, chemical elements and drugs, including hormones, to meet the patient's needs.

Metabolic units are very valuable but adherence to a strict food discipline requires a high degree of patient co-operation. A very high standard is also required from the staff; every item of food and drink must be weighed and analysed; every specimen of urine and faeces must also be measured and analysed—one mistake can ruin several days' work.

5

Nutritional Disorders

Nutritional disorders may occur either due to an inadequate diet or failure of absorption from the gastro-intestinal tract, or from both combined. In the past and, indeed, even now in many parts of the world, people's diets are grossly deficient; in particular they may be deficient in certain vitamins or in protein. The symptoms of vitamin deficiency are well known, but particularly deficiency of vitamin D, vitamin C and vitamin A may lead to serious orthopaedic disorders.

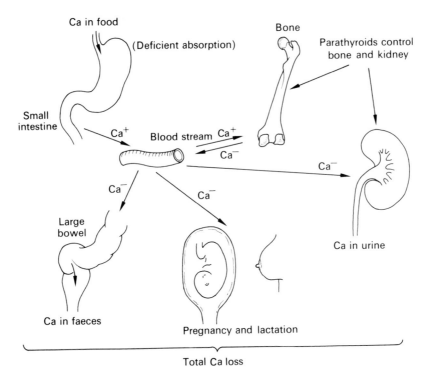

Fig. 5.1 Movement of calcium.

Avitaminosis D

Infantile rickets

Vitamin D is essential for calcification of bones and without vitamin D the pre-osseous tissue or osteoid cannot be converted into true bone and the condition of rickets develops (Fig. 5.2). Rickets is characterized firstly by the child's general malaise; he will be off colour, suffer from colds and restlessness, sweat easily and be irritable. If untreated the condition will lead

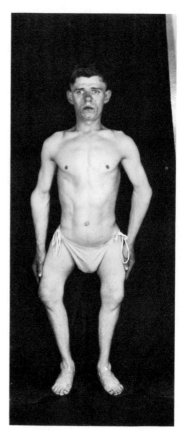

Fig. 5.2　An adult with the deformities caused by rickets during childhood.

to severe deformities of the limbs, either bow-legs or knock-knee, bowing of the tibiae, femora and humerii. In addition, the patient will have a large square skull, a narrow high arched palate and dental caries. The classical condition of rickets is seldom seen in this country nowadays, though it was seen frequently in the past and is still seen in many of the poorer parts of the world. Classical rickets is a disease of infancy, particularly in children under one year of age, but in the elderly a deficiency of vitamin D may lead to the analogous condition of osteomalacia. The bones become soft, fragile and deformed, the patient's back becomes kyphotic and will easily suffer fractures from minor injuries; there are typical appearances on the X-rays Figs. 5.3a, b and c.

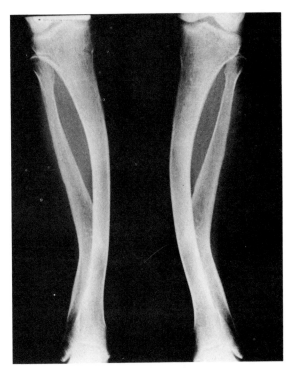

Fig. 5.3   (a) Rickets affecting tibia and fibula.

There is another form of rickets often called renal rickets (Fig. 5.3c), in which there is a failure of the osteoid tissue to calcify, leading to deformities. In this case the condition is not due to lack of vitamins but to a metabolic upset due to kidney disease. This takes two main forms—there is firstly the disease of the glomeruli which leads to a higher blood urea, acidosis, general dwarfing and usually early death of the patient. The treatment is to correct the acidosis by administration of alkalies to improve the excretion of nitrogenous matter, and to give adequate calcium and vitamin D.

The other form of renal rickets is tubular rickets in which there is a failure to re-absorb certain amino acids from the tubules of the kidney. The

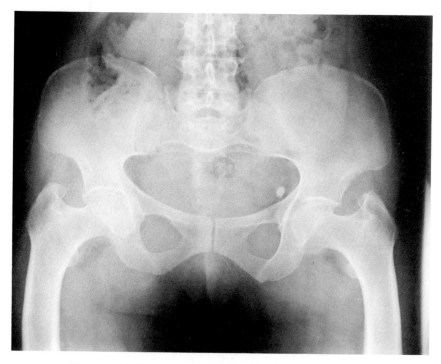

Fig. 5.3   (b) Coxa vara with flattened pelvis secondary to rickets.

patient is comparatively well, but the formation of bone from osteoid tissue is inhibited. In this case the prognosis is good, there is no acidosis and the treatment is to give large doses of vitamin D.

The adult

Osteomalacia. As already mentioned, osteomalacia or softening of the bones, may occur in elderly people due to a deficient diet, but it may also occur in disorders of the gastro-intestinal tract, of which the three most common are:

1   *Post-gastrectomy.* Following a gastrectomy there may be a deficient diet and deficient absorption of food, and some ten years after a gastrectomy it is not uncommon for a patient to suffer from bone pain, softening of the bones and deformity, particularly kyphosis and multiple compression fractures of the vertebrae. The treatment is to ensure that the patient takes a diet containing plenty of protein, vitamin D and calcium.

2   *Steatorrhoea.* In addition, chronic diarrhoea, either tropical or non-tropical, with an associated steatorrhoea may lead to defective absorption

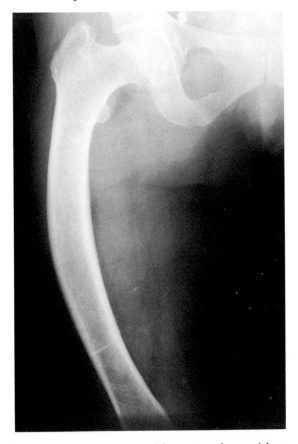

Fig. 5.3 (c) Lateral bowing of femur secondary to rickets.

of calcium and vitamin D, leading to softening of the bones and deformity as outlined above.

3 *Miscellaneous.* There are a number of other syndromes characterized by deficient absorption, of which gluten sensitivity is the most important. In this condition the child is abnormally sensitive to gluten and if gluten is included in the diet, he will have chronic diarrhoea and deficient absorption, particularly of vitamin D. The treatment is to give him a gluten-free diet.

Scurvy

Lack of vitamin C in the diet gives rise to the condition known as scurvy, which is characterized by anaemia, multiple haemorrhages, particularly in the gums and into the skin, leading to petechia, and in severe cases the teeth may fall out. There will also be a tendency to bleed into the subperiosteal tissues, leading to swelling of the bones and subperiosteal ossification.

The important thing is to suspect the condition and if it is suspected, adequate amounts of vitamin C must be given.

Avitaminosis A

Lack of vitamin A may cause night blindness and failure of ossification. Equally, excessive vitamin A may lead to hyperostosis. In ordinary clinical practice, deformities and orthopaedic conditions due to lack of vitamin A are rare.

Beri-beri and pellagra

Lack of vitamin B may give rise to a number of syndromes including peripheral neuritis and cardiac myopathy. Again it is unusual for lack of vitamin B by itself to cause deformity or orthopaedic conditions, though if a patient complains of unexplained pain and weakness, the possibility of vitamin B deficiency must always be considered.

In order that bone should be adequately formed, it is first of all necessary for the body to form what is known as osteoid, or pre-osseous tissue; and secondly, for the osteoid to be turned into bone by the deposition of calcium hydroxyphosphate, in the matrix of the osteoid tissue. In order to lay down bone it is necessary for there to be an adequate supply of protein, calcium, phosphate and vitamin D, and it is also necessary that there should not be any condition like acidosis which will interfere with the biochemical mechanism by which calcium salts are deposited in the osteoid matrix.

Osteoporosis

Osteoporosis, which may be defined as loss of bone bulk without a disturbance of the osteoid bone ratio—i.e. the soft tissue/mineral ratio in the bone remains unchanged—but the total bulk or density of the bone is less than it ought to be (Fig. 5.4). Osteoporosis may be caused by a number of conditions: for instance, following prolonged bed rest, immobilization of a fracture or where there is paralysis of the muscles.

In addition, osteoporosis is likely to occur adjacent to an inflamed joint

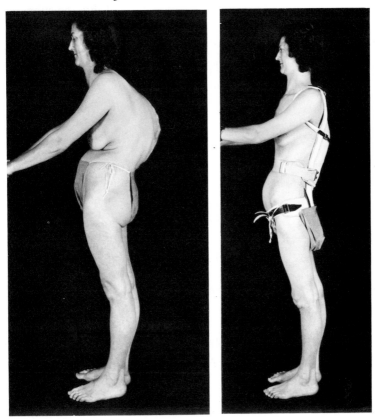

Fig. 5.4 Patient with osteoporosis (a) before correction and (b) after correction and wearing a spinal support.

—e.g. tuberculosis, or rheumatoid arthritis, or it may occur due to local disease of bone. Commonly a certain degree of osteoporosis is seen in elderly people. In some cases this appears to be due to lack of sex hormones, as it is more common in women following the menopause. But the exact cause of senile osteoporosis is unknown. Probably there are a combination of a number of factors—diminished use, diminished sex hormones, poor intake of protein and calcium, may all play their part. This is a very common condition leading to multiple pains, deformity of the spine, collapse of vertebrae, and spontaneous fractures. It is usual to investigate such patients by performing calcium balance tests and if it is shown that the patient is excreting more calcium than is being taken in, steps must be taken to correct this imbalance.

Osteoporosis as well as osteomalacia may occur in association with diseases of the gastro-intestinal tract—e.g. after a gastrectomy or in association with any chronic diarrhoea or other intestinal disorder. In particular, atrophy of the mucous membrane of the small intestine may lead both to osteomalacia and osteoporosis and this should be suspected and investigated in any patient with evidence of osteoporosis.

Obesity

Food taken into the body is required for many purposes; one is the production of energy to enable the body to work and perform exercise. Some disabled people are extremely limited in the amount of exercise and work they can do. As a result, there is a danger that reserves of nutrition taken in a diet may be deposited as fat in the body with subsequent increase in weight. People who are confined to bed or to wheelchairs for much of their time ought to restrict their diet to prevent this happening. In addition, boredom may lead a person to eat more than is needed in order to maintain health. In the Western world many people with sedentary occupations eat too much. People who are ill also may suffer from distortion of their appetite and eat too many sweet things and too much carbohydrate. A correct diet, i.e. well balanced and of the correct quantity, is essential for health and recovery from illness or operation.

Management in endocrinal and nutritional disorders
(See also Chapter 4, page 33.)

1 Investigations and diagnosis

The clinical signs described in the first part of this chapter are often adequate to establish the diagnosis. Precise confirmation of the patient's condition will call for various forms of examination.

(a) *Radiography.* To ascertain the state of the skeleton of the patient, radiographs of the body may be required. Generally all bones of the body are involved and, if they are not examined radiologically, increase or decrease in density, hairline pathological fractures, or the less obvious deformities may be missed.

The radiographs must be taken with the correct exposure necessary for the production of a good image if less obvious lesions are to be seen.

(b) *Blood chemistry*. Pathological examination of the blood will reveal abnormal quantities of calcium, potassium or other constituents. It is essential that the pathology department are aware of the provisional diagnosis so that they will extend their tests to include all possible chemical abnormalities.

(c) *Faecal analysis*. The patient may not absorb some of the essential constituents of his diet. The presence of a bulky fatty stool for example, may mean that the patient is discarding fat-soluble vitamins in his diet and thus is not making use of vitamins A, D, E or K.

(d) *Urinalysis*. This examination is very important in estimating what is being discarded and not used by the patient. The usual laboratory specimen bottle supplied may not be sufficient and a twenty-four hour specimen may be required by arrangement with the pathology laboratory.

2 Dietary management
This requires full collaboration by the medical, nursing and dietetic staff. A thorough enquiry is necessary to find out the previous dietary regime of the patient; what factors contributed to the inadequacies in nutrition that caused the disease? What are the patient's fads, likes and dislikes? Did these create the nutritional problem? What social factors influenced the problem; perhaps the death of the wife or the loss of false dentures?

Once all this has been established, these findings plus those resulting from the laboratory tests, will guide the team in providing the most suitable feeding regime for the patient, both in hospital and after rehabilitation. The likes and dislikes of the patient must be taken into consideration and alternatives found to replace any items in the diet which are necessary but are not acceptable to the patient. If more complicated investigations are required, these are done in a special metabolic unit (see Chapter 4).

3 Social work
The social worker has much to contribute to the care of these patients. The background of the patient is investigated when malnutrition is found and the cause sought and remedied for the future; the remedy may be relief of financial stress with welfare funds or grants.

4 Psychological or psychiatric problems
Sometimes nutritional disorders are caused by psychiatric disturbances; e.g.

anorexia nervosa. The psychiatrist and psychiatric social worker may be of assistance in caring for patients with nutritional disorders.

The patient with a nutritional disorder may also be irritable, apathetic or depressed. This is a notable feature in avitaminosis C (scurvy). Once treatment is commenced, improvement in attitude by the patient may be related to his improved physical state.

5 General nursing

In the active stages of any nutritional disorder affecting the skeleton and muscles, bed rest may be an important aspect of management. The patient is prevented from standing or sitting until the nutritional disturbance is remedied by dietary or medical means.

Sunlight and exposure of the body to other forms of ultraviolet light are beneficial, provided the amounts of both natural and artificial ultraviolet rays are regulated.

In addition to a full range of general nursing care the patient with nutritional problems will require consistent psychological and emotional support from nursing staff to tolerate a regime which may be tedious.

Section B

Acute Orthopaedic Conditions

6

Principles of Orthopaedic Treatment

The general aims are:
1   To restore or maintain function.
2   To prevent deformity.
3   To correct deformity if it already exists.
4   If some loss of function or permanent deformity is inevitable, to develop the patient's powers of compensation and adaptation.

In addition to what may be termed general and medical measures—which include encouragement and explanation—specific orthopaedic treatment is traditionally classified as conservative and operative. These are not antagonistic; operation—if it is indicated—is only one item in a carefully thought out programme of treatment in which conservative measures are employed before and after operation.

Conservative treatment

Active exercises. Normal function depends on good muscular control, therefore active exercises are an essential part of the treatment of any orthopaedic condition. Specific remedial exercises directed to one muscle or group of muscles will be required:
(a) If these muscles are weak and deformity is likely to occur due to unopposed action of the antagonistic muscles.
(b) If muscles are weak following direct injury or injury to their nerve supply.
(c) If a lesion of the brain or spinal cord has caused impairment of muscle control.
(d) Following tendon injuries.
(e) To restore joint movement.

Passive movements, or manipulation. These are usually combined with active movements when they are known as assisted movements. They must

always be gentle. They are used:
(a) To correct deformity, e.g. in treating a club foot.
(b) To restore joint movement.
(c) To relieve muscle spasm in certain lesions of the central nervous system.

Frequently gentle movements, in which the therapist's sensitive fingers respond to the 'feel' of the joints and muscles are essential. Violent tearing manipulations invariably do more harm than good.

Splinting
Splinting is used:
(a) To relieve pain.
(b) To diminish muscle spasm.
(c) To prevent undesirable movements, e.g. stretching of weak muscles.
(d) To hold fractured bone ends in position until the fracture is united.
(e) To maintain the position after reduction of a dislocation until the joint capsule has healed.

Operative treatment

(a) On bones. 1   Division or osteotomy to alter the shape and correct deformity.

Osteotomy may be linear (transverse or oblique) or cuneiform (Figs. 6.1 and 6.2).

2   Internal fixation with plates, screws or nails, either for fractures or after osteotomy (Figs. 6.4–6.6).

3   Bone grafting, either for non-union (Fig. 6.3) after a fracture or osteotomy or after excision of a tumour.

Bone grafting is used:
(a) to replace defects in bones
(b) to aid the arthrodesis of damaged joints
(c) to help in the correction of deformed bones—usually combined with division of the bone (osteotomy)
(d) to secure union of ununited fractures or to speed union in fractures which are known to unite slowly.

Bone grafts are of three types:
(a) Autografts taken from another bone of the patient.
(b) Homografts taken from another human being (dead or alive).
(c) Heterografts or allografts taken from the bones of another species.

Every bone graft has, at any rate potentially, a complex function. If it

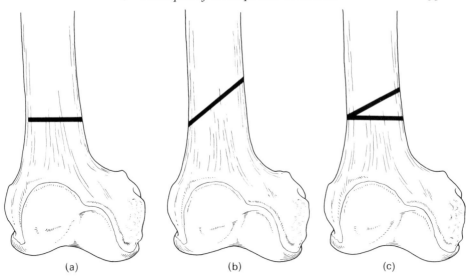

Fig. 6.1   (a) Transverse linear osteotomy. (b) Oblique linear osteotomy.
(c) Cuneiform osteotomy.

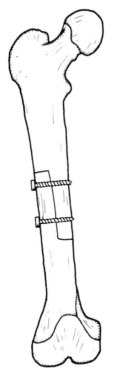

Fig. 6.2   Transverse osteotomy in leg shortening.

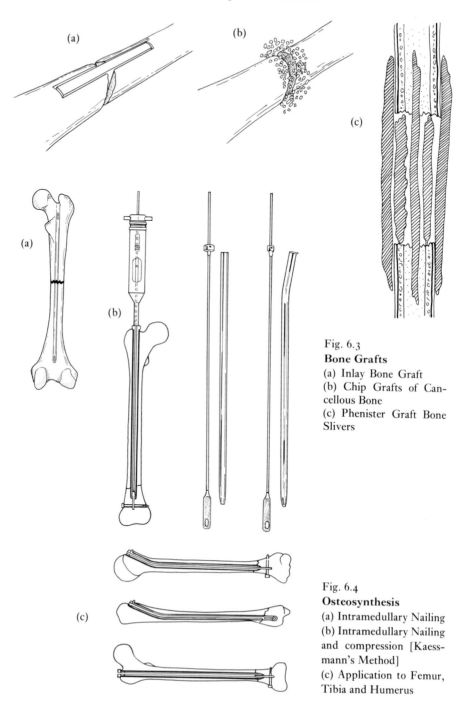

Fig. 6.3
Bone Grafts
(a) Inlay Bone Graft
(b) Chip Grafts of Can-
cellous Bone
(c) Phenister Graft Bone
Slivers

Fig. 6.4
Osteosynthesis
(a) Intramedullary Nailing
(b) Intramedullary Nailing
and compression [Kaess-
mann's Method]
(c) Application to Femur,
Tibia and Humerus

Fig. 6.5
(a) Plating of Fracture
(b) Intramedullary Nailing
(c) Latch Graft
(d) and (e) Plating and
intramedullary Grafts

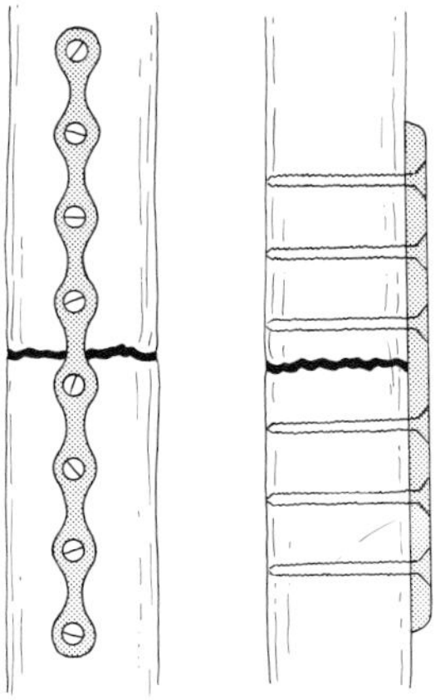

(a)

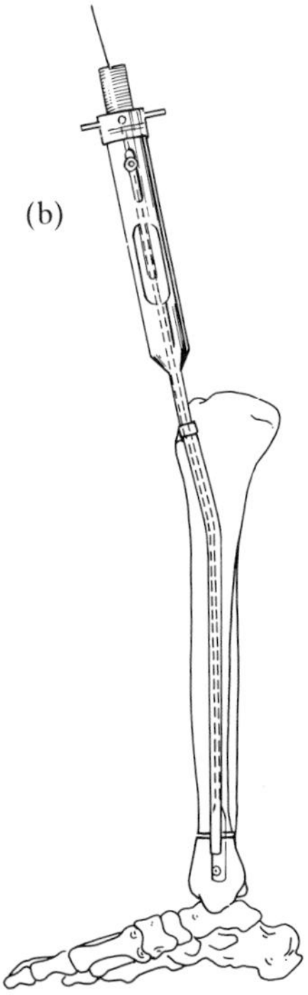

(b)

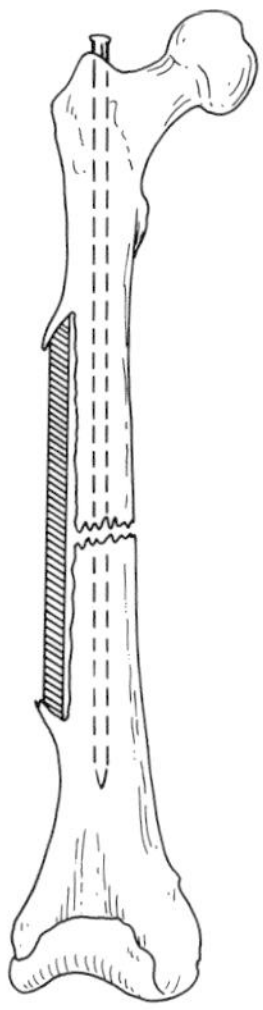

(c)

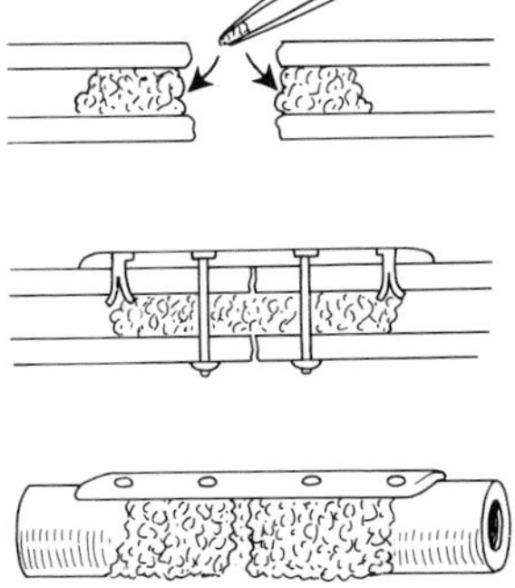

(d)

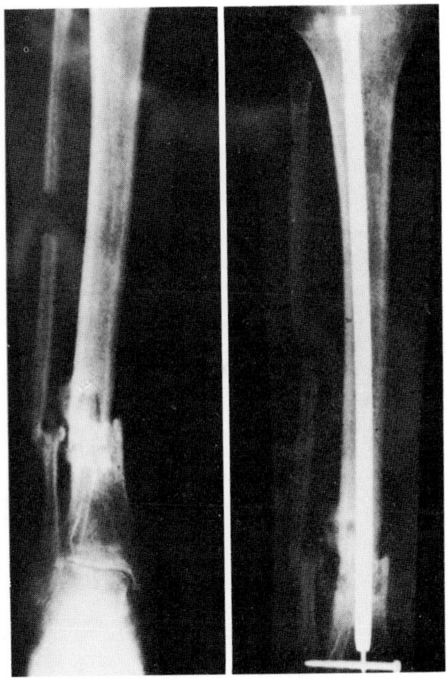

(e)

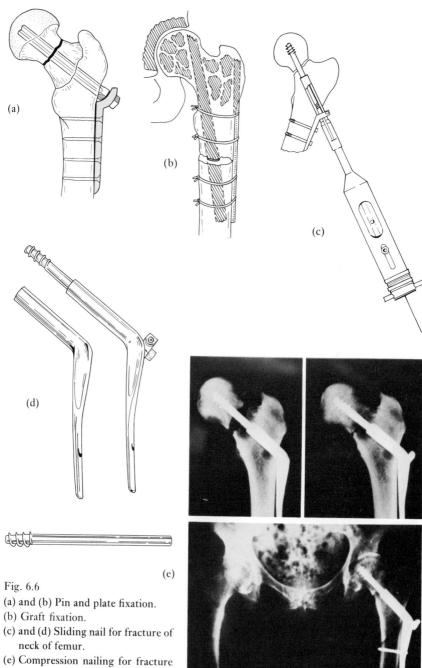

Fig. 6.6
(a) and (b) Pin and plate fixation.
(b) Graft fixation.
(c) and (d) Sliding nail for fracture of
     neck of femur.
(e) Compression nailing for fracture
     of femur.

contains cortical bone it can act as a mechanical splint. If it contains cancellous bone this is an ideal scaffolding into which the cells of the recipient or host area can grow, proliferate and lay down new bone. Therefore, it is important that the bone graft should be placed in a healthy bed, free from infection and fibrosis and with a good blood supply. An ideal bone graft could at any rate theoretically possess three properties:

(a) It could contain living, potentially osteogenic (bone forming) cells which could grow, divide and proliferate.

(b) It should contain chemical agents which stimulate the conversion of mesenchymal (primitive connective tissue) cells into bone forming cells.

(c) It must not connect harmful antigenic substances which stimulate antibody formation and cause graft rejection.

'Autografts' certainly possess the last two qualities and under favourable circumstances some osteogenic cells may survive though it is uncertain whether a sufficient number do so to make a significant contribution to new bone formation.

'Homograft' cells do not survive and, unless specially treated, homografts are likely to cause undesirable antigen/antibody reactions. These can be diminished by special treatment such as freezing, freeze drying, preserving in epoxy resin, etc.

'Heterografts' only act as a physical scaffolding and will cause undesirable antibody reactions unless their protein content is removed.

It is often desirable to use a combined graft—auto, homo and hetero with bone marrow cells from the donor (Chaklin). In addition bone grafts have been combined with various plastics so that a conglomerate is formed with the application of ultrasonic energy.

4   Removal of pieces of bone, either for histological examination (biopsy) or because there is excess of bone pressing on an important structure or causing pain.

5   Operations for bone infection, e.g. removing dead pieces of bone (sequestrectomy) or draining abscesses.

(b) On joints.   1   Division of capsule or fasia to correct deformity.

2   Excision of pathological synovium either as a curative measure or for biopsy.

3   Removal of intra-articular 'loose bodies', e.g. torn menisci or osteocartilaginous 'joint mice'.

4   Excision of a joint to secure movement (pseudarthrosis).

5   Fixation of a badly damaged and painful joint (arthrodesis).

6   Refashioning of a damaged joint (arthroplasty).

7   Stabilization of a flail joint or where recurrent dislocation is occurring.

(c) **On muscles and tendons.** 1   Suture for division of these structures.
2   Division to correct deformity or prevent deformity when it is due to muscle imbalance or contracture.
3   Tendon transplant to restore function and prevent recurrence of deformity when important muscles are paralysed or damaged.

(d) **On nerves.** 1   To suture divided nerves.
2   To free nerves from pressure by fascia, ganglia, callus or tumours.
3   To divide nerves supplying overactive muscles.

(e) **For skin loss and deficient blood supply.**

(f) **Amputation** if the limb is useless and/or painful, or the site of a disease which is dangerous to life and no other treatment is available.

Joint replacement

During the last 20 years there have been noticeable advances in the construction of artificial joint implants to replace damaged joints. These can be applied to a wide variety of arthritic conditions—rheumatoid, degenerative, post traumatic and post infective. There are a considerable variety of appliances which differ both in the design and the material from which they are constructed.

Sepsis is a major problem in joint replacement. The slightest infection and disaster ensues usually leading to removal of the prosthesis. Deeper joints, with inherent stability, such as hip joints are not quite so vulnerable as more superficial joints such as the knee.

Another problem is to find suitable materials which do not wear out and produce irritating debris and have a low coefficient of friction. Some debris from the wearing out of prostheses may be toxic.

On the whole, a combination of a plastic (high density polyethylene) acetabular component cemented into the acetabular socket and a stainless steel femoral head prosthesis also cemented into the bone has proved most successful. It is very important that the components be aligned and orientated accurately otherwise they may dislocate. Venous thrombosis and pulmonary embolism are another consideration. More recently, ceramics have been used as material for joint replacement. They have a low coefficient of friction but are more brittle than other materials.

Finger joints. For finger joints there are two main types of prostheses, one being made of silastic rubber, whilst the other is a hinged metallic prosthesis. In both cases fixation is obtained by inserting the ends of the prosthesis down the intramedullary cavity after excising the joint ends. After operation splinting and physiotherapy are very important.

Hip joints. If the acetabulum articular surface is still relatively intact it is sufficient to remove the head and neck of the femur and insert a substitute which can be made of metal, plastic or, ideally, a combination of metal and plastic in which a small metal head is surrounded by a plastic skin, movement occurring both between the metal head and the plastic skin and the plastic skin and the acetabulum (Monk) (Fig. 19.21c). If, however, the articular surface has been damaged or the shape of the articular socket is abnormal, it is necessary to replace both the head of the femur and the acetabular socket. Many systems use the combination of a metal head and a plastic socket (Fig. 6.7), but some surgeons (Ring) use a metal socket as well as a metal head. Components can be fixed in the bone by screws or a filling material, sometimes called cement, which also serves as a 'grouting' agent between the prosthesis and the bone, so that the pressure between the two is evenly distributed.

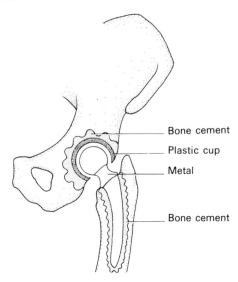

Bone cement
Plastic cup
Metal

Bone cement

Fig. 6.7   Total hip replacement.

Other joints, particularly the knee, elbow and shoulder can also be replaced by artificial implants. In each joint the problems of shaping, designing, choice of material and fixation to the chosen bones have to be considered separately. No doubt in the future there will be advances in the development of more suitable materials and improved methods of fixation but above all it is important to avoid infection, have good facilities for redeveloping muscle control and in certain cases employ temporary splinting to ensure stability. Ideally the material should be non-irritant, should not be adversely eroded by the body fluids, should be capable of firm bonding with the chosen bone and the coefficient of friction between the two joint surfaces should be low.

Knee. Three main types of prosthesis are used
1   The Mackintosh,
2   Hinged prostheses,
3   Covering femur and tibia.

One of the problems of knee prostheses is that the knee has no inherent stability as does the hip. If the knee ligaments are lax, as often occurs in rheumatoid arthritis, the prosthesis must either have stability in the coronal plane as in hinged prostheses or sufficient bulk of prostheses must be inverted to tighten the ligaments. Most hinged prostheses secure fixation by intramedullary stems; considerable strain is thrown on these and the adjacent bone which may later develop stress fractures at the level of the tip of the stem (Fig. 6.8).

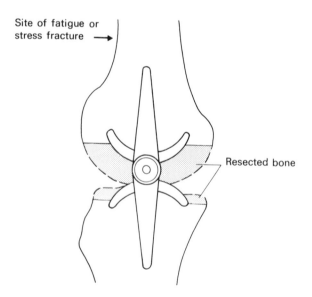

Fig. 6.8   Hinged knee prosthesis.

There are also a variety of shoulder and elbow prostheses which are mainly used in rheumatoid arthritis. Although the strain is less on upper limb joints than on lower limbs the shoulder has no inherent stability and the prosthesis must provide this by a cup and ball design (Fig. 6.9).

Most elbow prostheses are hinged with intramedullary stems as for the knee (Fig. 6.8).

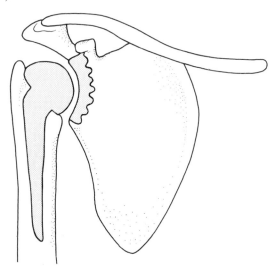

Fig. 6.9   Shoulder prosthesis (ball and socket joint) made from metal and plastic.

7

Multiple Injuries

Introduction

The 'multiple injuries' patient is a phenomenon of the present day. In the past, serious accidents happened and patients acquired more than one injury but not as commonly as they do today; if they did receive multiple injuries they often died.

The main reason for the rise in the number of persons affected by multiple serious injuries is the increase in the speed of transport and increasing mechanization in factories and at building sites. Whereas in the past people stayed within a limited area, often near their birthplace, now the majority of people, particularly in an affluent society, can expect to take at least one journey in their lifetime on a fast plane, and to make many journeys in fast cars. The problem is increased as the number of people per aircraft increases. The supersonic airliner of the future will carry hundreds of passengers on each journey; it follows therefore, that when such a vehicle crashes, hundreds of people will be killed or injured on that single occasion.

To reduce this to an everyday commonplace occurrence, in a single incident on our roads involving a pair of cars (the type of incident that occurs many times every day), at least two drivers will be killed or injured, probably seriously injured, and if the cars are fully laden, probably eight.

Road transport research

The prevention of accidents and multiple injuries calls for major research into the best design for cars and the roads on which they move. Such research has already been in progress for a number of years and continues. But the main cause of road accidents is hurry and impatience. Until human beings learn patience there will be accidents.

Research into casualty management

Another form of research, which must proceed, is into the best methods of collecting casualties, transferring them to hospital and sorting the many patients quickly into priorities for treatment. The most suitable ambulance vehicles, the training of personnel, catastrophe schemes in cities and other areas, and the design and provision of adequate casualty clearance and treatment centres in our hospitals requires much reappraisal in the light of the number and seriousness of our modern multiple injuries victims.

The development of two way radio transmission between ambulance and casualty department has been a notable advance. The staff at the hospital can be alerted as to the number and the gravity of the various accident victims. At the same time the hospital staff can give advice about roadside resuscitation if the ambulance staff need it, or if someone is trapped a team can go out from the hospital.

Another development in rural districts is the general practitioner emergency accident service. At any time one of a group of general practitioners is immediately available on call and equipped with all necessary resuscitation apparatus—intravenous infusions, respiratory aids, etc.

The 'multiple injuries' patient

The patient who suffers multiple injuries requires rapid transport to the most suitable centre for the unusual nature of his injuries. The main problems to be considered if his life is to be saved are: chest injuries; shock, related to blood loss; head injuries; abdominal injuries; spinal injuries, and pelvic injuries.

Chest injuries

Chest injuries are fairly frequent; they may not be recognized at the time of the injury, and an unconscious or semiconscious patient will not complain of pain. It is therefore important to examine the chest carefully in every multiple injury patient, and particularly to take X-rays, as it is possible for a patient to fracture several ribs and have a haemothorax or pneumothorax without this being clinically detectable. In addition to impairing movement of the chest wall, fractured ribs may be associated with damage to the underlying pleura and lungs, and sometimes even to the heart. It is therefore important to exclude any associated lesions, such as haemothorax or pneumothorax. In extreme cases, extensive damage to the chest wall may lead to a flail chest with the phenomenon of paradoxical respiration, i.e. the flail segment of the chest is sucked in when the patient attempts to breathe in, and blown out when the patient attempts to breath out. This means that relatively little air enters and leaves the lungs at each attempted breath. If steps are not taken either to stabilize the chest wall, or to provide artificial respiration for the patient, he will die of cyanosis and anoxia. This serious injury is usually treated nowadays by a tracheotomy and intermittent positive-pressure ventilation by the use of a suitable machine.

Occasionally a chest injury may be associated with direct damage to the heart, and in extreme cases, this may lead to cessation of the heart beat, and death.

Shock

Shock is defined as a clinical condition characterized by low blood pressure and a rapid weak pulse; the patient is pale and may even be cyanosed; he is cold and clammy; he may be apathetic or restless. Usually the breathing is rapid and shallow but occasionally it is slow and sighing. This is a serious condition in which the effective circulatory blood volume is diminished and the effective circulation, particularly to the extremities, is poor. If shock is allowed to continue it become irreversible and fatal damage is sustained in the most vulnerable tissues, namely the heart, brain and kidneys.

There are five main causes of shock (these may be combined):

1   *Oligaemic shock.* Firstly, there is blood loss—such as occurs due to haemorrhage, either external or internal. In external haemorrhage, the bleeding can be seen and the amount can be assessed. It is an important duty of whoever sees a patient suffering from an external haemorrhage that all soiled clothing and extravasated blood should be collected so that an accurate assessment can be made of the patient's blood loss. If the haemorrhage is internal, it will naturally be more difficult to assess blood loss, but one knows empirically that certain conditions, e.g. fractures of the pelvis, or fractures of the femur are usually associated with a considerable loss of blood (Fig. 7.1).

A similar oligaemic cause of shock is when plasma is lost as, for instance, after severe burns. Immediately after a severe haemorrhage the volume of circulating blood is reduced, but the haemoglobin concentration remains normal. After some hours blood dilution occurs, the haemoglobin concentration falls, and an estimation of the haemoglobin then indicates the seriousness of the condition.

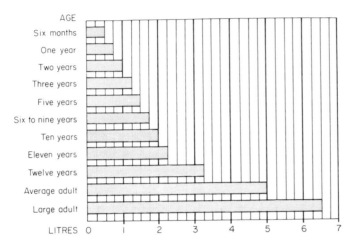

Fig. 7.1 Relationship of blood volumes to size of body.

2 *Toxic shock*. The second important cause of shock is toxic shock. This may occur due to an overwhelming septicaemia and in particular when the septicaemic condition affects the adrenal glands the patient will be severely shocked. Other toxic causes of shock are the absorption of toxins, e.g. in association with an area of gangrene or where there is any major ischaemic lesion. Included among these would be the so-called crush syndrome, where following crushing of muscle, toxic products from the crushed muscles are absorbed leading to a condition of shock which may well be fatal, especially as there can be a very deleterious effect on the kidneys. A similar condition can occur if a tourniquet is left on a limb for more than six hours and is then released.

3 *Cardiac shock*. Severe cardiac infarction may lead to a state of shock called cardiac shock. This is often the case in severe coronary thrombosis. This is primarily a medical condition but when a surgical patient suddenly collapses, this possibility must be borne in mind. Similarly, if there is passive pulmonary embolism there is a reflex inhibition of the heart action, leading to profound shock.

4 *Anaphylactic shock*. Allergic reactions may also lead to shock and for this reason great caution must be taken in giving injections such as tetanus antitoxin, which is notorious for producing anaphylactic shock. Sensitized patients may also suffer from severe shock after what would otherwise be

relatively trivial incidents such as wasp stings, or following the administration of antibiotics or drugs to which they are sensitive.

5 *Neurogenic shock*. A temporary fall of blood pressure may be caused by a purely reflex neurogenic mechanism as is seen in the common faint, and this may be precipitated by an emotional shock. A severe blow to the solar plexus or a head injury may cause neurogenic shock.

Nursing management

The first duty of the nurse when confronted with a patient in a state of shock, is to stem any external bleeding and make sure that a good airway is maintained. If the patient is restless it is nearly always wise to arrange for him to be given a sedative, for instance, an injection of morphia, but care must be taken if the diagnosis is uncertain, or if there is an associated head injury as under these circumstances morphia may be very dangerous. Once these first aid measures have been instituted it is important to do three things: namely, to ascertain the bloodgroup of the patient in order to prepare for an emergency blood transfusion; secondly, to take the necessary steps to diagnose the cause of the shock, in particular to see if there is any evidence of internal haemorrhage, or gross swelling of one limb, or damage to the pelvis, spine or ribs; and thirdly, to assess the amount of external blood loss, basically the responsibility of the doctor in charge, but in a case of difficulty he will require X-rays of the chest, pelvis and head, and perhaps an electrocardiogram.

It is the nurse's duty to maintain the airway and to keep a constant record of the pulse rate and blood pressure; a rising pulse rate and falling blood pressure are extremely sinister signs. In fact, the ratio between pulse rate and blood pressure is one of the most important guides to the patient's condition. The respiration rate is more variable and is in general a less reliable guide, though extreme slowing of respiration rate may be a valuable sign of increasing cerebral pressure.

Shock and the micro-climate

When a patient is suffering from shock or is seriously ill from any cause, he should not be subjected to any undue stress. Noise and bright light are obviously harmful. Equally, extremes of temperature or humidity may increase the metabolic rate with harmful results.

Recently the concept has been developed of controlling the patient's environment by pumping air at a controlled temperature and moisture content through a special mattress so that the micro-environment of the patient is always optimal. The concept is similar to that of putting an ill neo-natal infant in an incubator. The aim is to reduce the patients metabolic rate and ensure that blood and oxygen supplies are maintained to essential organs.

Head injuries

After considering shock, the next and most important organ to be considered in a patient with multiple injuries, is the head. Head injuries are most important, not only because of the possibility of severe damage to the brain, but also because there may be severe haemorrhage from the scalp which is a very avascular organ, and there may be associated injuries particularly to the eyes, ears, nose, face and jaws. It is very easy to fail to notice one or other of these and to find that although the hospital team may have saved the patient's life, he is later either deaf or blind, or has some difficulty in eating. It is therefore important to make a systematic examination of the eyes, ears and jaws in any patient with multiple injuries, particularly if he is semi-conscious or unconscious.

Nursing management

In general, in the management of head injuries, apart from the obvious measures of maintaining an airway and stopping external bleeding, the most important thing is to keep a careful note of the state of the patient's consciousness, the condition of his pupils, his pulse rate, his blood pressure and his respiration rate. Various degrees of disturbance of consciousness are recognized. At one extreme there may be slight lethargy, the patient can answer questions but does not talk or move spontaneously; this may later be associated with amnesia for this period, and a patient may appear to behave fairly normally and have no recollection of what has happened or what he was saying when he 'comes to' a few hours later. A rather deeper state of unconsciousness is when the patient is listless but can just answer simple questions such as giving his name, or obeying simple commands like, 'Open your eyes' or, 'Close your fingers'. A still deeper state of unconsciousness is indicated if the patient does not answer or obey commands, but his reflexes are still present and, for instance, if his arm or leg is pinched or pricked he withdraws it. The most serious state is when the patient is deeply unconscious or comatose; breathing is stertorous, the reflexes are absent, and he does not even respond to pricks or pinching by any movement. In certain cases of head injury where there is progressive bleeding inside the skull, the doctor may decide that an operation is indicated, but in the majority of head injuries, attention to respiration and treatment of the patient's general condition will yield the most satisfactory result.

Spinal, abdominal and pelvic injuries

Injuries to the lumbar spine, abdomen and pelvis, are of special importance. If there is damage to one of the important intra-abdominal organs, particularly damage to the spleen, this may cause a fatal haemorrhage. Delayed rupture of the spleen following an abdominal injury is a well known complication which is extremely difficult to detect, but may lead to rapid death of the patient if it is not diagnosed. In addition, there may be lacerations of the liver, tears of the intestine, or damage to the bladder or urethra. Therefore, in any abdominal or pelvic injury, it is important to exclude damage to these essential organs.

Finally, in this section it should be noted that in case of injuries to the spine, there is often reflex spasm of the abdominal muscles leading to an immovable abdomen which is board hard, similar to the board hardness seen following a perforation or intra-peritoneal haemorrhage. This may make diagnosis extremely difficult and, in the presence of a spinal injury the diagnosis of intra-abdominal injury may be impossible without recourse to laparotomy.

Wounds

In general, the first-aid treatment of wounds is to stop haemorrhage. Secondly, to decide if there are any important underlying structures, and thirdly to clean the wound, remove all dirt and foreign bodies, and to sew up the wound. In addition, where it is considered necessary, the appropriate antibiotic is given.

Tetanus and gas gangrene
There are two specially serious complications of wounds—namely, tetanus and gas gangrene. These are both caused by spore-forming micro-organisms.

Tetanus. It is possible to give prophylactic inoculations against tetanus by tetanus toxoid, and it is fortunately a common practice to give such prophylactic injections to children when they are receiving prophylactic injections against other infectious diseases. If the patient has already had a course of tetanus toxoid prophylactic injections, he should be given a 'booster' dose if he sustains a severe laceration.

If the patient has never had a course of toxoid immunization, there is some conflict of opinion about the best course of action, but most surgeons nowadays advise that the wound should be thoroughly cleaned, all dead and contaminated tissue excised, and the patient given a course of an anti-biotic such as penicillin. In the past it was customary to give anti-tetanic serum as a routine to all patients with cuts and lacerations, but it has been found that there is a considerable complication rate following the admini-stration of anti-tetanic serum and it is probably better not to give it as a routine measure.

Gas gangrene. This is another serious complication of wounds, especially where there is extensive destruction or ischaemia of muscle. It can be avoided by careful excision of all dead tissue. If gas gangrene is diagnosed, the two most valuable measures are (1) to give the patient a high concentration of oxygen—as in a hyperbaric oxygen chamber, and (2) to administer large doses of an antibiotic such as penicillin.

Compound fractures

The association of a wound and a fracture when there is communication between the wound and the fracture is known as a compound fracture. The danger is that micro-organisms may enter the bone from the surrounding skin, clothing or air, leading to chronic infection of the bone and osteo-myelitis. This is a very serious complication which may lead to prolonged crippling, non-union of the fracture, stiffness of joints and ultimately even to amputation or death; it is therefore important that every compound fracture be most carefully treated, firstly by excising all dead and dirty tissue, secondly by careful attention to skin healing and the administration of the appropriate antibiotic.

Burns in multiple injuries

Some patients with multiple injuries often suffer from burns. If the burns are extensive, these are extremely serious not only because of shock due to loss of plasma, but because an extensive burn usually becomes infected and the patient may die of toxic absorption. The older the patient the less their resistance to burns. Young patients have survived burns which would certainly be fatal in old patients. In general, the outlook for survival is very doubtful if more than 40% of the body surface is burnt. The main treatment of burns in the early stages is (1) to treat shock and to try to prevent infection by covering the burnt area with a sterile dressing, and (2) to admit the patient to a special sterile ward or cubicle so that infection is avoided if possible.

Crush injuries

If there is extensive crushing of a limb, particularly if there is crushing of muscles, this may lead to tissue necrosis; toxic products from the dying muscle are then absorbed into the blood stream and may give rise to severe shock and damage to the kidneys, liver and other organs. The treatment is firstly to prevent this by excising damaged muscle, if the crushing is extensive or if a tourniquet has been left on too long (that is, more than six hours) it is dangerous to remove it. Unfortunately the only safe advice is to amputate the limb above the tourniquet, otherwise toxic products of muscle decomposition will lead to renal failure and death.

If a patient is crushed and trapped by a falling building, beams or masonry, immediate amputation on the spot may be necessary to free the patient and prevent probably fatal absorption of toxic products from the crushed muscles.

The multiple injuries unit

Ideally this is a special unit entirely used for the reception of patients with serious and multiple injuries. Its prime function is to ensure survival of the patient until he can be moved to a conventional nursing unit in the hospital; it follows that the patient remains in the unit either only for a few hours or a few days, depending upon his needs; once he is out of immediate obvious danger of death, he is transferred to another ward to clear the unit for other casualties. The multiple injuries unit may be part of an intensive care unit.

The siting of the unit

The unit should be (a) relatively close to an area where serious accidents are likely to occur; for example, near a complex of motorways; (b) where ambulances can reach it most expeditiously. The entrances and road must be kept free by prohibited parking. There should be a turning area for ambulances to reverse to the doors. A helicopter landing area is a useful asset. (c) It should be close to or part of a general hospital in which a full range of specialist treatment, operating theatres and ancillary units are available. A blood transfusion bank is essential.

The design and organization of the unit

The unit should be compact and suffice for the care of a maximum of six patients at one time. Conventional beds are less desirable in the unit than the special emergency casualty trollies which enable the radiographer to take X-rays without transferring the patient to another surface; they can also serve as efficient operating tables.

Direct access to the ambulance parking area is important; this avoids any delay in starting to treat the patient as soon as the ambulance arrives.

Ample hand washing sinks, electric points, piped oxygen points, suction points and storage space with working surfaces are needed. Local control of the heating and ventilation of the unit is also desirable.

The equipment must be comprehensive both for applying simple procedures and for more advanced measures such as tracheostomy. A full range of sterile packs for all the most likely forms of emergency treatment should be permanently maintained in the unit. Anaesthetic equipment and accessories are supplied as standard equipment.

The unit is staffed by a sufficient number of highly experienced nursing and medical staff so as to provide a twenty-four hour service. A scheme must exist for calling out extra personnel when the occasion demands it.

Liaison with ambulance personnel

Full collaboration between the ambulance staff and the staff of the unit is needed for the welfare of the patient. An intelligent and relevant report on what occurred at the site of the accident is most helpful to the doctor. The estimation of blood loss, if any, and if the patient has been unconscious are two examples of vital information.

Most ambulances are provided with emergency respiratory equipment, for example, hand operated resuscitators and other means of maintaining the patient's respiration until hospital is reached. Most ambulance drivers are very skilled in first aid and are also skilled in assessing the amount of blood the patient has lost, and the patient's condition; they can give invaluable help in making an exact diagnosis, which may well be life-saving.

Emergency treatment in the unit

First priorities—1 *Respiration:* Restoring and maintaining the airway of the patient by intubation, tracheostomy and intermittent positive pressure-ventilation, if necessary stabilizing fractures of the walls of the thorax or immobilizing a flail sternum, closing penetrating wounds of the chest walls, and correcting paradoxical respiration. Maxillo-facial injuries receive a high priority if they impede breathing.

2   *Exsanguination:* Arresting the loss of blood by control of wounds. Replacing lost blood to its full volume at a speed relevant to the condition of the patient. Treating shock. Emergency surgery such as splenectomy for a rupture of the spleen.

3   *Cardiac massage:* This may be either external or internal.

4   *Head injuries:* Carefully recorded observations of the patient will indicate the need for either cranial operations, for example, increasing intracranial pressure causes lowering of the level of unconsciousness and slowing of the pulse and respiration.

*Later priorities—*1   *Fractures:* Stabilization of broken limbs by external splintage, either temporary or permanent. This may be a measure necessary to enable the surgeon to attend to the first priorities.

2   *Wounds:* Surgical toilet and suturing of wounds, (a) to prevent the entry of infection; (b) for cosmetic reasons; and (c) to increase the speed of healing.

Treatment of eye and ear injuries
The specialized treatment of this form of injury will require consideration, by the relevant consultant.

Relevant notes on emergency tracheostomy
As part of the urgent treatment in a patient with serious and multiple injuries, an operation on the trachea may be required either to create an alternative airway when the normal route, through the nasal cavities or mouth, is obstructed by severe injuries to the face, nose, jaw and mouth; or to provide a means of inflating and deflating the chest by artificial means when crush injuries of the thorax prevent the natural respiratory action.

Usually the passage of an intracheal tube by a skilled anaesthetist will be enough to maintain respiration for a time.

The decision to perform a tracheostomy can then be made 'at leisure' but if no anaesthetist is available or there is no laryngoscope it may be wise to perform an emergency life-saving tracheostomy if the patient is in any type of respiratory distress.

With the patient's neck extended and straight, the surgeon makes a mid-line incision into the trachea below the larynx. The opening is dilated by special dilators; a tube is introduced into the opening to permit the entry and exit of air into the respiratory tract of the patient.

The tube may be made of metal, polyethylene or rubber. The latter may have an inflatable rubber cuff to serve to close off the trachea to the passage of air by any route except through the tube; if the patient must be ventilated by mechanical means this may be essential.

When emergency tracheostomy with ventilation is required, the anaesthetist plays a major role in ensuring that the patient is receiving an adequate volume of air at the rate most suited to his needs. This requires some means of estimating these factors. The measuring is done by (a) a spirometer on the machine which indicates the quantity of air passing into and out of the patient, this is related to his size and weight; (b) by a series of blood chemistry tests which indicate the carbonic acid level of the blood and report if it is lowered or raised; (c) by the colour and general appearance and condition of the patient.

Nursing management for tracheostomy patients. The nursing management of the tracheostomy patient requires:

(a) *Careful observation and recording of the observations.* In a multiple injuries patient this process is routine and the tracheostomy of the patient will be covered in the general observations.

(b) *Care of the tracheostomy tube and wound.* The tube must be kept clear and free from mucus. A replacement for the tube and a pair of tracheal dilators must always be at the bedside. In the event of obstruction of the tube, replacement may be required urgently. The wound is dressed and cared for as any surgical wound.

(c) *Suction.* By observation it is possible to see and hear any fluid or other obstruction in the respiratory tract. Bubbling and other noises or cyanosis and anxiety if the patient is conscious, would indicate the need for aspiration of secretions in the trachea. This is an aseptic procedure and the special Pinkerton's catheter must be sterile when it is inserted. The catheter is connected to the suction tube and constricted with the fingers before insertion; it is passed down the trachea for eleven or twelve centimetres and the fingers release the constriction. It is unnecessary and unwise to 'jiggle' the tube; altering the position of the patient by raising the foot of the bed will carry the fluid to the opening of the tube. By turning the tube-opening towards one bronchus and then to the other the fluid obstruction can be extracted. The tube is again constricted before removal.

(d) *Humidification.* The function of the nasal cavities is to warm and moisten the air before it passes down into the lungs. If the nasal cavities are by-passed it is necessary to warm and moisten the air before it enters the tracheostomy tube. This is achieved with special humidification apparatus supplied by firms of surgical appliance makers.

(e) *Removal of the tube.* When the reason for the tracheostomy no longer exists, the tube may be removed. This may require simple removal of the tube, permitting the patient to breathe in the normal manner, or by 'weaning' him from the tube over a period of days.

The wound may require surgical toilet and closure, or it may be allowed to heal by itself, depending upon the decision of the surgeon.

(f) *Communication by the patient.* The unconscious multiple injuries patient has no need for communications. If however the patient is conscious then a writing block and pen, or some other system of signalling must be provided as he cannot speak normally.

Relevant notes on blood transfusion

In 'multiple injuries' patients a large amount of the total volume of blood in the body may have been lost before admission to the unit, and enquiry from ambulance personnel is necessary regarding this. Ambulance personnel should whenever possible bring blood-stained clothing, sheets, carpets, etc. which give a useful indication of the amount of blood lost. The obvious clinical signs of shock with a lowered blood pressure and rapid pulse will indicate an urgent need for blood replacement. In patients who have not obviously lost a large amount of blood externally there may be 'static blood' which is out of circulation at some situation in the body, either in dilated splanchnic veins or due to internal bleeding.

Most multiple injuries patients will require varying amounts of blood and other body fluids to replace the loss and to provide a reserve for any operation which may be necessary.

The pathologist and his staff are essential members of the multiple injuries unit team and an early action in the care of the patient is to obtain a specimen of his blood for cross-matching with blood from the blood transfusion bank.

Before the grouping and cross-matching can be completed, however, it is often necessary to proceed with intravenous infusion. This may be achieved with stored plasma (this is dehydrated plasma to which sterile pyrogen-free distilled water is added), or group 'O' Rhesus negative blood. Previous cross-matching of blood is always preferable however.

In patients with multiple injuries it may be necessary to put blood into the circulatory system at a very fast rate. This is done only by the surgeon in charge and some form of positive pressure may be applied to the air inlet of the blood transfusion bottle.

In severely collapsed and shocked patients the veins may be so constricted that the conventional intravenous infusion needle cannot be entered into the vein. Surgical venesection and the insertion of a plastic polyethylene cannula into the vein may be performed; this is also considered a wise move in those patients who will require continuous transfusion over several days.

Adequate transfusion is an essential feature of all modern surgery. A patient who has received adequate blood replacement will recover more quickly. He will demonstrate this by an improvement in his general condition, efficient wound healing and improvement in the state of his tissues, and an increased resistance to infection.

These notes are not intended as a comprehensive document on the nursing management of patients on blood transfusion.

Spinal injuries

Spinal injuries are a common feature of fast transport accidents, gunshot wound incidents and catastrophes when buildings have fallen on the occupants. Such injuries are a major facet of modern orthopaedic care. They require much more discussion than is possible as a section of this chapter and the reader is referred to Chapters 10, 16 and 31.

8

Fractures and Dislocations of the Upper Limb

Fractures and dislocations of the upper limb usually occur from a fall but they may also occur through direct injury, e.g. in road traffic accidents, or through the arm or the hand being caught in revolving machinery. They are mainly of significance in so far as they may lead to loss of function of the limb and in this sense damage to nerves, vessels, joints, skin and muscles is of paramount importance. These affections are described in other chapters, therefore in this chapter we will restrict ourselves to certain of the more common bony injuries to the upper limb, reminding the reader that associated injuries to the soft structures are important in every case.

Relevant applied anatomy and physiology

The shoulder, arm, forearm and hand together constitute a precision instrument which responds to instruction from the brain (Fig. 8.1). The function of this upper extremity is to serve as a prehensile unit capable of being placed in any reasonably required position at the exact point required for a given purpose. It is able to handle and use a tiny object such as a sewing needle as well as grip firmly and strike with a heavy object such as a sledgehammer. The human hand is most adaptable.

An important function of the upper limb is to reach and attend to any part of the head, e.g. to comb the hair, clean the teeth and put food in the mouth, remove obstructions from the ears, nose or eyes, protect the head and neck from injury when falling; all of these are essential for independent existence and loss of ability to do these things means severe hardship to the individual. The orthopaedic surgeon has this in mind when he treats lesions of the shoulder, elbow or forearm; thus if an ankylosis of the elbow is likely to occur or arthrodesis may be necessary, the surgeon will arrange to fix the elbow in a flexed position so that the face can be reached.

If for any reason both elbows are ankylosed one should be flexed 20 degrees above a right angle the other extended 20 degrees below a right

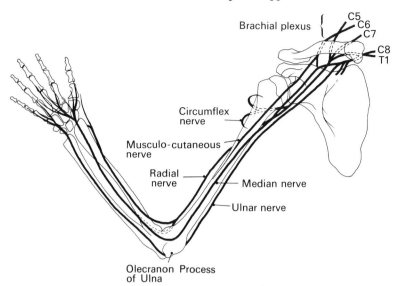

Fig. 8.1   Main nerves of the upper limb.

angle. Fortunately the development of elbow prostheses has made this a rare occurrence.

The bones of the upper limb are lighter in weight and therefore easier to move than the lower limb bones. The joints have as wide a range of movement as it is possible to find in an animal joint. The forearm has the wonderful ability to pronate and supinate, a most useful attribute in writing, typing, dressing, sewing and the many other tasks which man can perform but other animals cannot. The hand can be poised in thousands of different postures because of the large number of freely movable joints and active muscles. Trauma or serious infection may impair its function. Although the upper limb has such a superb structure, no structural or functional feature is wasted. The ball and socket joint at the shoulder (Fig. 8.2) is ideal in that situation so that flexion, extension, abduction, adduction, medial and lateral rotation and circumduction are all possible. These movements are aided by the joints at each end of the clavicle. Where such a wide range of movement is provided it is also necessary to have an equivalent set of muscles not only to cause the movements, but also to restrain them and hold the joint in the desired position. The shoulder is controlled by a large number of muscles. The elbow joint is also ideally adapted for its position. The actions of flexion and extension ensure maximum reaction compatible with the ability to bring the hand to the face. The action of pronating and supinat-

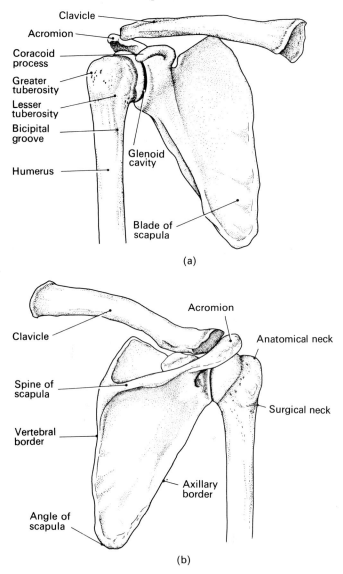

Fig. 8.2   (a) and (b) Bones of the pectoral girdle.

ing the forearm and hand makes for maximum flexibility in this limb. This movement depends on there being two bones in the forearm—the radius and ulna, and that these two are related as the axle (the ulna) and the other as the rim (the radius) of a wheel. Thus, these two bones are related to each other at three important points: the superior radio-ulnar joint in the elbow capsule; the interosseous membrane which connects the bones along the length of the shaft; the inferior radio-ulnar joint in the capsule of the wrist.

A serious injury to the elbow, or the mid-forearm, or the wrist carries the possibility of loss of pronation and supination and thus considerable disability.

As in any part of the body the upper extremity must have an excellent blood supply and nerve supply. There are large blood vessels and nerves passing down the whole length of the limb from neck to fingers. They may be damaged in fractures, dislocations, deep incisional or contusional wounds, with resultant paralysis. These nerves will be discussed in greater detail in Chapter 11.

Relevant first aid

As in any other part of the body, a fracture of the arm is a painful and un-pleasant experience. The patient will be in distress with pain and anxiety and will often give a history of feeling and hearing the bone break. The patient therefore requires just as much gentle handling and sympathy as the patient with a lower limb injury who cannot stand.

First-aid measures consist of efficient immobilization of the whole limb, using the trunk as the support for the fractured limb. The use of a large arm sling with a number of padded wide bands of material passing around the arm and trunk is the simplest method when there is a reasonable expec-tation that the patient will be treated in hospital fairly soon.

The positioning of the broken limb is important. Most examples of upper limb fractures can be immobilized with the elbow flexed to 90 degrees; the exception is in elbow injuries and supracondylar fractures of the humerus. When the latter is suspected, flexion of the arm may cause the ends of the fracture to close on an artery, resulting in ischaemia of the muscles of the forearm. It is therefore better to fix the arm to the side with the elbow extended beyond 90 degrees.

(a) Fractures of the clavicle
These are commonly due to a fall on the outstretched hand, though they may be due to a direct injury. Curiously enough, complications of fracture of the clavicle are relatively few, and in particular damage to the brachial plexus and subclavian artery only occurs on rare occasions.

The classical deformity is dropping of the shoulder, haematoma over the clavicle, and an obvious protrusion of the inner half of the bone (Fig. 8.3). Basically this fracture is self-healing; it does not require elaborate splinting;

in children a simple sling with local support for comfort is often enough. However, in adults and particularly young girls, in whom the appearance may be of great importance, slightly more elaborate measures may be necessary. Of these, undoubtedly recumbency is the easiest way of securing

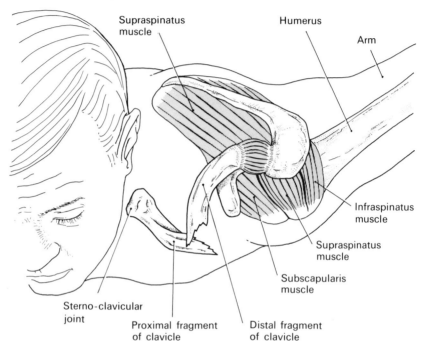

Fig. 8.3 Fracture of the clavicle.

a perfect anatomical reduction and of maintaining the bones in this position until they have united. However, such drastic treatment is seldom necessary and conventionally the use of a sling to support the elbow and a padded figure-of-eight bandage to control the position of the fragments and restrain their movements, is the most usual method of treatment (Fig. 8.4). The bandage must not be applied so tightly that it presses on nerves or blood vessels. The fracture usually unites in three weeks; following this, simple exercises to restore shoulder movement are all that is necessary. On very rare occasions non-union may result (see Chapter 2), and there is also a rare congenital type of pseudarthrosis of the clavicle.

The nursing management of a patient with a fracture of the clavicle. Although the treatment of these patients is so simple, there is a need for nursing supervision; as they are usually treated as out-patients, the patient must be asked to report to the fracture clinic at suitable intervals. The nursing staff must check that:

1   the fixation is adequate—neither too loose nor too tight;

2   there is no complaint of 'pins and needles' or tingling or numbness in either arm or hand;

3   that the skin under the bandages is free from excoriation or cuts. Washing and powdering of the skin is performed at examination.

When the fixation is applied, the wool padding or foam-rubber placed around the shoulder and axillae must be adequate. The wool must be orthopaedic splint wool, which contains a proportion of oil and therefore does not absorb perspiration; if surgical absorbent white wool is used it becomes saturated with perspiration in this region and changes from soft

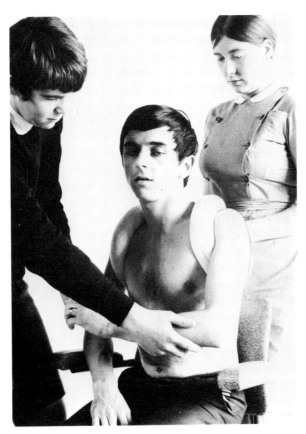

Fig. 8.4   Padded bandage to control position and restrain movements of fragments in a fractured clavicle.

material into tough inflexible bands which damage the skin and constrict nerves and blood vessels.

(b) Fractures of the scapula

These are usually due to direct injury and are associated with widespread bruising of muscles and not uncommonly with fractures of the underlying ribs. Although painful, there is usually little displacement. The only treatment necessary is to rest the arm in a sling until the pain has disappeared, and as a general rule there is full restoration of movement and function.

(c) Dislocation of the shoulder

This is one of the most common of the upper limb injuries and almost certainly the most common dislocation. It may be associated with damage to the nerves and, on rare occasions, to the blood vessels, therefore the condition of the arm should always be carefully examined before reduction, otherwise the doctor who reduces the dislocated shoulder may later be blamed for damaging the adjacent nerves which actually had been damaged at the time of injury.

The appearances are characteristic with flattening of the tip of the shoulder; the most prominent part of the shoulder becomes the acromion (Fig. 8.5) and there is also a fullness anteriorly. However, in very fat people

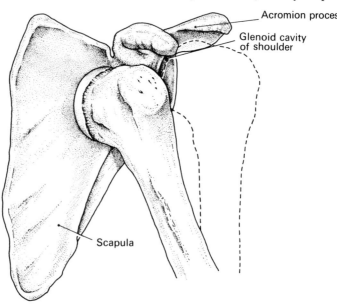

Fig. 8.5   Dislocated shoulder.

these signs may be difficult to elicit; there is of course, inevitably limitation of movement, particularly of abduction. Dislocation of the shoulder may be associated with a fracture of the humerus.

Treatment is to reduce the dislocation as soon as possible; for this purpose a general anaesthetic with full relaxation is usually necessary, though in cases of habitual dislocation, or where the patient is seen immediately after the injury, it may be possible to reduce the dislocation without an anaesthetic. There are numerous manoeuvres described in order to reduce a dislocated shoulder, but probably the most successful is the traditional Hippocratic method of applying traction to the arm with counter pressure in the axilla by the manipulator's fist or foot (Fig. 8.6). In all cases it is important to check that the dislocation has been satisfactorily reduced by an X-ray and also to observe whether there are any associated fractures.

After-treatment varies with the age of the patient. In young people the risk of habitual or recurrent dislocation is fairly high and so it is usually wise to immobilize the shoulder, e.g. a collar and cuff with the arm bound at the side—for some four to six weeks (Fig. 8.7). In the older patient, e.g. over fifty, the risk of recurrent dislocation is minimal but the risk of stiffness of the shoulder is very considerable and in such patients it is usually wise to start with gentle active and assisted movements as soon as the patient can tolerate them. In older patients it may be difficult to secure full movement and in such patients a course of treatment for a stiff shoulder may be required.

When the arm is fixed to the side under clothing there are two skin surfaces in direct contact; perspiration on both surfaces will occur and the result is unpleasant for the patient as the skin is constantly moist and may smell unpleasantly.

Unless some member of the patient's family is willing to be trained in the re-application of the bandage, the patient must be brought under some nursing care; either in the hospital, or by the visiting district nurse. The bandage is removed whilst the limb is held in its correct position by another person. The skin of the arm, axilla and chest wall is thoroughly washed and powdered with talc. This is done at fairly frequent intervals or at least twice weekly.

(d) Fractures of the humerus
The humerus may be fractured in four main sites:

1   *At the upper end or through the neck.* This is a common injury in adolescence. At first sight the appearances suggest a dislocated shoulder with fullness in front of the shoulder joint and a hollow just below the tip of the

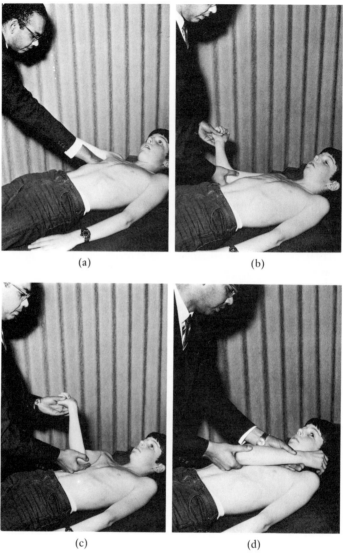

(a)   (b)

(c)   (d)

Fig. 8.6   Methods of applying traction for the treatment of a dislocated shoulder:

(a) Hippocratic method: the head of the humerus is lifted into place using the fist in the axilla as a fulcrum and the arm as a lever. Classically the unbooted foot was used as the fulcrum but the hand is safer and more sensitive.

(b) Gentle external rotation to stretch the subscapularis muscle, care must be taken not to fracture the humerus.

(c) Adduction of the arm till the head of the humerus lies in front of and lateral to the glenoid.

(d) Internal rotation to reduce the head into the glenoid.

(b, c and d) Kocher's method.

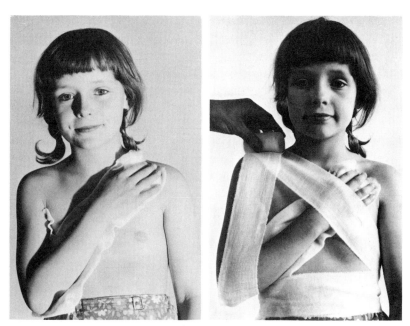

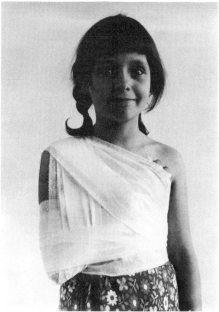

Fig. 8.7   Stages shown for immobilization of the arm of a patient. After reduction of a dislocated shoulder.

shoulder. Careful palpation will, however, show that the point of the shoulder is still formed by the greater tuberosity of the humerus, not by the acromium (Fig. 8.5). This injury can usually be treated satisfactorily by putting the arm in a collar and cuff and applying an external splint. Even though the X-ray may have looked very unsatisfactory, this simple conservative treatment usually yields a perfectly satisfactory result, both functionally and cosmetically. Occasionally the displacement of the fragments is so great that either non-union or a very ugly arm would result. In these cases open operation may need to be undertaken, but the surgeon will realize that the scar of open operation may be more disfiguring than a slight bump, which usually disappears in time; it is not necessary to treat these injuries by routine open operation as some surgeons have suggested.

In fractures where the head of the humerus is completely displaced and dislocated as well as the complete fracture its blood supply has been cut off and it will undergo avascular necrosis. Prosthetic replacement may be the best treatment, the alternative is removing the head leaving a pseudarthrosis.

2 *Fractures of the shaft of the humerus* are chiefly important because they may be associated with damage to the musculo-spiral nerve and wrist drop (see Chapter 11, page 164). Again these fractures can usually be treated ex-

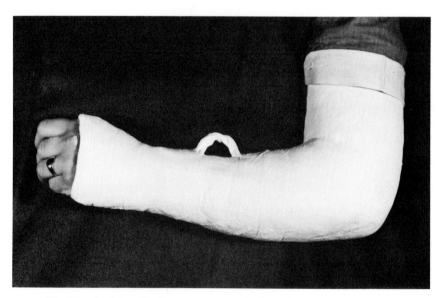

Fig. 8.8 A plaster for the management of a fractured forearm or of simple fractures of the upper third of the humerus.

tremely successfully by simple conservative measures, e.g. a collar and cuff and the application either of three gutter splints or a hanging plaster (Fig. 8.8). Although these do not secure complete immobilization, they rest the limb in a satisfactory anatomical position and this allows union to occur with a good cosmetic and functional result. In this fracture over-treatment—particularly distraction of the fracture—must be avoided at all costs as this will inevitably lead to non-union. In a small percentage of patients, for reasons which are not clearly understood, no callus is formed and the fracture enters into a state of non-union, in which case bone grafting will be required (see Chapter 6).

Fractures of the humerus are relatively easily treated in ambulant patients or in those who can sit up. If the patient has multiple injuries and particularly lower limb fractures so that he must lie in bed it is much harder to control a fractured humerus by conservative external splinting and this may be an indication for internal fixation.

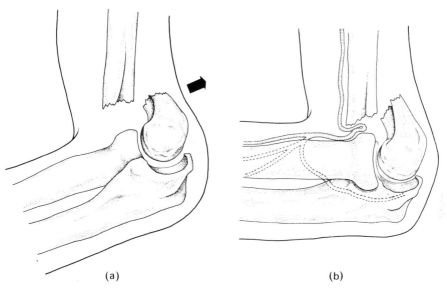

(a)   (b)

Fig. 8.9   (a) Supracondylar fracture showing direction of force, and (b) trapping of the brachial artery.

3 *Supracondylar fractures* (Fig. 8.9) are mainly important in children between the ages of 6 and 14 and are due to a fall on the outstretched hand. Their chief importance is that they are often associated with damage or kinking of the brachial artery which may lead to Volkmann's contracture (see Chapter 21, Fig. 21.4). Therefore, however, when the injury is treated,

the circulatory condition of the limb is the most important aspect to which attention must be directed. These fractures are usually fairly easily reduced by direct traction and manual pressure on the displaced fragment. The diagnosis is usually obvious with prominence of the elbow at the back but the condition must be differentiated from a dislocated elbow (Fig. 8.14).

After reduction, it is wise to put the arm in a collar and cuff sling with the elbow flexed to just above a right angle, but a very careful watch must be kept on the circulation and if there is the slightest risk of circulatory impairment, the arm must be extended and nursed in one of the ways described under Volkmann's ischaemic contracture (Chapter 17, see also Figs. 8.10a and b). If the surgeon fails to secure a satisfactory position it may often be wiser in the absence of circulatory complications, to accept a poor radiological position rather than perform repeated manipulations, as it is well recognized that repeated manipulations are one of the factors that may

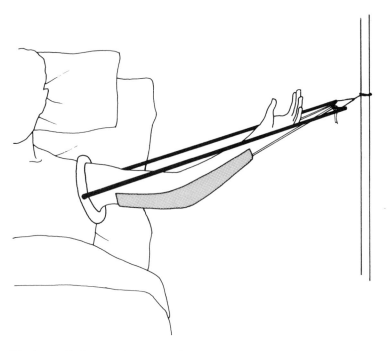

Fig. 8.10   (a) A method of supporting the arm using a Thomas arm splint which is a good method of treating injuries with avascular complications.

precipitate ischaemia. In young children especially, the powers of bone remodelling are very considerable, and even a severely displaced fracture

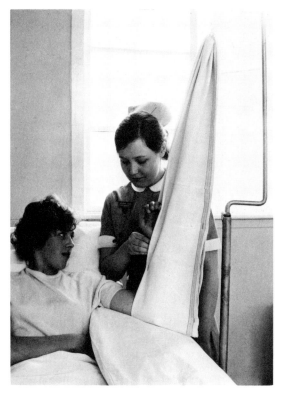

Fig. 8.10   (b) A method of supporting the arm in a roller towel during observation of the circulation to prevent complications.

which has united with an appalling X-ray picture, may ultimately become virtually normal as time passes.

Nursing supervision of these patients during the early stages of treatment is very important. Careful observation of the wrist pulse and colour, plus temperature of the hand are made and charted at short intervals. Admission to hospital for twenty-four hours at least is nearly always necessary, particularly for child patients or when there is doubt about the patency of the brachial artery.

4   *Fracture of the olecranon.* This is usually due to a direct fall which causes the olecranon to fracture. The pull of the triceps muscle displaces the fragments, the patient is unable to extend the elbow actively and a gap can be felt between the olecranon and the rest of the shaft. This fracture is usually best treated by open operation and either fixing the two fragments together,

which may be achieved either by a special type of lag screw or by a long intramedullary nail; alternatively if the separated fragment is small it may

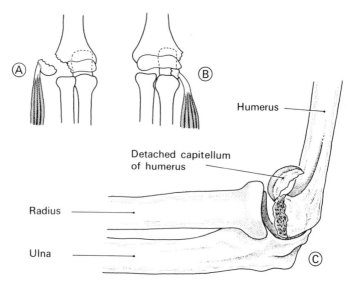

Humerus

Detached capitellum of humerus

Radius

Ulna

Fig. 8.11 There are three different fractures shown:
(a) Fracture of the capitellum in children, or more correctly the capitellar epiphysis.
(b) Trapped medial epicondyle in the joint such as occurs with a dislocated elbow.
(c) Detached fractured capitellum such as occurs in adults.

be excised and the triceps tendon re-attached to the end of the ulna.

Excision is not advisable if the fragment is large and the elbow has been dislocated.

Following the reduction of the fracture and fixation, in the reduced position, the patient's arm is put in a sling with his elbow at a right angle and active movements are encouraged.

5   *Fracture of the capitellum.* This is characteristically an injury that occurs between the ages of 4 and 6 years when the capitellar epiphysis and a small fragment of the adjacent shaft are avulsed. The pull of the attached extensor muscles causes the fragments to be displaced and rotated (Fig. 8.11). It is extremely difficult to reduce this fracture by closed manipulation and, even if it is reduced, it is very difficult to maintain the fracture in a reduced position. If the fracture is left in the displaced position, non-union and progressive cubitus valgus are likely to arise (Fig. 8.12), producing an ugly, weak and painful elbow, with ulnar neuritis as a secondary complication. For this reason this fracture is one of the few fractures in children where it is

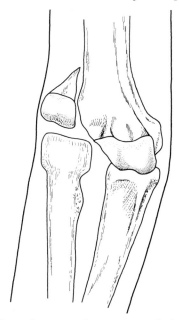

Fig. 8.12 Cubitus valgus, secondary to an ununited capitellar fragment.

usually necessary to do open reduction and internal fixation. Fracture of the capitellum in adults consists mainly of articular surface and adjacent bone. It is usually wise to excise the loose fragment (Fig. 8.11c).

6 *'T' shaped fracture of the lower end of the humerus.* This is usually due to direct violence. There is considerable comminution of the bony fragments

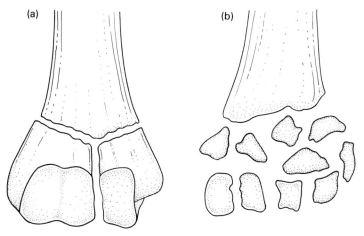

Fig. 8.13 (a) 'T' shaped fracture of the lower end of the humerus. (b) Comminuted fracture of the lower end of the humerus.

and damage to the articular surface. It is a difficult fracture to treat; the elbow is grossly swollen and painful and is often described as a 'bag of bones' (Fig. 8.13).

There are two views on treatment: one is that one should accept the fact that the bony fragments cannot be restored to their proper position but one should try to develop what joint movements are possible. This is done by putting the limb in a collar and cuff and commencing gently early active movements. Another school of thought believes in open reduction with internal fixation. There are many different methods employed for trying to hold the fragments afterwards, they all have the disadvantage that they are likely to lead to extensive fibrosis of the muscles and peri-articular tissues, and ultimately to stiffness of the elbow joint. As a general rule a better functional result is obtained purely by conservative treatment, even though the X-rays continue to look extremely unsatisfactory. In general, the more comminuted the fractures the less satisfactory are the results of the operative treatment. A clean break involving the articular surface can usually be successfully treated by operation.

If there is severe limitation of function at a later date total joint replacement may be considered.

All injuries of the elbow joint are liable to the complication of myositis ossificans.

(e) Dislocated elbow

This is a fairly common injury. The diagnosis is usually obvious with gross prominence of the ulnar bones and alteration in the shape of the elbow (Fig. 8.14). As a general rule, reduction is easy—the elbow is flexed over the

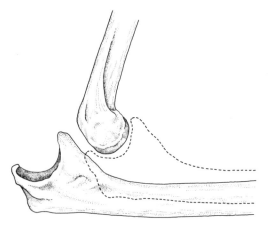

Fig. 8.14   Dislocated elbow.

surgeon's knee and, providing there has been adequate muscular relaxation, the bones can be felt to slide into place (Fig. 8.15). It is important to check the reduction with an X-ray.

After a dislocation, full recovery of movement is notoriously slow and in adults, if the dislocation has been unreduced for more than a few hours,

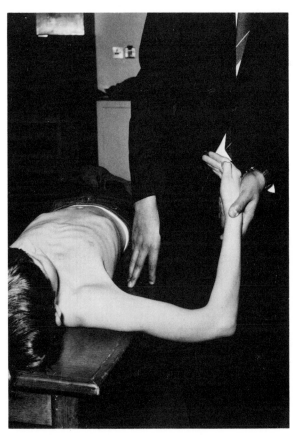

Fig. 8.15   Reduction of dislocated elbow by traction and flexion over the surgeon's knee.

considerable permanent diminution of movement is usually the result. Forced movements and manipulation are notoriously harmful in the case of the elbow and inevitably lead to further reduction of movement.

In early adolescence a dislocation of the elbow may be associated with avulsion of the epiphysis of the medial epicondyle and after reduction may become trapped in the joint. If left untreated after the initial reduction this will lead to stiffness and degenerative arthritis and it is important therefore that an X-ray should always be taken to exclude this condition. If present in the joint, the medial epicondyle must be removed by open operation. (Fig. 8.11b)

(f) Fractures of the radius and ulna

1   *Fractures of the head of the radius* commonly occur as a result of a fall on the outstretched hand. If the bony fragments are very comminuted, it is usual to excise the fragments, especially in adults. When the damage is less extensive there is a considerable difference of opinion between those who treat the condition purely conservatively by resting the limb in a collar and cuff for a few days, and those who advise excision. It should be pointed out that in all cases the ultimate prognosis depends on the amount of damage to the joint articular cartilage, and that if severe damage was done at the time of injury, some permanent limitation of extension of the elbow is almost inevitable. It is also worth pointing out that it is usually undesirable to excise the head of the radius in children, as this may lead to subluxation of the inferior radio-ulnar joint and progressive shortening of the radius.

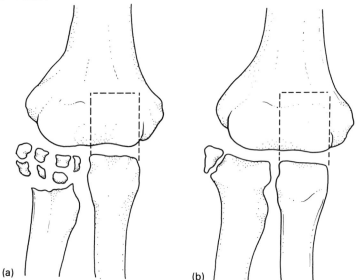

Fig. 8.16   (a) Unsuitable for conservative treatment. (b) Suitable for conservative treatment.

2   *Fractures of the radius and ulna* lead to obvious deformity of the forearm: in children these may be greenstick fractures, i.e. the bones are bent but there is no displacement of bone ends; such fractures can usually be treated

by simple manipulation and splinting. Even if the position is not perfect, further growth will usually restore normal anatomical appearance and it is almost unknown for an adult to have disability due to malunion of a fractured forearm in childhood. There is, however, one curious complication— namely, that the child is liable to re-fracture the bones of the same forearm some two or three months afterwards. This often gives rise to great anxiety on the part of the parents. The treatment, however, is to reassure the parents, re-reduce the fracture and splint the limb as previously.

In adults the position is very different; these fractures are usually asso- ciated with considerable displacement and, as a general rule, open reduction and internal fixation are desirable—for instance, the radius may be fixed by the application of a plate and the ulna fixed by inserting an intramedullary wire. If left displaced in adults, these fractures lead to a certain amount of de- formity and also gross limitation of the rotation movements of the forearm. As with other fractures of the forearm, there is a risk of ischaemic damage to the forearm muscles, leading to severe loss of function of the hand.

3   *Fracture of the ulnar together with dislocation of the head of the radius* is comparatively rare, but is, however, extremely difficult to treat. It is often known as the Monteggia fracture-dislocation. In children this can usually be treated conservatively—namely, by reduction and splinting—but in adults, open operation with reduction of the head of the radius and main- taining it in the reduced position by reconstruction of the orbicular ligament, together with fixation of the ulna in anatomical alignment, are usually necessary (Fig. 8.17).

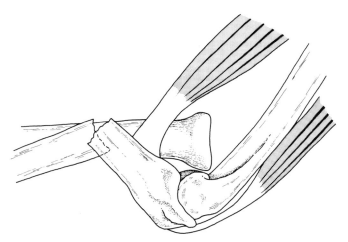

Fig. 8.17   Monteggia fracture.

Isolated fracture of the radius—often known as the Galeazzi fracture—is an important injury because it frequently occurs in adults and, if treated purely conservatively, is likely to lead either to non-union or malunion; it is therefore one of the fractures for which open operation is usually desirable, and this can be most easily achieved by the application of a fixing plate.

4 *Fractures of the lower end of the radius* are traditionally associated with the name of Colles and are known as Colles' fractures. These fractures frequently occur in elderly women; the deformity is characteristic with the hand displaced posteriorly, and is often described as a dinner fork deformity (Fig. 8.18). Reduction is usually easy but maintenance of reduction is not so simple. For this reason a number of complicated procedures involving the wrist being fixed in a distorted position have been suggested. However, the adverse affect on the function of the hand of the more extreme positions is now well recognized, and it is better to have a slight deformity and a normal hand, than a beautiful wrist and a stiff hand. Accordingly, most surgeons employ either simple splints or a below-elbow plaster of Paris cast to hold this particular fracture in position (Fig. 8.19).

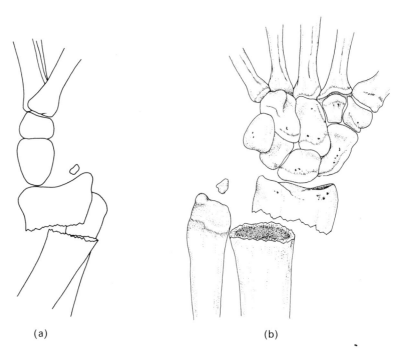

(a)   (b)

Fig. 8.18   Colles' fracture of the radius (a) side view, (b) anterior view.

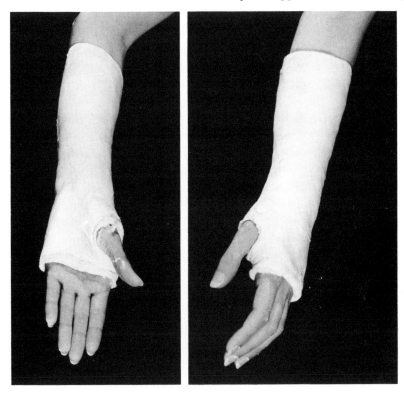

Fig. 8.19   Colles' wrist plaster.

Perhaps the most important thing about this fracture is that the patients should preserve full movement of their fingers and thumb, and active exercises of the hand, elbow and shoulder throughout treatment are more important than perfect reduction.

There are two common injuries to the wrist:

(i) *Fractured scaphoid.* This occurs due to a fall on the outstretched hand. The patient complains of pain and there is some local tenderness in the 'anatomical snuff box', but this is basically a radiological diagnosis and it is important to realize that the fracture of the scaphoid may not be obvious on first X-ray but may only become apparent some three weeks after injury. Therefore, if after a fall a patient complains of persistent pain, his wrist should be re-X-rayed. If left untreated there is considerable risk of non-union and this, in its turn, will eventually lead to degenerative changes in the wrist in a large percentage of patients. It is therefore usual to immobilize scaphoid fractures for some 8 to 10 weeks in plaster of Paris. If, at the end of this time, the fracture is still not united, the surgeon has three alternatives: (i) he can advise the patient to accept non-union; (ii) he can continue with immobilization, or (iii) he can advise a bone grafting operation. In young people this last alternative is usually desirable; in older people the first alternative is the best. It is seldom justifiable to continue with immobilization of the wrist for more than three months.

(ii) *Dislocation of the lunate*. This bone is usually dislocated forwards and presses on the median nerve, leading to symptoms and signs of median neuritis. It is therefore important in any wrist injury if there is a swelling or fullness anteriorly and the patient complains of pain in the median distribution, to have good X-rays taken (Fig. 8.20). If seen immediately it may be possible to reduce the dislocated lunate by direct pressure, but if some days have elapsed, this will usually be difficult, in which case open reduction is necessary. There is some risk that following open reduction

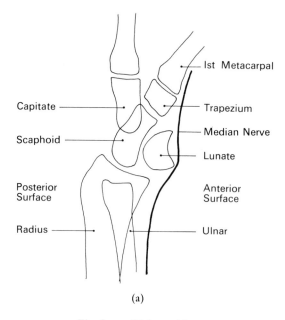

(a)

Fig. 8.20   Dislocated lunate.

the blood supply to the lunate will be disturbed and a condition of osteochondritis or Kienbock's disease may result. This may lead to permanent pain and stiffness of the wrist and, in extreme cases if prolonged conservative treatment does not bring relief, it may be necessary to perform an arthrodesis of the wrist.

(g) Bennett's fracture

This is a fracture of the base of the thumb metacarpal bone and is usually associated with slight subluxation of the metacarpo-phalangeal joint. (Fig. 8.21). The signs are swelling and limitation of movement. Many ingenious methods have been described for the treatment of this fracture, but in fact the ultimate functional result of relative 'non-treatment' is usually good. In other words, a simple supporting bandage or light plaster cast until the period of acute pain has passed, followed by progressive active movements, will usually yield a satisfactorily functional result even though there may be some permanent swelling at the site and the X-ray shows some residual deformity. The more complicated methods, such as open reduction, or prolonged traction, all have disadvantages and are seldom indicated.

(h) Fractures of metacarpals

Fractures of the other metacarpal bones do not usually require any elaborate treatment; even though there is some residual displacement the ultimate

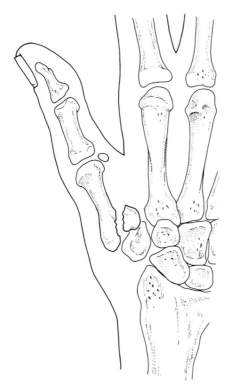

Fig. 8.21   Bennett's fracture.

appearance and functional result is usually good following a short period of splinting with active movements of the fingers throughout.

(i) Fractured phalanges

These have given rise to considerable controversy about the best method of treatment. In many cases where the displacement is relatively slight, a short period of splinting on a curved gutter splint followed by active movement will give the best functional result, even though it may result in some deformity of the finger. However, where there is gross displacement and especially in fractures of the proximal phalanx, it is well known that these may lead either to stiffness of the finger or to gross deformity, and in selected patients, open operation with internal fixation may be desirable both in the interests of appearance and in order to allow the patient active movements from an early date. Naturally, fractures of the phalanges may be associated with other injuries; e.g. damage to the tendons and digital nerves, or extensive damage to the pulp of the fingers. Multiple compound injuries to the fingers are likely to lead to permanent stiffness and deformity, and especially in a working man this may mean that the best treatment is to amputate the finger, as a stiff deformed finger is a risk and a nuisance, especially if the patient works with machinery.

Splints for the upper limb

The Thomas' arm splint

This is occasionally used for exerting fixed traction along the length of the humerus, alternatively it serves to provide a support for the arm when it is elevated for reducing oedematous swelling of the limb, or to provide the best means of observing a limb (Fig. 8.10a). It may be used for fractures of the humerus where the patient must remain recumbent e.g. due to associated fractures of the lower limbs.

It shares some similarities with the Thomas's bed-knee splint; but the ring is hinged at its union with the side bars. It may be used with a flexion piece so that the elbow is flexed, allowing the forearm to deviate from the direction of the traction on the humerus.

For ordering the splint the following measurements are needed:
(a) The circumference of the arm at the axilla;
(b) The length of the inner side of the arm to the finger tips, plus ten inches.

Littler-Jones arm abduction splint

The optimum position of rest for the shoulder is with the arm in abduction at 90 degrees to the median line; the function of this splint is to provide a support, for the limb, in such a position. This may also be achieved by a plaster of Paris spica (see Fig. 8.26).

The abduction splint is made of a lightweight metal frame with canvas straps and leather slings. When the splint is applied it is fixed to the trunk

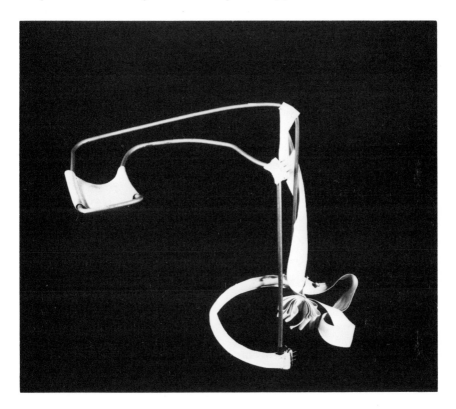

Fig. 8.22 Littler-Jones abduction splint.

by buckled canvas straps at shoulder level and pelvic level. The arm then rests on the platform of leather slings provided by the splint (Fig. 8.22). When ordering the splint the following information is required:
(a) Position of the limb which the surgeon requires.
(b) Whether left-sided or right-sided.
(c) Length of the arm from the shoulder to the palm of the hand.
(d) Circumference of the pelvis.

(e) Distance from the suprasternal notch to the shoulder.

(f) Distance from the symphysis pubis to the suprasternal notch.

Fitting the patient with the splint. The skin is washed and dried; the limb is supported in the desired position by one nurse who is seated, as is the patient.

The body portion of the splint is firmly buckled on to the patient with one strap over the unaffected shoulder and the other around the pelvis.

Using splint wool and bandages, the arm is fixed to the splint with the fingers clear for exercise.

Elbow cage (Fig. 8.23).

The purpose of this splint is to control a weak or unstable elbow joint, if this is required. It is made by the splint maker on a positive cast of the arm of the

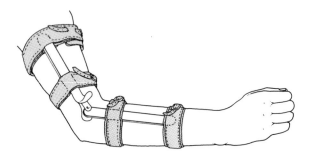

Fig. 8.23 Elbow cage.

patient (see Chapter 30). The hinge is adjusted to give the range of movement required.

Cock-up splints (Fig. 8.24)

These are probably the most commonly used splints of the upper extremity. The short cock-up splint supports the wrist in thirty degrees of dorsiflexion but leaves the fingers free for exercise. The long cock-up is only used when it is necessary to immobilize the fingers as well as the wrist, usually after crushing injuries to the hand or similar conditions or as a temporary measure after tendon surgery.

These are normally in stock in a hospital. They are covered with a layer of adhesive orthopaedic felt before they are fitted to the patient and then bandaged into position.

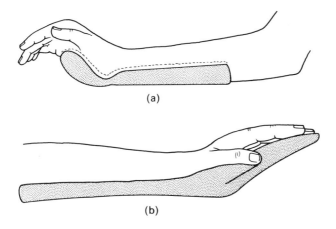

(a)

(b)

Fig. 8.24   Cock-up splints. (a) Supporting wrist only. (b) Supporting whole hand to fingertips.

Wrist straps (Fig. 8.25)
These are made for each patient by the splint maker. They are made of soft leather to support the wrist. A thong passes from the strap over the thenar eminence between the thumb and the index finger.

For working splints and other nerve palsy splints, see Chapter 11.

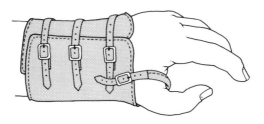

Fig. 8.25   Wrist strap.

Plaster of Paris splintage for the upper limb

(See also Chapter 30.)

The usefulness of plaster of Paris splintage is in its speed of application and the adaptability of the material to varying positions and shapes. Most forms of splintage for the upper limb can be made in this material.

Shoulder spicas:

Requirements. Plaster wool   three rolls.
                Plaster bandages   15 cm wide—eight.
                Plaster slab   15 cm wide—6 layers, 90 cm long.
                Grey felt   two circles, 10 cm diameter; one
                                   circle, 5 cm diameter.
                A stockinette vest.

The shoulder spica serves the same function as the Littler-Jones abduction splint, namely, to hold the shoulder joint in abduction in the optimum position of rest with the elbow flexed and the hand towards the mouth. The desired position for the limb is maintained by the doctor in charge of the procedure until the spica is completed (Fig. 8.26).

Position of the ambulant patient. The patient either sits or stands for the application. The posture of the trunk is important and the patient must be positioned with the spine erect.

Method. A stockinette vest is applied to the trunk and a thin layer of wool roll is arranged over the limb. Felt is used to pad the iliac crests and the medial epicondyle of the humerus on the affected side.

The spica is made in two parts; a trunk section and an arm section. The trunk section is made first; it extends from below the iliac crests to the nipple line around the circumference of the trunk. From the trunk section the plaster is continued on down the shoulder and arm. Slabs may be used to strengthen it. The arm section ends below the heads of the metacarpal bones so that the fingers and thumb are left free. A window is cut into the anterior of the trunk section to permit greater abdominal movement.

Position of the anaesthetized patient. The method is the same but the patient is supported on an orthopaedic operating table or props to permit passing the plaster bandages around the patient.

The shoulder spica can be converted into an open abduction splint by removing the upper portion of the arm and shoulder section.

Although the patient is probably ambulant, nurses should always appreciate the discomfort of any patient whose thorax and abdomen are totally enclosed in plaster.

The 'U' plaster for humeral fractures (Fig. 8.27)

This is used in the treatment of patients with fractures of the shaft of the

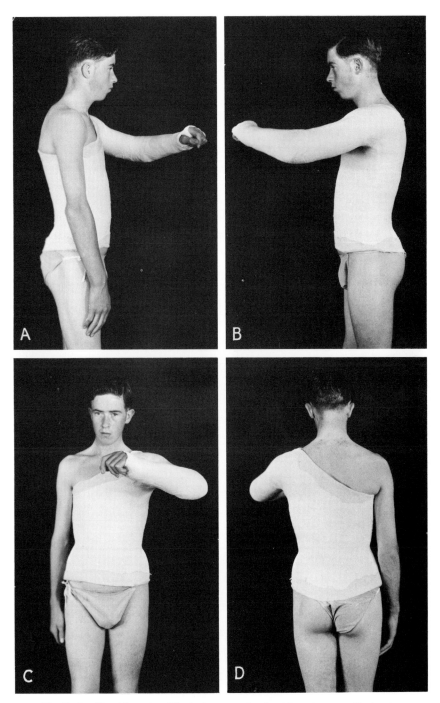

Fig. 8.26　Shoulder spica. The jacket part of a shoulder spica must fit closely round the pelvis as the main support is from the iliac crests. It is difficult to secure a well fitting shoulder spica when the patient is anaesthetized.

humerus. The weight of the cast serves to distract the overlapping fragments and align the ends of the bone (see page 86).

Requirements.

	Plaster wool	one roll.
	Orthopaedic felt	two 5 cm circles.
	Splint wool	small pad
	White open wove bandages	7·5 cm wide—three.
	Plaster slab	15 cm wide—six layers, 1 metre long.
	Narrow arm sling	

Method. A slab of several layers of 15 cm bandage is measured from the axilla of the patient down the inner side of the arm, over the flexed elbow and up

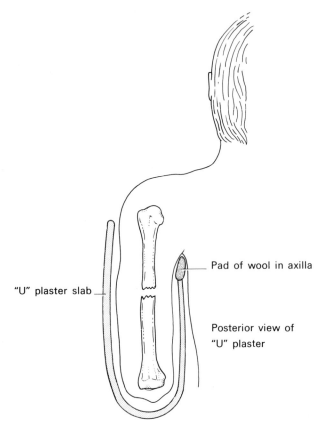

"U" plaster slab

Pad of wool in axilla

Posterior view of "U" plaster

Fig. 8.27 'U' plaster (posterior view).

the outer side of the arm to the base of the neck. The bony prominences of the epicondyles and the point of the ulna are protected with felt and some thin padding arranged at the site of the fracture. The slab is then soaked with water and applied, and moulded firmly to the skin of the patient.

A wet, white, open-wove bandage is then used to hold the U-shaped slab in position. The axilla is protected with a pad of wool and the narrow arm sling accepts the weight of the wrist.

Elbow plasters: (a) plaster slab

Requirements.   Plaster wool   two rolls.
                  Plaster bandages   10 cm wide—two; 15 cm wide—three.

Position of patient. Seated on a stool.

Method. A 15 cm wide plaster slab placed over a layer of padding extends down the lateral surface of the flexed arm from the middle of the deltoid muscle at the shoulder to the wrist. In some cases it may be necessary to continue it to just below the heads of the metacarpals. A wet 7·5 cm white open-wove bandage is used to hold it in place. This is applied in two parts; on the upper third and lower third of the slab, leaving the middle third clear of obstruction for observation of the elbow.

(b) Complete plaster (Figs. 8.8 and 8.28)

This encircles the limb and is therefore *not* suitable for the treatment of recent injuries of the elbow when observation of the part is required. It is applied over a sleeve of stockinette with the bony prominences protected with pieces of felt.

In both plasters the weight of the splint is taken by a narrow arm sling.

Forearm plasters

Requirements.   Plaster wool   one roll.
                  15 cm wide slab   six layers.

In controlling a fracture one established principle is to include the joints above and below the site of fracture. The forearm plaster must therefore include the wrist and elbow joints.

Position of the patient's limb. The plaster is applied with the surgeon holding the limb in the position he considers most suitable. Commonly this is with the elbow at a right angle; the hand neither pronated or supinated, and the wrist is dorsiflexed. The radius and ulna are thus parallel.

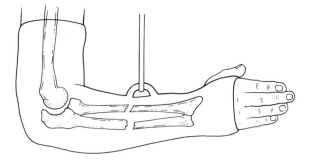

Fig. 8.28   Forearm plaster.

Method. An even layer of padding of either stockinette or wool roll is applied. The plaster can best be made up of a slab of 10 cm wide bandage which extends from below the heads of the metacarpal bones to the level of the neck of the humerus; this is moulded to the shape of the arm. The slab and arm are then encased in plaster bandages which are rolled on.

The plaster should be supported in a narrow arm sling.

Wrist splints

The cock-up splint described on p. 102 may also be simulated in plaster of Paris. Removable slabs made of 10 cm or 15 cm wide bandages can be made to fit the wrist in any position. They are made over a stockinette sleeve which is then split down the back along its length and pasted back over the edges of the splint. These are then bandaged in position when they are dry. They are useful splints for resting the joints of patients with rheumatoid arthritis. Commonly they are used as night splints.

Colles' plaster

Requirements.   Plaster wool   one roll.

Plaster bandages   10 cm wide—two.

Position of the patient's limb. Forearm pronated; wrist flexed with ulnar deviation; the hand is held by the surgeon maintaining traction on the thumb with one hand, and on the index and middle fingers with the other.

Method. The wool rolls are rolled on from below the heads of the metacarpal bones to the head of the radius.

A plaster slab is then placed on the dorsal surface extending over the same area mainly on the radial side of the arm and enclosing the first meta-carpal bone (Fig. 8.17). The slab is trimmed whilst wet.

The slab may be held on with wet, white, open-wove bandages or the plaster may be completed with encircling 7·5 cm wide plaster bandages. This depends upon the wishes of the surgeon; if the injury is new the former; if all swelling has subsided, the latter.

Scaphoid plaster (Fig. 8.29)
Requirements.   Stockinette
Plaster bandages   7·5 cm wide—three.
5 cm wide—one.
15 cm wide—one.

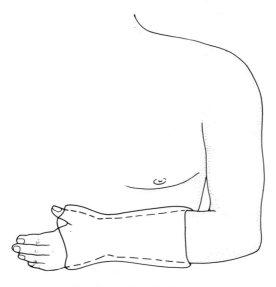

Fig. 8.29   A scaphoid plaster.

Position of the limb. The wrist is in 30 degrees of dorsiflexion with slight radial deviation. The thumb is held in abduction with the elbow resting on a table. An effective scaphoid plaster must be close-fitting and immobilize the thumb.

Method. Stockinette is rolled on to the limb from below the heads of the metacarpal bones to the head of the radius; a hole is made in it for the thumb. A thin layer of wool is arranged around the thumb.

A slab is made of the 15 cm wide bandage and this is soaked and applied to the palmar surface of the hand and forearm. Great strength is required in the area of the palm of the hand.

The cast is completed with first the 5 cm wide bandage around the thumb and the 7·5 cm wide bandages around the hand, wrist and forearm.

To include a finger in a hand plaster an extra slab is required. This is 5 cm wide and 5 cm longer than the patient's finger.

Nursing management. These patients are usually treated as out-patient casualties who will not be admitted to hospital and will return home after treatment. There is some danger in such an approach and certain precautions must be taken.

In the stress of coping with large numbers of patients (this is a particular problem in large city hospitals) the handling of the patient may be too rapid and too superficial. The nursing staff must guard against insufficient enquiry into previous and present illnesses of the patient; if the patient is diabetic, for example, special care is needed for anaesthesia. The nurse must also enquire into the circumstances that the patient must return to on departure from the centre; is the patient elderly? alone at home? living on an upper floor with the need to carry fuel? Is she a mother with a young baby or family to manage alone? There are cases where admission to hospital is better than immediate departure for home with a wet plaster on the limb and unwell after an anaesthetic. Special follow-up by a visiting nurse or the patient's doctor may be adequate.

For all patients who are to have anaesthesia the hospital is legally and morally responsible for obtaining written consent for the procedure and for ensuring that a reasonable clinical examination is carried out and urine testing routinely performed. The patient must be permitted to empty the bowel and urinary bladder before an anaesthetic and must be disrobed of clothing which may be soiled with plaster or which constricts the thorax or abdomen. At least four hours must elapse since food was taken to ensure that the stomach is empty.

Transportation home with a relative as an escort is a matter for the hospital staff to arrange. It is particularly important that a responsible relative or friend receives instructions about the drying of the plaster and the dangers of constriction of the limb if swelling should occur inside the plaster. These should additionally be given to the patient in a printed form with instructions about the next attendance at the fracture clinic. Under no circumstances should a patient be allowed to drive a car after an anaesthetic.

Physiotherapy and exercise

Particularly in upper limb injuries when plaster and other splints have been applied, care must be taken to ensure that the limb is maintained in good condition by exercise of all the joints and muscles that can be moved. The physiotherapist is an important member of the team caring for the out-patient.

The physiotherapist should be present at all consultations and must decide upon the most suitable regime for each patient. The more intelligent patient, perhaps with limited time available, will probably be taught exercises to practice at home. In some circumstances it may only be possible to deal with the patient in the physiotherapy department.

All patients with limb plasters must be instructed to use the fingers and thumb as much as possible; sewing, knitting, writing, are all useful exercises. There is a danger that the shoulder and elbow may stiffen through lack of use even though they were not involved in the injury. Such activities as hair brushing and dressing call for full use of these joints; the patient must be encouraged to perform these tasks and the next of kin discouraged from helping too much.

Cross references from this Chapter

Chapter 17: Page 266, ischaemia.
Chapter 11: Peripheral nerve lesions.
Chapter 21: Hand deformities.
Chapter 29: External splinting.
Chapter 30: Plaster of Paris technique.

9

Fractures and Dislocations of the Lower Limb

Relevant applied anatomy and physiology

In comparison with the structure of the upper limb with its lightness of weight plus wide range of movement, the lower limb has larger bones and muscles, and joints that are stronger, even if the range of their movement is less. This is because, in the human subject, the function of the two extremities, upper and lower, is different. The hand is prehensile (capable of grasping) and the function of the upper limb is to put this hand where it needs to be. The lower limb has the foot with the function of providing a suitable appendage for supporting the body in the upright position on two limbs.

The lower limbs must be capable of supporting the whole weight of the body, plus any weight carried by the body. Thus a man carrying a two hundredweight sack of fuel on his back transfers the whole weight of the contents of the sack plus that of his body on to the single limb that is resting on the ground as he walks. Thus a great deal is required of the lower limb, particularly in people who bear heavy weights. The lower limb structure therefore presents a nice balance between the ability to move and that of bearing great weight.

Included in the classification of the bones of the lower limb is the innominate bone, which is part of the pelvis, the femur or thigh bone, the patella or knee cap, the tibia or shin bone and the fibula which is a slim supporting bone (so called in ancient times because of its similarity in shape to a brooch-pin), the tarsal bones, metatarsus and phalanges of the foot.

The innominate bone is large and solid; forming part of the bony pelvis and the hip joint. The pelvis is a complete ring of bones forming a solid support upon which the main portion of the body rests. An important function of the pelvis, with the innominate bone, is protection of and support for the urinary bladder, the rectum and colon, the female internal genital organs, and nerves and blood vessels.

The hip joint (Fig. 19.1) is a ball and socket joint with a deep socket receiv-

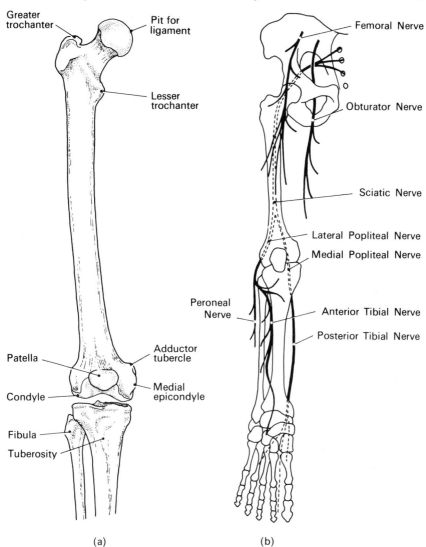

Fig. 9.1 Diagram of the lower limbs. (a) Bone structure. (b) Main nerves.

ing a large head placed on a strong neck. The capsule of the joint is made up of a fibrous capsule with a complete support of extracapsular ligaments and another support of muscle tissue from the cuff of hip muscles surrounding it. These muscles are essential for the strength and stability of the joint as well as the range of movement it can permit.

The knee joint is also a strong joint with ample support from surrounding ligaments. This is a hinge joint which can be moved from complete extension at 180 degrees to flexion of about 5 degrees. For efficiency it requires pieces of cartilage shaped like a meniscus, and two internal ligaments, the cruciate ligaments, to maintain the congruity of the distal end of the femur and the proximal end of the tibia. The patella is a sesamoid bone which is embedded in the tendon of the quadriceps group of muscles as it passes over the front of the knee; it forms a synovial joint with the front of the knee to improve the action of quadriceps in extending the knee.

The ankle joint depends for its efficiency upon a number of ligaments which secure the talus (one of the tarsal bones) of the foot against the distal end of the tibia and fibula. Rupture of these ligaments or a fracture of the tibia or fibula will result in an unstable ankle joint.

The muscles which move the ankle are situated on the leg below the knee. They operate the movements of the ankle by contracting against long tendons which are attached to the foot and toes some distance away from the muscle.

The lower limb has several large nerves and blood vessels passing down it. These are directly adjacent to the bones and joints at most of their length. Fractures and dislocations of the limb may be complicated by involvement of these vital structures (Fig. 9.1b).

Prevention of accidents to the lower limb

There will never be a time when fractures and dislocations of the lower limb will not occur. Man is an adventurous creature and he will climb mountains, enter the sports arena, drive fast racing cars and perform many of the hazardous activities which may result in broken bones if things go wrong. There are certain precautions which can reduce these incidents however. Throughout the development world there is an epidemic of trauma. With increasing affluence people buy motor scooters and cars. Industrialization and mechanization lead to more accidents.

Impatience and the desire to make more money quickly lead to neglect of safety precautions. Education and self-control are the only sure means of reducing accidents but technical considerations such as better design of machinery, cars, motor cycles, etc., mitigate the effects of accidents.

Road transport design
Many driver and front-seat passenger victims of road transport accidents

sustain broken legs. This may be the result of concertina force on the car and victim as the engine is crushed against the legs (Fig. 9.2). In the case of drivers of heavy goods vehicles, the legs may be fractured around the upright steering column. Much research goes on into better safety factors to be introduced in the design of new vehicles; a bulkhead between the engine and the passenger seat and collapsible steering columns, for example.

Motor-cyclists are probably the most vulnerable of all transport users; their body protection is minimal, the legs are usually completely unprotected. Suitable leg-guards in the design of motor-cycles would help to protect the lower limbs.

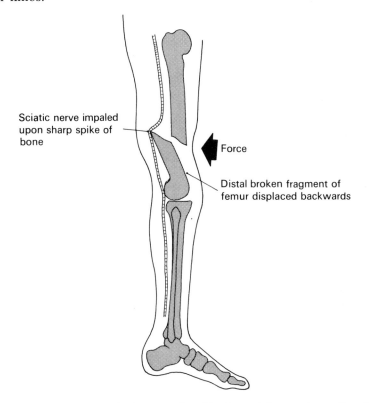

Sciatic nerve impaled upon sharp spike of bone

Force

Distal broken fragment of femur displaced backwards

Fig. 9.2   Fracture of the femur produced by direct violence and complicated by involvement of the sciatic nerve.

Flooring surfaces

Youth and adaptability enable younger folk to cope with slippery flooring or irregular surfaces without falling. In the older person, these become serious hazards. On wet streets and wet tiled or rubber flooring an unstable old person, with poor balance, raised blood pressure and dizziness, may fall and fracture bones which are osteoporotic and brittle. Research into the provision of flooring which absorbs moisture and retains a non-slip surface, even when wet, has been in progress for many years; such surfaces are in use in geriatric units.

Industrial hazards

It is difficult for an employer to remove all possible hazards to his workers. The work must continue and heavy objects must be transported and turned. The provision of footwear with metal toecaps is advocated and safety officers are employed in factories, building sites and mines to train workers in methods which reduce the hazards to broken limbs.

Sports injuries

Most sportsmen disdain the use of padding and protection yet these are essential, particularly in fast games such as ice hockey and football. When fast, hard balls are used, in cricket for example, pads to the legs are necessary.

The principles of first aid in lower limb fractures

Symptoms and signs

A broken leg causes shock in a patient because bleeding into the periosteum from the site of the fracture may be great and this then becomes static blood —that which is out of circulation and lost from the blood vessels. In fractures of the femur, for example, the patient will be severely shocked for this reason.

Additionally the patient will have all the local signs and symptoms of a fracture which are:

1   Pain.
2   A history of the type of injury which could cause a broken bone.
3   A story of feeling and hearing the bone break.
4   Obvious deformity of the limb, both at the site of the fracture and in the general alignment of the limb.
5   Shortening of the limb by comparison with the opposite uninjured limb; abnormal lateral rotation of the affected limb as the patient lies on the ground.
7   Swelling and discoloration at the site of the fracture—this gives the appearance of bruising and blueness of the area.
8   Inability to bear weight on the limb or stand; but of course, the patient must not be asked to try to bear weight!
9   If the fracture is compound there will be a wound at the site of fracture, with bleeding.

First-aid treatment

The positions and types of fractures affecting the lower limbs are many and varied, but certain principles of first-aid management exist for all of them and can be applied to all patients. These are:

1   Do not move the patient from the area in which he is lying before the limb has been immobilized, unless he is in danger from other factors, which cannot be controlled such as fire, or falling buildings and debris.

2   Arrange for one assistant to apply steady manual traction along the length of the limb and a second to place a hand above and below the site of the break to reduce movement whilst the limb is being immobilized.

3   Use the unaffected limb of the patient as a support to immobilize the broken limb. Only when both legs are broken is it necessary to use timber or other improvizations as splints.

4   Move the unaffected limb towards the affected leg rather than move the broken limb.

5   Pad the hollows and spaces between the legs to provide an even surface against which the affected leg can rest. This is to avoid angulation of the fragments of the bone at the fracture site. Soft garments or wool will serve for this purpose.

6   Fix the legs together at the following points:

(a) At the feet and ankles with a figure of eight bandage arranged over the footwear.

(b) Around the knee joints with padding under the knot to avoid causing a sore. The area below the knee must be avoided to prevent compression of the lateral popliteal nerves.

(c) Around the hip joints at the level of the great trochanters of femora.

7   The site of the fracture must be effectively immobilized. This can be done with pieces of corrugated cardboard or box wood extending for some inches above and below the site of the fracture and held in place with bandages at the top and bottom of the supporting splintage.

The shock to a patient who has a fracture of the femur or tibia and fibula can be great. Warmth, using coats or blankets, careful lifting and handling, and transfer to hospital as quickly as possible are obvious needs; no fluids or food may be given because an anaesthetic may be required soon after admission. An important factor in prevention of shock in limb fractures is immobilization of the part as soon as possible.

If both limbs are fractured it is necessary to apply external splintage. The same bandaging as described above is used, but lengths of wood extending from the axillae to beyond the feet must also be incorporated.

Plaster of Paris emergency packs for splintage are now available for use in centres where fractures are commonly occurring such as on sports fields. Inflatable polyethylene splints are also sold commercially and have their uses in accident centres and first-aid posts. Being radiotranslucent an X-ray can be taken without their being removed. Care should be taken not to over-inflate and impair the circulation.

Fractures of the lower limb

Fractures of the pelvis
These are usually due to direct violence, though in elderly people with soft bones they may occur following a minor fall. Their main importance is the

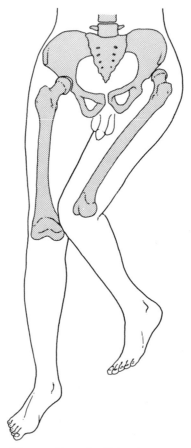

Fig. 9.3   Posterior dislocation of the hip.

possibility of there being associated damage to the pelvic organs, particularly the bladder, urethra, rectum and on rare occasions the female genital organs and the sciatic nerve. These complications are, however, rare; in general, fractures of the pelvis do not require accurate reduction or open operation and are fairly simply treated by a rest in bed with a firm binder, allowing the patient to become mobile as soon as their pain subsides. The more complicated procedures which were used in the past, including extensive plaster jackets and so on, are usually unnecessary, but for nursing purposes it may be convenient to treat the patient in suspended slings.

Blood loss in association with pelvic fractures may be considerable. This is a so-called silent area in which there may be no external signs of internal bleeding. In unexplained shock following an injury the possibility of a fractured pelvis should always be considered. Occasionally a major artery or vein is torn in association with a pelvic fracture; immediate surgery to stop bleeding and save life is then required.

Fractures of the acetabulum

These are of three main types: there is first of all the posterior lip fracture of the acetabulum which is usually associated with a posterior dislocation of the hip joint and often with a sciatic nerve lesion (Fig. 9.3). Open reduction is usually required with internal fixation, as otherwise the hip will re-dislocate and severe arthritis will develop.

There is, secondly, the crack fracture of the pelvis which involves the acetabulum. This is usually of relatively minor significance, especially if it does not involve the main weight-bearing area.

Thirdly, there is the stove-in acetabulum—sometimes referred to as a central dislocation of the hip though this is actually a poor descriptive name (Fig. 9.4a). Here the important thing is to try to ensure that the head of the femur is reduced to its correct position under the main weight-bearing portion under the acetabulum (Fig. 9.4b). To do this, lateral traction on the hip for instance, by means of a Steinmann's pin inserted through the great trochanter and with weights over the side of the bed, is a useful measure. It is surprising what excellent function eventually results, even with an indifferent X-ray picture, provided the head of the femur comes to lie under the weight-bearing portion of the acetabulum. Some surgeons have endeavoured to perform major acetabular reconstruction by open operation and internal fixation, but these operations are difficult and have not gained general acceptance. Some patients require a hip replacement at a later date.

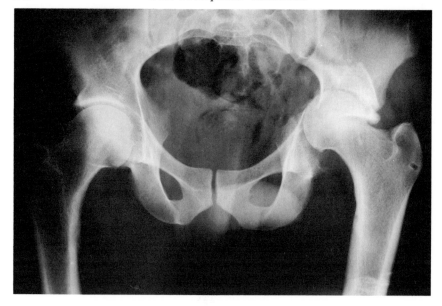

Fig. 9.4   (a) A 'stove-in' acetabulum.

Dislocation of the hip

Traumatic dislocation of the hip is commonly a posterior dislocation; this may occur either in association with a fracture of the posterior limb of the

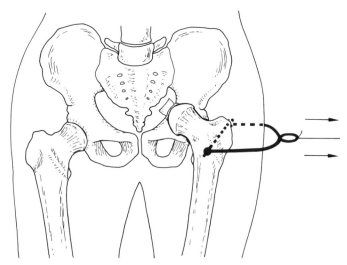

Fig. 9.4   (b) Lateral traction used in the treatment of a 'stove-in' acetabulum.

acetabulum, due to direct force imparted up the femur when the hip is in the flexed position, or it may be due to abduction, in which case the head of the femur dislocates inferiorly and then assumes the posterior position. The classical signs of a posterior dislocation are shortening, adduction, internal rotation and flexion. This dislocation is usually reduced quite simply by anaesthetizing the patient, lying him flat on his back and then by flexing the knee and the hip to a right angle, and with one assistant holding the pelvis, the operator lifts the hip gently forwards until the head of the femur is felt to enter the acetabulum, when the leg can be extended and externally rotated (Fig. 9.5).

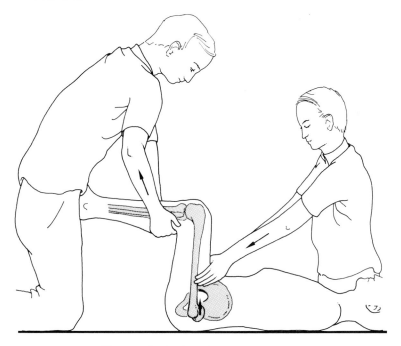

Fig. 9.5   Reduction of a dislocated hip.

Following this, the dislocation is stable providing there has not been an associated fracture of the acetabulum. Opinion varies as to the after-treatment which is necessary. It is well recognized that after a dislocation of the hip, some 25 to 30 per cent of patients develop aseptic necrosis of the head of the femur due to interference with the blood supply. Most surgeons, however, believe that no treatment can alter the incidence of this condition, therefore, after 10 days or so of traction in recumbency there is no reason why the patient should not start gentle non-weight-bearing exercises, and as soon as muscle tone has been restored, resume partial weight-bearing, e.g. 3 to 4 weeks after the injury. On the other hand, some surgeons believe that prolonged recumbency for 3 months diminishes the incidence of avascular necrosis and that this is necessary after every dislocation of the hip. Up-to-date there are no available figures which can prove or disprove this latter contention.

Fractures of the neck of the femur

This is a very important injury which is extremely common in frail old ladies. It is often associated with a considerable degree of osteoporosis. The classical features are that the patient trips over and has pain in the hip with shortening, adduction, external rotation and slight flexion. These patients are of an age where prolonged recumbency and incarceration in bed are badly tolerated, and therefore it is nearly always necessary to perform operative fixation of the hip.

Unfortunately at the time of injury the blood supply to the head of the femur is disturbed in some 40 per cent of cases, and this is likely to lead to avascular necrosis (Fig. 9.6) with all its disastrous complications. At the moment there is no known method whereby avascular necrosis can be

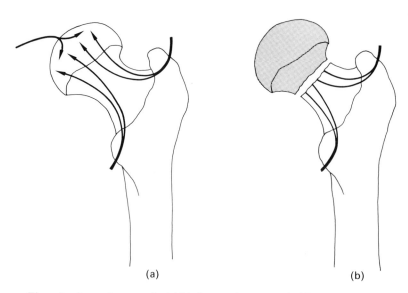

(a)   (b)

Fig. 9.6 Avascular necrosis. (a) Unfractured upper end of femur with blood supply ascending up head to neck. (b) Fractured neck with interruption of blood supply and avascular necrosis of head of femur.

avoided, but it is believed that the more efficient the internal fixation, the less chance there is of this complication. It is also known that the greater the degree of displacement of the fracture the greater the likelihood of aseptic necrosis. Much effort therefore has been spent on ensuring that such fractures are perfectly reduced and then firmly fixed. If the proximal fragment is small and the bone is soft, this is by no means easy and the overall failure rate is considerable. In addition, one must bear in mind that many of these patients are in poor general condition with multiple cerebral, cardiac, pulmonary or renal pathology and, even with the best treatment, mortality within a year of the accident is very considerable. Even among those who survive, a considerable degree of residual disability is unfortunately only too common. This is often known as the 'unsolved fracture' and indeed, in view of its great economic and humanitarian importance in this country, it is not surprising that so much effort has been spent in hitherto rather ineffectual attempts to solve the problem. Some surgeons believe that the results of internal fixation are so poor that an immediate replacement arthroplasty is the correct treatment, but even this is not without its complications in such an age group. In general, a high subcapital fracture which is badly displaced should be treated by prosthetic replacement.

Intertrochanteric fractures

These are common in elderly people and are usually due to a fall. Although such fractures can be treated conservatively with success from the point of view of fracture union, they usually occur in people in whom prolonged rest in bed would be undesirable, therefore they are usually treated by internal fixation by means of a pin and plate (Fig. 9.7).

The complication of avascular necrosis of the head of the femur is very rare but these fractures commonly unite with considerable varus deformity due to the fact that the lesser trochanter has usually been avulsed from the femur. This means that there is no effective action of the psoas muscle and the uncompensated action of the gluteal muscles produces a coxa vara deformity. Attempts have been made to overcome this by weakening the abductor muscles at the time of operation by dividing them at their point of insertion into the greater trochanter.

The clinical features of this fracture are, of course, pain, inability to walk, adduction and external rotation of the limb, together with extensive bruising in the hip region.

Internal fixation is least satisfactory in comminuted fractures in patients with some osteoporosis. Under these circumstances Hamilton Russell

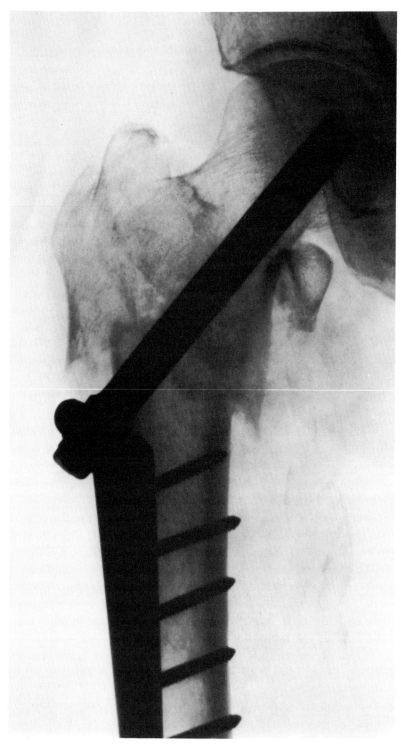

Fig. 9.7 Internal fixation of intertrochanteric fracture with pin and plate.

traction gives a better functional result if the patient's general condition is good enough.

Sub-trochanteric fractures
In children, these fractures do not present any special problem and can be treated on a Thomas' splint. But in adults there is a greater tendency for the proximal fragment to be flexed; this results either in union with deformity, or malunion. Accordingly, in adults it is customary to fix the bones either by a pin and plate or by an intramedullary nail.

Fractures of the shaft of the femur
These fractures are fairly common at all ages and are usually due to direct violence (Fig. 9.2). In children such fractures are best treated on a Thomas' splint and the results are excellent—that is to say, union in good position with full restoration of function is achieved in a comparatively short time. Opinions differ about the ideal treatment in the adult. While the majority of these fractures can be satisfactorily treated in a Thomas' splint, this requires a fairly long period in bed and may result in stiffness of the knee. Although this usually disappears in time, in severe fractures it may be permanent. Accordingly, some surgeons believe that these fractures should be treated by open operation; internal fixation with an intramedullary pin is the most popular treatment (Fig. 9.8). It has the advantage that, if successful, the patient is able to move far sooner and is not confined for such a long period to bed. Knee stiffness is also less of a problem. But this method has the disadvantage that if infection supervenes, a chronic osteomyelitis of the femur results with very serious consequences. Also, the fixation is not one hundred per cent, especially in relation to rotation movements, and the instance of non-union following operative treatment is higher than that following conservative treatment. Some surgeons believe that these fractures should be treated by the application of two long plates at a right angle. This involves considerable muscle stripping which is undesirable. If image intensifiers are available closed intramedullary nailing is the treatment of choice if the fracture is in the shaft and is not comminuted.

If internal fixation is used a right angled blade plate is the best but even with this if the bones are soft it is necessary also to use external splinting.

Supracondylar fractures of the femur
These are difficult fractures in the sense that it is hard to hold the fragments in good position and that stiffness of the knee is very much more common. While attempts have been made to treat these fractures by internal fixation,

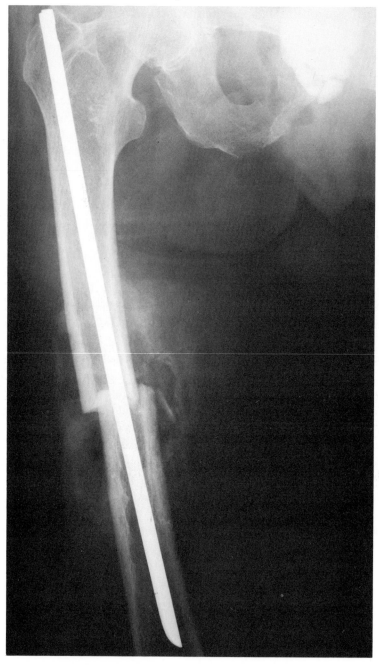

Fig. 9.8   (a) Internal fixation of the shaft of the femur with an intramedullary
pin (Kuntschner nail).

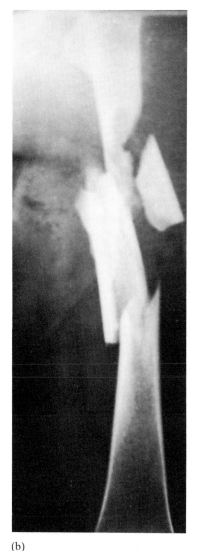

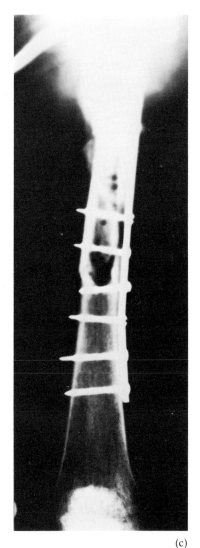

(b)   (c)

Fig. 9.8   (b) Fracture of the femur before plating.

Fig. 9.8   (c) Plating of a fracture of a femur.

this is not entirely satisfactory and non-union and malunion are not infrequent. On the whole, the fracture is best treated by the application of
traction with a Steinmann's pin inserted into the tibial tubercle with the
knee bent to some 60 degrees with a Pearson Knee-flexion attachment and
ordinary Thomas' splint (Fig. 9.10). This will result in union in a satisfactory

position but knee stiffness will be a problem and may even require a quadricepsplasty or freeing of the patella at a later date.

Fractures of the patella

There are two main types: first of all there is the stellate comminuted fracture which is usually due to a direct blow. In this type of fracture there is no failure of continuity of the quadriceps mechanism and the fracture can be treated successfully by conservative means, this may, however, result in considerable irregularity of the patello-articular surface demanding an excision later, as for chondromalacia of the patella. In order to prevent this some surgeons advise immediate excision of the patella.

The other type of patellar fracture is the transverse fracture which is usually due to indirect violence in which the two fragments are separated. If left untreated this would result in non-union or fibrous union with considerable weakness of the knee extension mechanism. It is therefore customary to perform an operation to restore continuity of the quadriceps mechanism; this can either be by suturing fragments of the patella together, or by exercising the fragments and affecting a repair of the quadriceps mechanism.

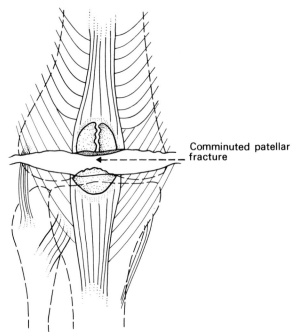

Comminuted patellar fracture

Fig. 9.9 Transverse fracture of the patella with associated tearing of the lateral expansions of the quadriceps and wide separation of the fragments. If untreated, permanent weakness and limitation of extension results.

Dislocation of the knee

This is usually due to direct violence and it may be associated with pressure on the popliteal vessels. It is therefore essential that the dislocation be

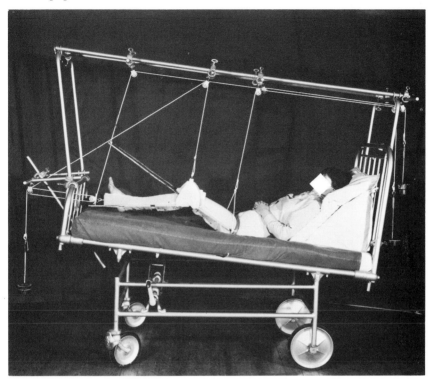

Fig. 9.10 (a) Patient in Thomas' splint with Pearson knee-flexion piece.

reduced at the earliest possible moment. Curiously enough instability of the knee is relatively rare; the main problem is permanent stiffness of the knee.

Following reduction of the dislocation the knee is held in a plaster cylinder or in a Thomas' splint for some three weeks, after which active movements are commenced.

Rupture of the collateral ligaments

A varus strain will produce rupture of the fibular collateral ligament often with an associated lesion of the external popliteal nerve. A valgus strain will produce rupture of the medial collateral ligaments. Minor degrees of rupture may be treated purely conservatively, but if there is complete rupture, operative repair is usually indicated. In order to assess the degree of rupture it is customary to examine the knee under anaesthetic applying the approp-

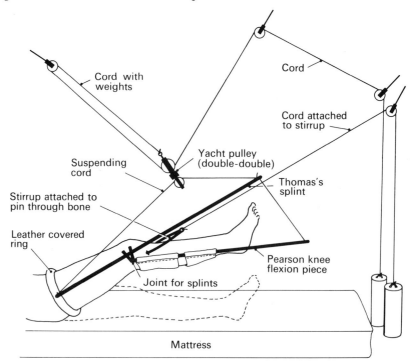

Fig. 9.10   (b) Detail of Thomas' splint with a Pearson knee-flexion piece and applied traction.

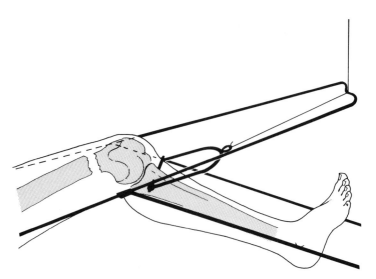

Fig. 9.10   (c) Pearson knee-flexion piece, showing skeletal traction. .

riate strain, either varus or valgus. If the ligaments are repaired straight away the ultimate prognosis is good, but if they are allowed to unite with lengthening, weakness and some instability of the knee usually results which may lead to severe degenerative arthritis at a later stage.

Torn ligaments are often associated with tears of the corresponding meniscus, therefore at operation this should be examined and if it is found to be hopelessly torn it should be excised.

Tears of the cruciate ligaments are usually due to a direct blow on the upper end of the tibia. They lead to considerable instability of the knee, in particular when the knee is flexed it is possible to glide the tibia backwards and forwards in relation to the femur—the so-called 'draw' sign. Repair of the cruciate ligaments is difficult and is much more likely to lead to arthritis of the joint at a later date. On the whole it is best to treat this lesion conservatively, laying particular emphasis on the development of the powerful quadriceps muscles. In spite of this there is likely to be appreciable residual disability in the shape of instability of the knee, leading ultimately to degenerative arthritis. Late repair of lax ligaments is usually unsatisfactory whereas the results of immediate repair are good. Prompt diagnosis and treatment are essential.

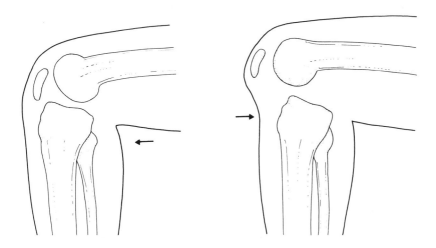

Fig. 9.11   Drawer sign in ruptured cruciate ligaments.

Fractures of the tibial plateau

These are common and are usually due to a varus or valgus strain with depression of the corresponding plateau—that is, following a strain there is depression of the lateral part of the tibial plateau and *vice versa* for a varus strain; depression of the medial part of the plateau. Minor degrees may be left relatively untreated—that is to say, after a short period of rest in a back splint and aspiration of any associated haemarthrosis, active non-weight-bearing movements are started as the major risk is stiffness of the knee. However, if there is gross deformity which would lead to permanent genu valgus or genu varum, it is customary to operate, elevate the fracture and pack chips of cancellous bone under the fracture so that the bone is held in the reduced position. This is a comparatively difficult operation and as the combination of operation and long external fixation is liable to increase the chance of stiffness to the knee, it is therefore important that mechanical fixation should be secure in order to allow early knee movement.

Fractures of the shaft of the tibia

This is the most common fracture and probably the commonest cause of prolonged disability in young adult males. As the antero-medical surface of the tibia is subcutaneous, the fracture is often open or compound and this frequently leads to chronic osteomyelitis, delayed union and even amputation. In addition, there is often damage to muscles and blood vessels.

In children, treatment is nearly always conservative—manipulative reduction and plaster fixation. Even though there is some shortening, this corrects itself with growth and provided there is good alignment, slight or moderate overlap of the fragments does not matter. It is however important that the fracture should not be allowed to unite with a rotational deformity.

In adults, treatment is far more difficult and there are wider differences of opinion on the best treatment.

Simple transverse fractures can usually be treated successfully by manipulation and plaster. Nevertheless, many surgeons believe that internal fixation with metallic plates—with or without compression—increases the speed and certainty of union. Other surgeons feel that there is a risk of infection and that this risk outweighs the advantages of internal fixation. The risks of infection are less if the plate is placed under muscles and not on the subcutaneous surface of the tibia.

External (Russian) splinting

The popular method of using compression plates has the disadvantage that they are usually applied to the subcutaneous surface and being bulky, wound closure may be difficult and skin healing may be delayed.

An alternative treatment is by the use of external splinting fixed to the bone by transfixion pins (preferably Kirschner wires). This system has been used extensively with great success on the Continent of Europe for some years. It is particularly indicated when there is skin damage.

Oblique fractures treated with plaster of Paris usually unite quickly but often with half to three quarters of an inch of shortening. This can be prevented either by open operation or by the application of continuous traction through the os calcis and placing the limb on a Bohler-Braun splint (c.v.) (Fig. 9.12). There is some evidence that os calcis traction leads to stiffness of the subastragaloid joint.

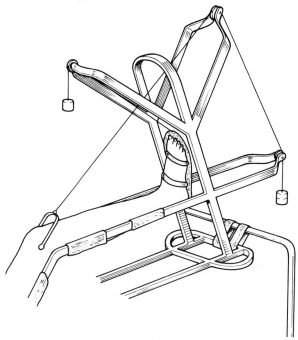

Fig. 9.12   A Bohler-Braun splint.

'Butterfly' and comminuted fractures are difficult to treat in a simple plaster cast and maintain perfect anatomical alignment. The choice lies between accepting a certain amount of deformity, skeletal traction (see above) and plate fixation. Most surgeons believe that, if plate fixation is used, the fixation should be as rigid as possible and to ensure this, fixation with compression is often employed.

Fractures of the fibula
Fractures of the shaft of the fibula alone are usually fairly trivial conditions due to a direct blow and do not require any special treatment. However, it is

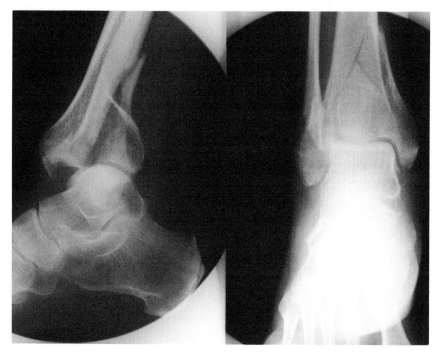

Fig. 9.13   (a) Fracture of the ankle.

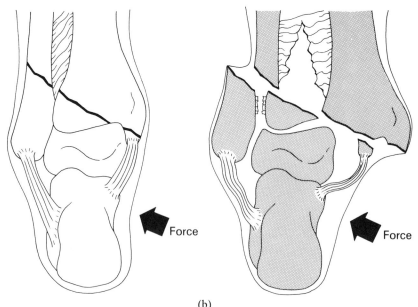

(b)

Fig. 9.13   (b) Force resulting in a fracture—dislocation of the ankle joint.

important to exclude associated fractures of the tibia or dislocation of the ankle.

The so-called Maisonneuve Fracture consists of a fracture of the upper end of the fibula with rupture of the deltoid ligament and lateral subluxation of the astraqalus. Every X-ray of the fibula should include the ankle.

Ankle fractures

These are traditionally associated with the name of Percival Pott, and it is common to group all fractures of the ankle as a Pott's fracture-dislocation (Fig. 9.13). In point of fact there are three quite distinct fractures with a different mechanism. There are first of all fractures due to an adduction injury. In its minor degree an adduction injury merely causes a sprain of the ankle or tear of the fibular collateral ligaments. This can be treated conservatively, provided there is no associated bony lesion, but in more severe examples there is associated fracture of the medial malleolus which is displaced. This fracture can be treated conservatively by reduction and fixation in plaster, but as operative fixation of the medial malleolus is a very simple and satisfactory procedure, this is usually advisable.

There is another group of fractures due essentially to an external rotation of the foot in relation to the tibia. This results in a spiral fracture of the tibia with either tearing of the deltoid ligament, or an associated fracture of the medial malleolus. It is important to determine how extensive the ligamentous damage is and whether the ankle is unstable. If the ankle is unstable, the fracture may be treated either by reduction and fixation with an above-knee plaster—a below-knee plaster does not control rotation forces—or alternatively, it can be treated by open reduction and the insertion of a screw between the tibia and fibula to hold the tibial fractures reduced. If there has been an associated fracture of the medial malleolus, this can also be fixed by a screw, preferably at the same time.

A pure abduction force may give rise to a fracture of the lateral malleolus, with either tearing of the deltoid ligament, or a fracture of the medial malleolus. In rare cases there may be complete disruption of the inferior tibio-fibular ligament, giving rise to the so-called Dupuytren's fracture. These fractures are usually best treated by open reduction if there is extensive damage to the medial side of the joint, but if the medial side of the joint is relatively undamaged they can be satisfactorily treated by reduction and fixation in a below-knee plaster.

Fractures of the talus

These are usually due to a plantar flexion force applied to the foot and were common in aviators in the earlier type of aeroplane. The blood supply to the talus is precarious and, following a fracture, may be cut off, leading to avascular necrosis, arthritis of the ankle and sub-taloid joint, and non-union of the fracture.

Treatment is difficult because although it is perfectly easy to reduce the fracture, there is a very real risk of the above complications. If avascular necrosis supervenes, the patient will have a painful and stiff ankle with considerable impairment in function. The question of treatment is extremely difficult; some surgeons believe that the fracture should be immobilized in plaster for a prolonged period, e.g. up to two years. Open reduction with internal fixation usually results in union but does not diminish the incidence of avascular necrosis. It has the advantage of obviating the need for prolonged external fixation which almost inevitably causes a stiff foot.

If avascular necrosis occurs it is difficult to treat as attempted arthrodesis of the ankle is often unsuccessful. The alternatives are wearing a moulded external support, astragalectomy with or without tibio-calcaneal fusion and, if all else fails, amputation.

Fractures of the calcaneus

These are usually due to a fall onto the feet from a height. The characteristic features are, pain, swelling, broadening of the heel and obliteration of the normal hollow under the lateral malleolus. There is always assumption of greater or lesser degree of damage to the sub-talar joint. Most surgeons

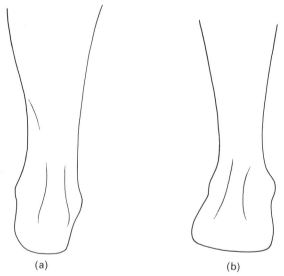

(a) (b)

Fig. 9.14 Calcaneal fracture. Showing (a) normal and (b) abnormal heels.

believe that it is impossible to reduce these fractures or to restore the sub-talar joint to normal, and that complicated methods devised to aid reduction nearly always fail and only serve to increase the deformity by creating stiffness of the other joints of the foot. Therefore this fracture is usually treated by elevation and the application of a firm bandage and early movement. There is also a rare avulsion fracture of the point of insertion of the tendo Achillis which requires operative repair.

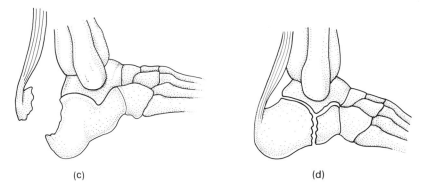

(c)   (d)

Fig. 9.14   (c) Avulsion of insertion of tendo achillis. (d) Crush fracture of oscalcis.

Fractures of the metatarsals and phalanges

Such fractures are usually caused by direct violence. There is often associated damage to the skin and blood vessels which may lead to Volkmann's ischaemic contracture of the foot or gangrene (Figs. 9.15 and 9.16). They nearly always require to be treated by elevating the foot and improving the circulation. Admission to hospital is often required even for apparently minor fractures of the phalanges and metatarsals. The damage and danger to the blood vessels and muscles is far greater than the osseous damage. Gangrene of one or more toes can occur after even an apparently trivial injury if it is neglected.

Splintage for fractures of the lower limb

Cross reference—Chapter 28: Traction; Chapter 29: External splintage.

Thomas' bed knee splint

This is commonly used for fractures of the shaft of the femur. In supra-condylar fractures of the femur it may be used with a knee flexion piece.

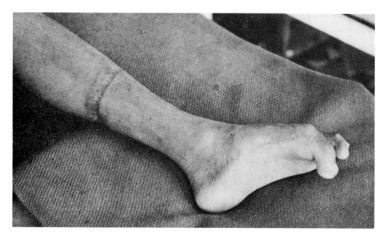

Fig. 9.15 Volkmann's contracture of the foot, secondary to a tourniquet. The mark of the tourniquet is seen around the calf.

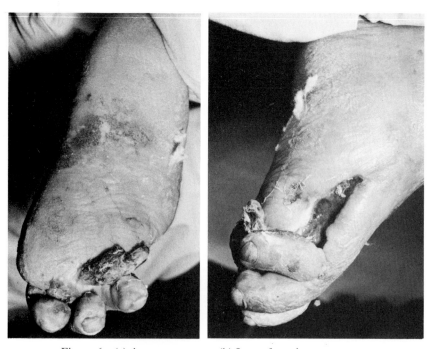

Fig. 9.16 (a) A gangrenous toe. (b) Loss of toe due to gangrene.

Thomas' walking caliper

This is a modification of the bed knee splint to allow ambulation of the patient who has been confined to bed with a fracture of the femur. The main modification is at the lower end of the splint where the bars are bent inwards to enter a tube socket fitted into the heel of the patient's footwear and opening on either side.

The length of the bars may be altered to suit the patient at an adjustable extension piece at the end of each of the bars. A leather back-strap and buckle holds the bars of the caliper into the heel of the shoe.

Leather knee shields and slings hold the knee and prevent flexion or hyperextension of the joint.

The length of the caliper is adjusted on the instructions of the orthopaedic surgeon to be either weight-relieving, when the weight of the body is taken on the ring of the splint with the heel of the patient's foot clear of the inside of the sole of the boot, or non-weight-relieving when the weight of the patient is taken through the leg and on the foot and sole of the boot. The function of the caliper in the latter case is to protect and support the knee.

Measuring for a Thomas' walking caliper

1   Around the thigh at the level of the adductor tendon;
2   On the inner side, from the adductor tendon in the groin to the level of the sole of the foot with the ankle at a right angle. 1·5 cm are added to allow for the depth of the heel of the boot. If the caliper is to be weight-relieving, a further 1·5 cm are added.

The patient's boot must be sent to the splintmaker when the caliper is ordered. Some surgeons require a new cloth boot to be supplied.

Applying the Thomas' walking caliper

The patient will have been on fixed traction with a Thomas' bed knee splint on his leg for a fractured femur. This will be the first occasion for release of this traction so that gentleness in handling the leg, and the maintenance of the traction manually are necessary until the walking caliper is fitted.

The nurse applying manual traction is seated at the end of the bed. The Thomas' splint and slings are dismantled and the extensions removed. The walking caliper is slipped on to the limb while traction is continued. The ring is made to fit comfortably around the thigh, and the boot is laced-up. The knee sling and shield are firmly fastened and the length of the caliper is adjusted at the extension fittings on the ends of the bars.

The patient may be required to wear the walking caliper and boot continuously whilst in bed until instructions are given for him to commence walking. The physiotherapist attends to improve the musculature of the limb during this time.

The care of the patient in this caliper is as for a patient wearing any type of splintage, and careful observation of the ring area and heel are necessary in case pressure on the skin in these areas should cause sores.

Plaster of Paris splintage of the lower limb

Cross reference—Chapter 30; Hip spicas.

Leg plasters
Above-knee plaster. This extends from groin to toes.

Requirements.	Wool roll	three rolls
	Plaster bandages	15 cm—twelve
		10 cm—three

The method. Applying an efficient plaster for a fracture of the lower part of the leg requires skill in ensuring that the fragments and the limb are properly aligned. It is essential that the surgeon in charge of the patient is present, and he will hold the limb in the desired position during this procedure.

The usual position for the limb is with the ankle at a right angle and the knee in a flexed position at five degrees. A knee bending block and pillow are useful assets in maintaining the position of the limb during the application; control of both knee and ankle as well as the fracture may be difficult however.

A thin layer of wool is rolled on from toes to groin. The plastering then begins. It is customary to make the cast in two parts: For a fracture in the lower part of the tibia and fibula, the limb is plastered from the toes to below the knee firstly. If the surgeon is satisfied with the position of the limb the plaster is then extended up over the knee to the groin.

If the fracture is in the upper region of the tibia, a cylinder is commenced above the ankle and finished at the groin. The foot piece is then added, when the surgeon is satisfied with the position of the fracture and the knee.

Wedging. Mal-alignment of a fracture of the tibia and fibula may be corrected by wedging the plaster. For this, the plaster is cut through around its circumference and then replastered in the corrected position. Pieces of cork may be used to open the jaws of the cut plaster in realigning the fragments. Radiographic control of this procedure is necessary.

Below-knee plaster. This extends from the toes to the neck of the fibula. The knee is supported on a knee bending block and pillow. The below-knee plaster may be used for strains of the ankle and for fractures of the tarsus and metatarsus, and fractures of the internal or external malleolus which are not severe. Severe and unstable fractures around the ankle require an above-knee plaster.

Methods. There are two alternatives:

Requirements for method A. Plaster wool   two rolls
Plaster bandages 15 cm wide—four
10 cm wide slab—one

Method A. A thin layer of plaster wool is rolled on first. The cast is commenced either at the toes or below the knee. As the plaster bandages are applied they are moulded to fit snugly around the heel and malleoli. If it is to be used as a walking plaster, a 10 cm wide slab is incorporated into the foot section along the base of the cast.

Requirements for method B. Splint wool, sheets   one
Plaster bandages 15 cm wide—three
10 cm wide—three

Method B. With the limb held in position, a layer of the splint wool is arranged down the back of the leg and under the foot. A 15 cm wide slab is then measured to extend from the level of the neck of the fibula to the heads of the metatarsus, down the back of the leg and under the foot. Cuts are made in the slab at the level of the bend of the heel. The slab is moistened and applied. It is moulded carefully to the heel using the slots in the slab to assist in this.

One 15 cm wide plaster bandage and one 10 cm wide are then moistened and applied from above down to enclose the slab and the limb.

With either of these plaster methods it is essential that:

(a) complete movement of the toes is permitted, and

(b) the knee can be fully flexed without hindrance from the top of the plaster.

If these movements are not possible the plaster must be trimmed.

Walking plasters

No attempt must be made to walk on a plaster until it is completely dry. It is necessary to give positive instructions to the patient that the plaster must be kept off the ground for at least five days. After this time has elapsed, a plaster boot which completely encloses the foot section of the plaster is supplied and fitted.

Plaster leg cylinders

These are used to immobilize the knee.

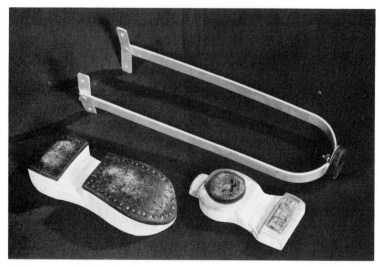

Fig. 9.17 Additional pieces for incorporation into walking-plasters. A walking iron and two foot pieces.

Requirements. Plaster bandages 15 cm wide— ten

Adhesive felt for ankle one strip
Stockinette to fit the limb one piece
Wool roll to protect the knee of thin patients one

Method. The stockinette is rolled on first and if the knee requires it, a layer of wool roll is applied. The plaster bandages are then moistened and rolled on, extending from the groin to 5 cm above the malleoli.

If the limb is thin, straight and cylindrical, the cylinder may slip down as the patient walks. This can be prevented by incorporating a stip of adhesive into the cylinder at its lower end.

When desired, the cylinder can be converted into a back-splint by removing a section from the front.

Cross references: Chapter 30: The principles of plaster of Paris technique; Chapter 22: Affections of the knee.

The nursing management of patients with fractures of the lower limb

Fractures of the pelvis

These patients are most usually treated with complete bed rest until the pain subsides, when mobilization is commenced.

During the early stages of treatment the patient may be enclosed in a tubigrip binder around the pelvic area, or he may be supported in a suspended canvas sling which is counter-balanced with weights, using a balkan beam with two single pulleys. This latter method assists nursing in raising the patient from the mattress for the purposes of attending to the skin or inserting a bedpan.

Nursing observations will include watching in the early stages for any involvement of the pelvic organs, but the surgeon in charge will usually recognize and treat such complications on admission to hospital. Urinary problems or constipation, or complaints of irregularities of this nature must be reported.

In all pelvic fractures the most important points are to look for evidence of internal bleeding, damage to the bladder and urethra, damage to the rectum or, more rarely, damage to the femoral or sciatic nerves. Visceral and cascular lesions take priority in treatment. Once these have been excluded or treated attention is paid to the bony injuries. The majority of pelvic fractures heal in satisfactory position with simple bed rest but there are exceptions.

Wide divarication at the symphysis pubis can be closed by suspending the patient in a canvas sling attached to ropes, pulleys and weights which cross (see Chapter 28: Traction).

Occasionally satisfactory repair of the bladder or urethra requires internal fixation at the pelvic fracture.

In young women, the stove-in pelvis may present a problem in parturition, and correction by lateral and longitudinal traction may be needed. The patient is usually too ill for a major operation apart from stopping bleeding.

Unilateral dislocation of the sacroiliac joint with upward displacement of that side of the pelvis often requires skeletal traction to the corresponding leg.

Fractures of the neck of the femur
This is most likely to be in an elderly patient, although patients in the younger age group may sustain such fractures.

The approach to treatment by the surgeon will be related to the complications which may ensue if the aged person is kept static in bed and every effort is made to internally fix the fracture and commence mobilizing the patient—firstly by sitting her out of bed and then walking as soon as feasible. Unless this is done the patient will deteriorate, despite active nursing and therapeutic methods, with the following possible complications:

lung and thoracic infections,
stasis in the tissues and pressure sores,
reduced urinary output with uraemia,
mental confusion with disorientation,
stiffness of joints,
muscle wasting,
incontinence of urine and faeces.

When surgical internal fixation of the fracture is not possible, because the patient is in a poor physical state due to other diseases, then Hamilton-Russell traction (see p. 424) may be the method of treatment and nursing.

Whether surgical reduction of the fracture or conservative methods of treatment are decided upon, dedicated nursing and physiotherapy of these patients are essential.

General management

1   *Clinical examination.* It must not be a supposition that the fracture of the neck of the femur is all that is wrong with the patient. The fracture may be the result of a fall when dizziness occurred, or the bone itself may be osteoporotic. Perhaps there is anaemia or uraemia.

All of these possibilities are eliminated by a thorough examination by the doctor and exhaustive blood, urine and other relevant pathological tests.

When secondary ailments are found, these are treated as part of the patient's regime. Blood transfusion or other intravenous therapy is often required.

2   *Psychological improvement.* Often these patients are demoralized—not only by the accident, but also from sustained loneliness, apathy, malnutrition and poverty. Social casework to improve their future prospects is needed, but in their immediate care the nursing staff can do much.

Optimism must be the keynote in dealing with the patient. Contact with younger people improves their state, as does meeting people of their own age who have recovered from a similar catastrophe. The next of kin and other relatives and neighbours must be encouraged to visit and given every opportunity to support the patient during her stay in hospital and after discharge.

Many old people who live by themselves are frightened that their homes will be taken away from them or be vandalized while they are in hospital.

The morale of the patient is also improved by a high level of cleanliness, personal hygiene, cosmetic appearance and dress. The patient should be encouraged to dress and groom herself to the best possible standard.

3   *Antibiotics, chemotherapy, drugs and nutrition.* Pharmaceutical advances mean that most conditions can be adequately treated and the conditions affecting the aged are no exception. Thus antibiotics may be used to overcome existing chronic infections and as prophylaxis; the vitamins supplied in concentrated form to combat anaemia and other examples of avitaminosis; raised blood pressure, uraemia and chronic coughs can all be treated.

An important aspect of treatment is to establish the patient on a balance between sleeping and waking. The patient may tend to sleep all day and lie awake and be noisy at night unless this is properly managed with correct sedation.

4   *Physiotherapy.* The physiotherapist will do much to rehabilitate this type of patient. Whilst the patient is bed-fast the physiotherapist will work to prevent joint stiffness and will give passive movements to all the joints of the body. Breathing exercises are also necessary to prevent hypostatic pneumonia.

When the patient is allowed out of bed the physiotherapist will teach her methods of walking and exercises to maintain the tone of the muscles.

5   *Diversional therapy.* A problem with aged patients always is to overcome a loss of interest with apathy. Diversional therapy of all kinds is needed to stimulate these interests. Radio, television, floral arrangement, colour in the environment, activities such as knitting and embroidery all play their part.

6   *Nursing.* See also Chapter 27 for surgical nursing.
The full regime of nursing care for any sick patient is essential. Additionally, however, these patients require constant alteration in position while confined to bed; a chart to indicate sequence of turning should be established.

A good intake of fluid is necessary and these patients must be made to drink plenty even though they may resist. A fluid balance chart must also be maintained.

One of the factors which have contributed to the admission of the patient to hospital with a fractured neck of femur may have been a dietary insufficiency; lonely old people often sustain themselves on a poor diet which requires little preparation. Nursing management requires that the patient is encouraged to take a high protein diet with plenty of dairy produce and other foods containing vitamins and chemical elements such as calcium, phosphorus, and potassium.

10

Fractures and Dislocations of the Spine

Relevant applied anatomy and physiology

The spinal column has the following functions:

1 Protection of vulnerable nervous tissue
The spinal cord passes down the neural canal of the vertebral column to the level of the first and second lumbar vertebrae. Below where this has terminated, nerves forming the cauda equina continue to the lowest point of the neural canal. The protection of this hard bony canal is necessary for this delicate tissue and its membranous surroundings.

2 Protection of visceral organs in the thoracic and abdominal cavities
The vertebral column forms a bony posterior boundary to both of these cavities.

3 Support for the trunk and head
The twenty-six bones placed one above the other, form an upright column. The cranium is the uppermost structure resting on this column. Movements of the head in any direction depend upon movements of the cervical vertebrae. Movements of the trunk in bending forwards, backwards or sideways require a mobile, healthy pain-free vertebral column. Distortion or deformity of the vertebral column results in a related deformity of the trunk.

4 Attachment for muscles
The strong column provides a reliable anchorage for many of the muscles of the neck, thorax, abdomen and pelvis through sheets of fascia, ligaments and tendons. Derangement of the spine affects the efficiency of these muscles. The diaphragm uses the column for part of its anchorage.

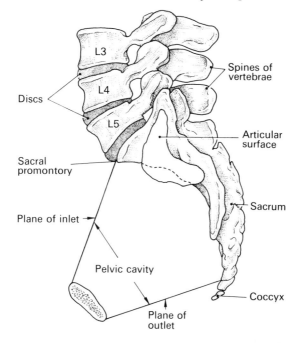

Fig. 10.1   Vertebrae with discs and showing the pelvic cavity.

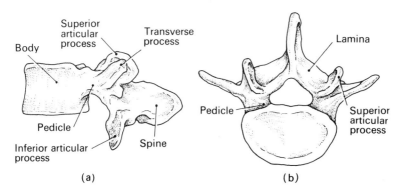

Fig. 10.2   Lumbar vertebrae (a) lateral view, (b) superior view.

5   Permitting movement of the trunk

We are endowed with an intervertebral disc between each of the twenty-six bones of the vertebral column. Each disc is a mixture of cartilaginous end plates, fibrous capsule and central gelatinous nucleus pulposus. These both act as shock absorbers and allow movement. These can be compressed at any point to allow bending in any direction; they will also spiral to permit rotation of one vertebra on another. In addition there are two synovial gliding joints on the posterior surface to each pair of bones in the vertebral column.

6   Limiting movement of the trunk

It is dangerous to have unstable, excessive motion in the trunk but it is also inconvenient to have reduced range of movement. The vertebral column serves to prevent acute angulation and kinking of the spinal cord by permitting only gradual bending along its length.

Relevant first aid in spinal injuries

The results of mismanagement of patients who sustain a fracture-dislocation of the spinal column can be awesome and irrevocable. Therefore as a first aid measure it is wiser to treat every patient with the slightest suspicion of spinal injury as if he has a severe injury until proven otherwise by medical examination and radiography. Relatively slight injuries (whiplash injuries to the neck in a transport accident, for example) can cause permanent paralysis of the whole body without any sign of a wound or bruising. It is always best to be safe and sure by the assumption that the neck or spine is fractured and dislocated when lifting and transporting these patients.

Methods of lifting

The patient can only be lifted by a number of people—four to six, working as a team. Rather than one or two people attempting to raise the patient from the ground it is better to cover him until more help can be obtained. A strong blanket or sheet is used to lift the patient.

The patient must be carefully rolled slowly and evenly by the team with the head and neck carefully aligned to the rest of the body by one member of the team who concentrates on this sole function throughout the procedure. The helper at the head is opposed by a person at the feet who pulls the ankles and legs to help maintain the patient's body straight. The ankles and knees should be fastened together.

Before moving the patient a blanket is rolled lengthwise for two-thirds of its width. When the team have rolled the patient towards one side, the roll of the blanket is placed on the ground under him. The patient's body is then rolled back across the roll and over to the other side when the roll of blanket is then drawn through to the opposite side. The blanket is then used to lift the patient evenly from the ground while a board or stretcher is slipped under the

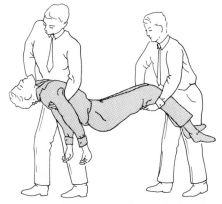

Fig. 10.3   Incorrect way to lift patient with spinal injury (cervical spine and thoracolumbar region unsupported and liable to further displacement).

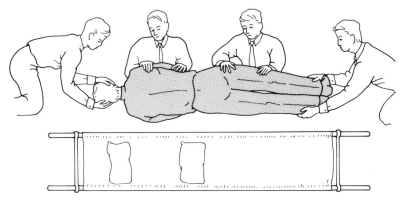

Fig. 10.4   Correct way to lift patient with spinal injury (patient is rolled onto blanket or stretcher with longitudinal traction on head and legs).

blanket and under the patient; at least three people to each side are necessary for this procedure.

Supports to the head in the form of a sandbag or small pillow at either side, and soft rolls of padding in the hollows behind the neck and lumbar spine are helpful in restricting movement of the patient's spine.

The patient should be moved to hospital with care to avoid severe jolting. The same careful, slow, but firm handling must, of course, be continued on arrival.

Spinal injuries

Spinal injuries are significant, firstly because of associated damage to the spinal cord and nerves: secondly, because such injuries may lead to

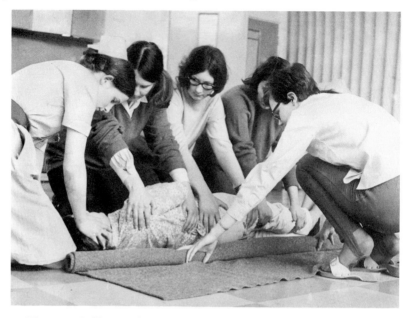

Fig. 10.5   Rolling a patient with a suspected spinal injury. The rolled blanket
is placed under the patient, who is lifted with it.

persistent pain, and thirdly because they may lead to persistent deformity.
Fourthly, spinal injuries may be associated with serious injuries to other
structures—particularly the head, heart, lungs and abdominal viscera.
Damage to the spinal cord can lead to a complete loss of function with complete paralysis and loss of sensation in all structures below the level of the
lesion. The treatment of paraplegia is dealt with in detail in Chapter 31.

General principles of treatment
Spinal injuries can usefully be divided into those that have immediate
major damage to the spinal cord and those in which there is little or no
damage. If there is immediate complete transection of the spinal cord, no
treatment will restore function and in general, treatment to the spine must
be secondary to treatment of the patient as a whole, e.g. prevention of
pressure sores, contractions, etc. (see Chapter 31). On the other hand, if
there is little or no damage to the spinal cord, it is important to ensure that
further displacement with possible subsequent damage to the spinal cord
does not occur. For this reason it is useful to divide injuries of the spinal cord
into those which are stable and those which are unstable. As a general rule,
crush injuries of the vertebrae are stable and rotation injuries with tearing of

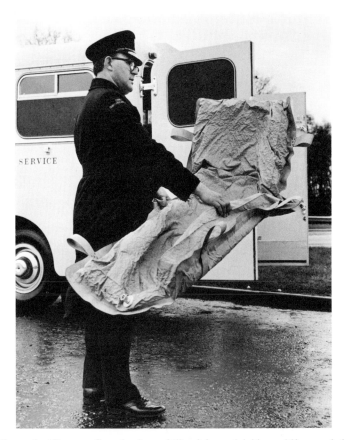

Fig. 10.6 'Egerton Casualty Immobilizer' forms 'rigid mould' around the patient; for transport to hospital. The Casualty Immobilizer consists of an envelope similar in shape and construction to an air bed but using a strong flexible cover and being partially filled with polystyrene foam pellets. The envelope has a valve enabling the air pressure inside it to be varied. It is laid out and the injured person placed on it. The weight of the casualty's limbs and body make their mould in the Immobilizer. The air is then evacuated from the envelope by means of a pump. As the vacuum increases, so the mould becomes more rigid until it is a solid cast. The injured person is then lying in the Immobilizer rather than on it and is completely immobilized and protected by it.

(By courtesy of Egerton Hospital Equipment Ltd.)

ligaments and joint capsules, are unstable. It may be impossible to make this differentiation with certainty until X-rays have been taken. Therefore, in the first-aid treatment of any spinal injury it should be assumed that the spine is unstable and the patient should be placed on a firm stretcher with a small pillow under the cervical and lumbar lordoses and he should not be moved until he has been examined by a competent doctor at a fully equipped hospital and the appropriate X-rays taken (Fig. 10.7).

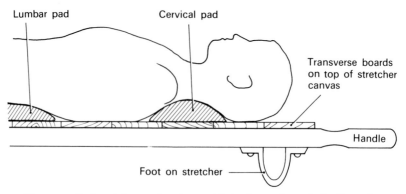

Lumbar pad

Cervical pad

Transverse boards
on top of stretcher
canvas

Handle

Foot on stretcher

Fig. 10.7   Patient lying on firm base with lumbar and cervical pillows for fractured spine.

If it is decided that a cervical injury should be reduced, the usual way to do this is by the application of skull calipers (see Fig. 28.18c). Occasionally if reduction cannot be obtained by this means, open reduction and bone grafting may be indicated, but usually, even if the spine is unstable, bone grafting is only performed some weeks afterwards and only for injuries which will not become stable on their own.

In the case of thoraco-lumbar dislocations, open operation and fixation may also be necessary, but in the vast majority of spinal injuries, early operation will do the patient more harm than good.

The different regions of the spinal cord have different anatomical properties and it is therefore convenient to consider spinal injuries on an anatomical basis.

Cervical spine injuries

Damage to the cervical spine takes three main forms:

1   Crush fractures

There may be a crush fracture of one or more vertebral bodies, often associated with a head injury, and sometimes associated with damage to intervertebral discs and damage to the spinal cord. These fractures are, however, stable in the sense that further displacement is unlikely to occur and it is pointless to attempt to reduce the fracture as, even if the crushed vertebra is pulled into a better shape, late collapse and return to its previous

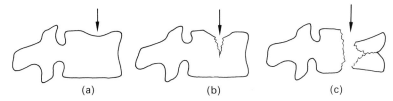

Fig. 10.8   Compression injury to spine. (a) Bulging at end of plate. (b) Split in vertebral body. (c) Bursting of vertebral body.

shape is inevitable. In general, simple crush fractures of the cervical spine in themselves do not require any ambitious treatment; rest in bed with a simple supporting collar, or light head traction for a few days is all that is required, though associated injuries either to the spinal cord or to the head may require more complicated treatment.

Severe bursting fractures of the cervical spine are usually associated with neurological damage. These are best treated by skeletal skull traction.

2   Fracture-dislocations

Fracture-dislocations of the cervical spine are common in young people and are usually due to rotation and flexion injuries. If there is a unilateral dislocation it is unusual for there to be significant associated damage to the spinal cord, but nipping of the corresponding nerve root with pain in the arm and paralysis of certain muscles, is fairly common. Unilateral dislocations should be reduced. This is most easily performed by the application of skull calipers with lateral traction of the neck, and then the application of a derotation force. It is important therefore, to determine the side of the dislocation and this is best done by obtaining adequate oblique views of the cervical spine (Fig. 10.9). Therefore, such patients must be treated in a hospital with good radiological facilities. Following reduction it is not infrequent to find that, due to extensive tearing of ligaments and joint capsules, the spine is unstable and, under these circumstances a localized spinal fusion may be required. This is in contrast to the crush fractures where spinal fusion is seldom, if ever, required. Bilateral dislocations are nearly always associated with complete tetraplegia and transection of the spinal cord. Although such dislocations can easily be reduced by skull traction, this does not improve the prognosis.

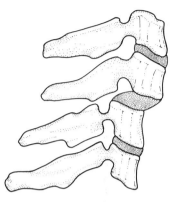

Fig. 10.9   Oblique view showing dislocated facets in unilateral dislocation.

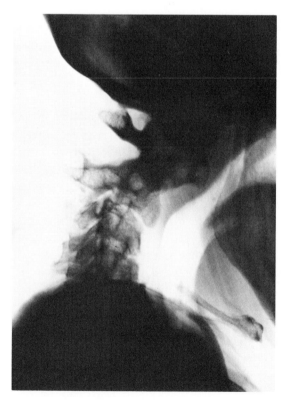

Fig. 10.10   Cervical spine showing the late sequelae of a spinal injury.

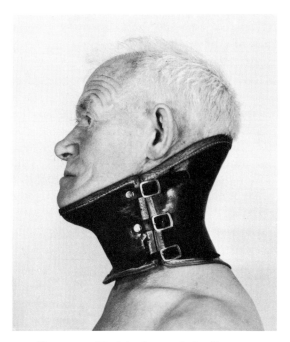

Fig. 10.11   Block leather cervical collar.

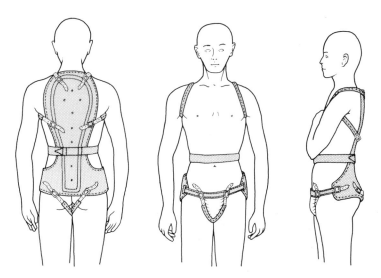

Fig. 10.12   Posterior spinal support.

3 Hyperextension injuries

The third class of spinal injuries—namely, hyperextension injuries—are common in elderly people, especially those with stiff or arthritic spines. There is usually a history of a fall on the face or a bang on the forehead, and often there is an associated cut or bruise on the patient's forehead. These injuries are usually associated with partial damage to the spinal cord and in particular with weakness of the arms.

The treatment is to hold the neck in a slightly flexed position by applying a simple collar (Fig. 10.11), and treatment for the associated paralysis of the arms is essential. Complicated measures such as skull traction or spinal fusion are contra-indicated. Some residual arm weakness is usual. Occasionally such extension injuries are associated with complete tetraplegia.

4 Whiplash injuries

During the last few years increasing attention has been paid to the so-called whiplash injury which classically occurs when a patient is sitting in a stationary car wearing a seat belt and another car runs into it. The patient's head is subject to a violent to-and-fro movement with greater or lesser degrees of ligamentous tearing. Occasionally the ligament tears are severe enough to produce vertebral instability which can be demonstrated by 'stress views' in the X-ray department—such views should always be taken. If instability is undiagnosed and untreated it leads to deformity later (Fig. 10.10). It is important that X-rays should include all the cervical vertebrae (this may be difficult).

Even in the absence of demonstrable instability, these whiplash injuries may give rise to prolonged pain, and require a supporting collar and physiotherapy.

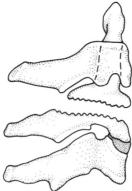

Fig. 10.13 Fracture of the second cervical vertebra typically found in 'blow to the face' injuries.

Another interesting cervical spine injury is the 'hangmans fracture' which occurs with a violent traction injury of the spine causing an avulsion fracture of the axis vertebra. Obviously it should not be treated by strong traction.

Injuries to the thoracic region of the vertebral column

A common injury in the thoracic region is a crush fracture of the vertebral body following, for example, a fall from a height, or injuries caused by an explosion. Usually, as with other crush injuries of the vertebral body where the ligaments are intact, such injuries are not associated with damage to the spinal cord. Reduction is pointless as the fracture is basically a stable one in the sense that further deformity is unlikely. The only treatment required is a short period of rest in recumbency, followed by redevelopment of the spinal muscles. Hyperextension jackets, posterior spinal supports, etc., are usually contra-indicated as, by causing stiffness of the uninjured parts of the spine, they do more harm than good.

Occasionally in association with injuries of the chest, a fracture-dislocation of the thoracic spine occurs. This is inevitably associated with complete paraplegia; the patient is always seriously ill. Reduction of the dislocation will not restore function to an irretrievably damaged spinal cord, and local operative treatment to the thoracic spine is normally likely to do more harm than good. Conservative postural reduction is usually the best.

Exceptions to this are high thoracic injuries with an associated sternal fracture and overlapping of the sternal fragments. These are associated with extensive tearing of the posterior ligaments, if unreduced by operation they lead to severe permanent kyphosis.

Thoraco-lumbar injuries

The common injury here is due to a rotation strain, producing a fracture-dislocation (Fig. 10.14). In this region damage to the nerve roots and cauda equina is common. This is basically an unstable fracture and further displacement is likely to occur. There is some evidence that partially damaged nerve roots may recover if they are not subjected to continual mechanical irritation. For this reason many surgeons believe that reduction of this particular dislocation with fixation—for example by spinal plates (see Fig. 10.15), is the wisest course of action. Alternatively, other surgeons believe that a closed reduction and fixation by skilled 'pillow nursing' is the best course (see Chapter 31).

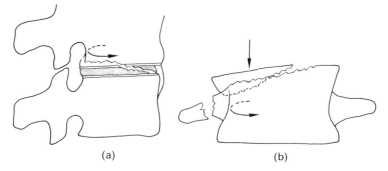

(a)   (b)

Fig. 10.14   Rotation injury to spine.

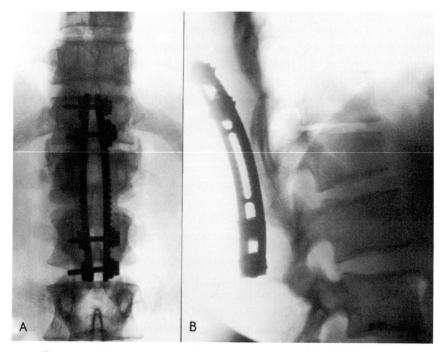

Fig. 10.15   Fixation of spine with plate. It is not always easy to maintain reduction by plates alone.

Lumbar spine injuries

A common injury here is a crush fracture due to a fall from a height or a similar injury. It is unusual for such injuries to be associated with neurological damage. They are perfectly stable; reduction is pointless; the only treatment required is a short period of rest in bed, with attention to strengthening the spinal muscles.

The nursing management of patients treated with skull traction

This is the method used to apply traction and counter-traction in the treatment of some patients with cervical lesions.

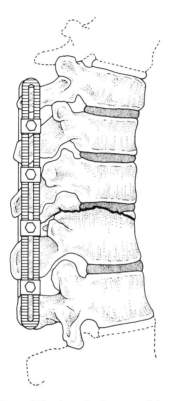

Fig. 10.16   Reduction and fixation of a fracture of the spinal column.

Setting up the traction
This is done by the insertion of skull calipers (Fig. 28.18c) into the cranial bones of the patient and applying the traction force through these. The skull calipers are inserted under local anaesthesia with the patient in the operating theatre. Until the skull calipers are inserted and traction is applied the patient must be handled with care and efficiency to ensure that the neck and head are maintained in correct alignment with the vertebral column. The head must be prevented from rolling or the neck being rotated by the use of

sandbags on either side of the head. In addition, a skilled nurse has the task of remaining at the head end of the bed or trolley to support the patient's head during all movements of the bed or trolley. Once the patient has been transferred to the bed on admission it is best to keep him on that bed until skull traction has been properly mounted. This means preparing the head and inserting the skull calipers with the patient still in his bed. If this is not possible, a large team of nursing staff are necessary to lift the patient from bed to operating table.

The patient is sure to be apprehensive and it is essential that an explanation is given to him as early as possible and his co-operation sought.

The head is shaved to remove all hair; skin preparation for surgery is performed.

After an anaesthetic (either local or general) has been given, a small incision is made on either side of the skull and drill holes made into the bones of the cranium for the insertion of the skull calipers. These wounds are dressed and treated as any surgical wound until removal of the calipers and healing has occurred.

Advance arrangements must be made for a single pulley on a projecting bracket to be installed on the head end of the patient's bed at the point where the line of the traction cord is most likely to occur. It is preferable that this is adjustable to suit the patient's and surgeon's needs. Radiographic control during the mounting of traction will also be needed.

The traction cord from the calipers is arranged over the pulley and a weight of 7 to 9 kg is attached to the traction cord. This may be reduced later according to the radiographic appearances of the spine and the wishes of the surgeon in charge.

Some surgeons prefer to apply traction by the halo device (see page 492).

Turning the patient
This is facilitated by the skull traction which helps to maintain the neck in correct alignment as the patient is rotated. In a dearth of adequate nursing staff for turning the patient, devices such as Stryker frames or Egerton Stoke-Mandeville beds (see Fig. 10.17) have their place. When sufficient nurses can be assembled to turn the patient however, the conventional bed with extra pillows is preferable.

Before turning, bedcovers, pillows and other accessories are removed to leave a clear field. The most experienced nurse stays at the head of the bed to control the head turning and traction weights, cord and pulley. She has a second function in giving clear and concise instructions to the other team members so that actions are in unison.

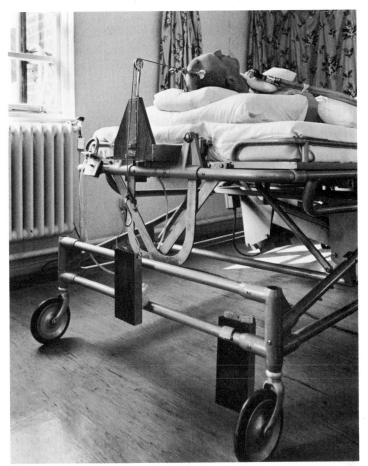

Fig. 10.17   Guttman Head Traction Unit may be used with either the Egerton-Stoke Mandeville Turning Bed or the Egerton-Stoke Mandeville Tilting and Turning Bed. This Unit allows constant accurate traction whilst the patient is turned from the supine to the lateral position. It also allows traction to be maintained whilst the patient is static in either of these positions (see also Chapter 31, page 504). Note endotracheal tube connected to respirator.

The turning routine is as follows:

(a) *From supine to lateral*

1   The leg away from the side to which the patient will turn is carried across the near leg.

2   The arms are arranged; they are best carried on the chest. If the patient can co-operate, he may fold his arms to control them.

3   The patient's body is carried over towards the side of the bed away from that which he will face on completion of the turn. A thin lumbar pillow which is in position in the hollow of the back is used to lift the trunk by two nurses, one on either side of the bed, who use the pillow as a sling to carry the patient. Another pair of nurses lift the legs and carry them over in line with the trunk. Care is taken to clear the buttocks of the patient from the undersheet so that the skin is not 'scuffed' as the patient is moved. During this move the nurse at the head carefully aligns the head and neck with the trunk.

4   The patient is now rolled slowly and evenly into the lateral position using the lumbar pillow as a device for rotating him.

5   The legs of the patient are now used to fix him in a stable position. The upper leg is placed straight down the bed on pillows with the ankle at a right angle. The lower leg is flexed at the hip, knee and ankle and adjusted so that the hip is flexed but neither abducted nor adducted.

6   The arms are placed comfortably so that they are not under the body. A pillow may be required to support the upper arm.

7   A bed cradle is placed over the patient's legs and the bed remade.

(b) *From lateral to supine.* The whole process is repeated except that:

1   At the start of the procedure the patient is rolled still further towards the prone position so that the undersheet and lumbar pillow may be checked and smoothed, or else replaced.

2   The patient is first rolled on to his back with the lumbar pillow held firmly against his spine; after this his body is lifted to the centre of the bed and the head traction re-adjusted.

3   The legs are arranged with both hips partially flexed and abducted, both knees slightly flexed and both ankles at a right angle.

The turning routines described above are applied to all spinal injury patients—whether on head traction or not. A similar procedure is also used for patients who are paraplegic or tetraplegic. In caring for any of these patients, a set routine of movement from right lateral to supine, and from supine to left lateral, at two hourly intervals must be maintained during the whole twenty-four hours of the day. A chart of these turnings must be kept and entered by the staff who carry out each turn.

Nursing observations of patients with spinal injuries

The patient with a stable fracture-dislocation or an unstable fracture-dislocation which has been surgically stabilised requires careful observation. Projecting through foraminae at the sides of the neural canal of the vertebral column are the spinal nerves. There are sixty-two of these which pass out in pairs at all levels of the vertebral column, to serve the viscera, the muscles, joints and skin of the trunk and limbs.

In injuries to the spine with any displacement of fragments, although the spinal cord may not be compressed or transected, these nerves may be constricted with subsequent related complications.

Nursing staff must therefore report to the surgeon:

1   Any complaint of pain, tingling, numbness, coldness or sweating in any part of the body, even though remote from the spinal column.

2   Any comment by the patient of difficulty in breathing, talking or swallowing.

3   Any gastric distress in the form of pain, distension with gas, difficulty in eructation or passing flatus or defaecation.

4   Urinary problems, either in micturition or unusual sensations in the bladder or genital organs.

Any spinal injury patients will be apprehensive in the period immediately following the injury and reassurance by nursing and medical staff is necessary. Once the shock of the injury has passed, with guidance from the surgeon the patient should be encouraged to increase the range of his activities daily in graduated stages. He must not be permitted to maintain helpless dependency for any longer than is necessary.

Cross references
Chapter 11: Peripheral nerve lesions.
Chapter 16: Lower motor neuron lesions.
Chapter 24: Low back pain and sciatica.
Chapter 25: Brachial neuritis.
Chapter 27: Comprehensive patient care.
Chapter 31: The paraplegic patient.

11

Peripheral Nerve Lesions

Definition of peripheral nerves

A peripheral nerve is a nerve trunk which communicates between the central nervous system (the brain and spinal cord inside the theca) and the periphery of the body (the parts outside the theca, e.g. muscles, and skin). The cranial and spinal nerves which together comprise the peripheral nerves, are the routes by which nervous impulses arising in the brain and spinal cord pass out to supply the skin, muscles, bones, joints, blood vessels, glands, sensory

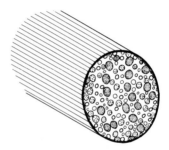

Fig. 11.1   Section through a peripheral nerve.

organs and other structures of the body. In the reverse direction, nervous impulses or action currents arising within these organs pass into the central nervous system. Damage to these nerves therefore results in an interruption in the communicating pathway connecting the brain and spinal cord with the periphery of the body. Such an interruption is what is meant by a peripheral nerve lesion.

The nerves which are classified as peripheral nerves are the twelve pairs of cranial nerves and the thirty-one pairs of spinal nerves. In this book a description of the cranial nerves is not relevant.

The spinal nerves
The spinal nerves arise at different segmental levels of the spinal cord (Fig. 11.2). There are eight cervical, twelve dorsal, five lumbar, five sacral and one

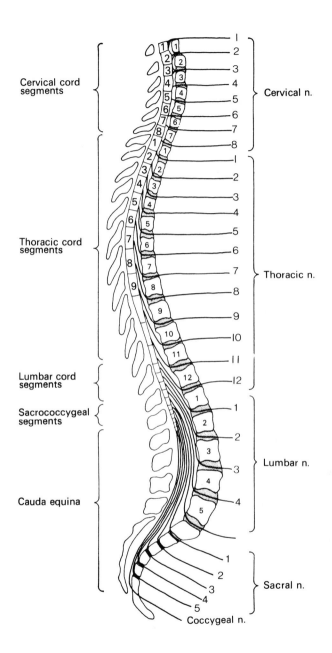

Fig. 11.2   The spinal nerves.

coccygeal pair. As the cord terminates at the highest part of the lumbar region the nerves leaving the lower part of the spinal cord must pass down inside the spinal canal before they pass through the spinal foramina and thence to the peripheral organs.

Each of the spinal nerves arise from the cord by two nerve roots on each side of the cord (Fig. 11.3). The root at the front transmits the impulses

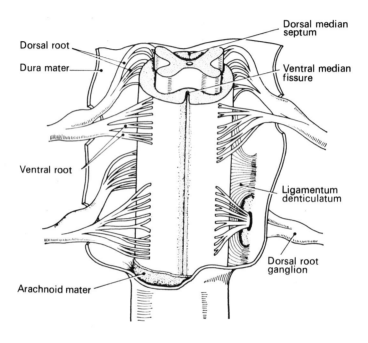

Fig. 11.3   Nerve roots of spinal nerves.

going out to the body (efferent or motor root), the root at the back transfers the impulses received from the body into the cord and brain (afferent or sensory root), although normally these roots are related to a pathway going up the cord to the brain (the posterior *sensory* root) or a pathway coming down the cord from the brain (the anterior *motor* root). Communication between the posterior root and the anterior root by communicating neurones within the spinal cord also occurs. The functional combination of sensory organ, afferent nerve, communicating neurone or neurones, efferent nerve and the muscle it supplies is known as a reflex arc. An automatic motor response elicited by stimulating a sensory end organ and utilising a reflex arc is known as a reflex action.

The plexuses. The spinal nerves are grouped together at certain levels particularly where they serve a limb. This grouping is the basis for the formation of many branches which supply a number of different structures arising from a few nerve roots. The main plexuses are:

1 *The cervical plexus.* This supplies the muscles and structures of the neck.

2 *The brachial plexus.* This supplies the upper extremity including the muscles connecting the thorax and the scapula, the shoulder, the arm and the hand. The plexus is situated in the infero-lateral part of the neck superior and medial to the shoulder joint, i.e. just above and behind the clavicle. It may be damaged by wounds or injuries in this area.

3 *The lumbar plexus.* This is situated at the back of the abdominal cavity on the side of the vertebral column. It passes forwards to supply the anterior, lateral and medial surface of the thigh and the anterior muscles of the hip and thigh. The femoral and obturator nerves derive from the lumbar plexus. It may be damaged by wounds of the abdominal cavity or back.

4 *The sacral plexus.* This is situated within the pelvis on the anterior surface of the sacrum. The largest branch, the sciatic nerve, passes out through the great sciatic notch at the back of the pelvis. It may be damaged in fractures and other injuries of the pelvis. The sacral plexus supplies the skin at the back of the thigh and the skin of the leg and foot below the knee. It supplies all the muscles below the knee and the back of the thigh and buttock. Branches from the sacral plexus also innervate the bladder and rectum.

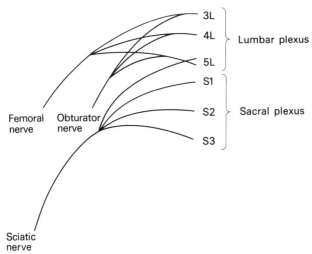

Fig. 11.4   A diagram of the lumbo-sacral plexus to show roots of the femoral, obturator and sciatic nerves.

Peripheral nerve lesions

A peripheral nerve is defined as a nerve which runs from the spinal cord to one of the peripheral organs, such as muscle, joints, tendons, skin, blood vessels, sweat glands. Each peripheral nerve consists of three types of fibres:
1   Motor or efferent fibres—i.e. the fibres which conduct nervous impulses from the spinal cord to the muscles.
2   Sensory or efferent fibres—which conduct nervous impulses from peripheral sense organs, e.g. sensory receptors in the skin, muscles, joints and tendons to the spinal cord.
3   Autonomic fibres—which conduct impulses from the spinal cord to the sweat glands, blood vessels and hairs.

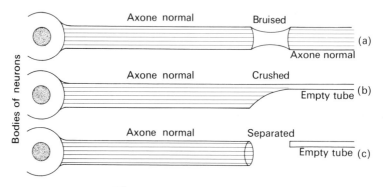

Fig. 11.5   Types of nerve lesions.

Lesions of peripheral nerves can interfere with one or all of these functions either completely or partly. Complete division of a peripheral nerve produces firstly, paralysis, and ultimately wasting, of the muscles supplied by that nerve; secondly, loss of sensation in the area of skin normally supplied by the nerve, and thirdly, absence of sweating and impairment of vasometer control in the same distribution as the area of sensory loss.

Wallerian degeneration

If a nerve has been completely divided and the ends become separated, the nerve fibres distal to the lesion degenerate, leaving empty Schwann tubes (Fig. 11.5c). However, if a nerve suture is performed, the proximal nerve fibres (or axones) will grow into the empty tubes and ultimately lead to restoration of function (Fig. 11.6). Naturally, recovery is better in children, in recent lesions, or in clean cuts; in elderly people, or in old standing lesions, or where there has been extensive bruising or impairment of the blood supply to the nerve, the prognosis is worse.

Modes of injury

Besides being cut, nerves may be bruised, have noxious substances injected into them, or be subjected to pressure from simple or malignant tumours for example, or scar tissue or callus, or they may be stretched (traction lesions).

In investigating a possible lesion of a peripheral nerve the first thing is to decide on the extent of the lesion; which nerve or nerves are involved, and the probable nature of the lesion. For example, in open wounds such as those from a knife, glass, bullets, etc., it is probable that the nerve has been divided and that the lesion is complete, whereas in closed wounds—those with fractures, it is probable that it has only been bruised. A bruised nerve will nearly always recover in time; a divided nerve will only recover after suture.

In certain situations—e.g. the buttock and the front of the elbow, it is easy to damage a nerve when giving an injection and special care must be taken to avoid such an occurrence. In other situations, for example, the brachial plexus, or the external popliteal nerve, closed injuries may apply a traction force to the nerve often causing extensive and permanent impairment of function. We can therefore classify peripheral nerve injuries as follows:

1   Clinical classification:
(i)   Concussion ⎤
(ii)   Continuous pressure ⎬ Closed injuries
(iii) Contusion ⎦
(iv) Division (Open injuries)
(v)   Injections
(vi) Traction

2   Pathological classification (see Fig. 11.4):
(i)   Neuropraxia (bruised)
(ii)   Axonotmesis (crushed)
(iii) Neurotmesis (separated)

3   Treatment:
(i)   Neurolysis
(ii)   Nerve suture
(iii) Nerve graft

1 *Clinical classification.* The causes of peripheral nerve lesions may usefully be divided into six.

(i) Concussion injuries—i.e. a temporary pressure effect from which there is usually a rapid recovery.

(ii) Continuous pressure effects—e.g. from a tumour, from callus formation, or from ligaments or other structures—for instance, the transverse carpal ligament at the front of the wrist not infrequently presses on the median nerve.

(iii) More serious blunt injuries which may be termed contusion or bruising injuries. These may cause intraneural haemorrhage which may lead to fairly prolonged paralysis due to interruption in the continuity of the neuraxone without breaking the nerve sheath itself.

These three causes may all be grouped together as being types of closed injuries and in them the prognosis for ultimate spontaneous recovery is very good.

(iv) Lesions due to division—These are usually due to open wounds— wounds by glass, knives or gunshot wounds. They are significant because they usually imply that part or the whole of the nerve has been divided and there is no prospect of spontaneous recovery without surgical intervention.

(v) Lesions due to injections—e.g. damage to the sciatic nerve—if intra- muscular injections are unwisely given into the buttock. Here the prognosis depends on the type of material injected. For instance, if a small amount of comparatively non-toxic is injected, there is likely to be temporary paralysis and ultimate recovery, but if a large amount (such as 10 ml) of a very irritant fluid is injected, a great segment of the nerve may be destroyed which will lead to permanent in- terference with function.

(vi) Traction lesions—these commonly occur either in the brachial plexus or in the lateral popliteal nerve in association with tears of the lateral collateral ligament of the knee. Here again, the prognosis varies with the extent of the lesion and the degree of violence. For example, minor traction lesions involving the upper trunk only of the brachial plexus, usually recover, but violent traction lesions involving the whole brachial plexus (especially if the roots are involved) seldom, if ever, recover and may indeed be associated with damage to the spinal cord, leading later on to spastic paralysis of the legs.

Lesions due to these last three causes in general have a bad prognosis.

2   *Pathological classification.* At the microscopic level, nerve lesions may be divided according to the condition of the individual nerve fibres. A nerve fibre may, for instance, be intact and conducting normally or it may be intact but temporarily concussed; this condition is often known as neuropraxia, or the axone may be divided—that is, there is degeneration of the neuraxone distal to the lesion but the sheath of the nerve is intact; this is often known as axonotmesis. Finally, both the neuraxone and the sheath may be divided, leading to neurotmesis (see Fig. 11.5c).

It is seldom possible to make an accurate diagnosis of the exact pathological condition of every nerve fibre without exploring the nerve surgically, but a good guess can be made by the type of injury and the clinical progress. For instance, if there is a closed lesion due to concussion or contusion and there is fairly rapid recovery, it is safe to assume that only minor damage has been done. On the other hand, if there is an open lesion—that is, if there is an open wound or cut or there has been an injection—and there is complete interference with nerve function with no sign of recovery, it is usually wise to assume that the nerve has been seriously damaged and an exploratory operation should be performed.

3   *Treatment of the nerve itself.* Exploration and trial section—in the first place, if there is evidence on clinical grounds that there is only temporary damage from which the nerve will recover, no special treatment is required. On the other hand, if recovery is delayed or there is a probability that the nerve has been seriously damaged, it is wise to carry out an exploratory operation. This may merely consist of an inspection and examination of the nerve, including, if a badly scarred area or a large neuroma is found, a trial section into the nerve to decide how much of the neuroma was nerve fibre and how much scar tissue.

Neurolysis—if the nerve is surrounded by scar tissue but is basically intact, then the simple operation of freeing the nerve from scar tissue (neurolysis) may be performed. This is specially effective if the nerve has been nicked, as for instance if it has been caught up in scar tissue near a fracture, or if the nerve is pressed upon by a ligament as commonly occurs with the median nerve at the wrist or with the ulnar nerve at the elbow.

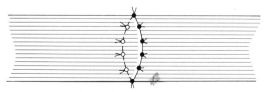

Fig. 11.6   Nerve sutures.

Nerve suture—if however the nerve has been completely divided, then it is necessary to perform a nerve suture. This must be preceded by removing any scar tissue at the ends of the nerve which would hinder the axones growth from the proximal and into the distal segment after suture. The scarred end of a divided nerve is called a neuroma. After suture it is wise to splint the limb so that no undue traction is put on the suture line until the two ends of the nerve have grown firmly together.

Nerve grafting—finally, if there is a large gap in the nerve, this may be bridged by means of a nerve graft, i.e. taking a piece of non-essential nerve from another part of the body and inserting it between the divided and separated ends of the affected nerve. Commonly the lateral femoral cutaneous nerve is used as a graft.

Care of the limb. In addition to the treatment of the nerve itself, one must consider the condition of the limb as a whole. Basically this consists of avoiding deformities, contractures and stiffness of joints by a combination of active and passive movements and 'lively' splinting. Secondly, it is important that the patient's skin, especially the anaesthetic areas, should not be injured by burns or other trauma, and the patient must be warned to avoid noxious stimuli such as excessive heat or cold or, in the case of the foot, pressure.

Lastly, every means should be taken to ensure that the circulation of the limb is maintained at an adequate level during the process of nerve recovery and this should include avoiding exposure to extremes of heat and cold or allowing the limb to hang down for a long period and thus become oedematous due to impaired vaso-motor control.

Theoretically the paralysed muscles can be maintained in good condition by frequent repeated galvanic stimulation. In practice this is often difficult to arrange and if it means that the patient has to stay away from work or has to make long and tiring journeys to hospital at frequent intervals, it is not worthwhile, though an intelligent patient can be taught to give himself galvanic stimulation at home.

Causalgia

Occasionally following injury to a nerve—especially the median nerve in the proximal part of the arm—the syndrome known as causalgia develops. It is characterized by intense, spontaneous, burning pain in the distribution of the nerve, accompanied by swelling, excessive sweating and blister formation; the hand often becomes pink or plum-coloured. The hand is extremely sensitive to the touch and the slightest stimulus—especially an emotional stimulus—precipitates an even more severe attack of pain. For example, anxiety, heat, vibration, noise or any other emotion makes the pain worse. Quiet and ice-cold compresses applied locally alleviate the pain slightly.

It is generally considered that this syndrome is due to a breakdown of insulation between the sympathetic fibres and the afferent pain fibres in the nerve. As a result, every time there is a discharge of impulses along the sympathetic fibres, the pain fibres are stimulated.

The treatment is to interrupt the sympathetic supply proximal to the lesion and, if this is completely successful, relief of the causalgic pain almost invariably occurs; if it has been a case of true causalgia. For this reason it is wise to reserve the term 'causalgia' for the syndrome described above and not apply it to everyone who has pain in the distribution of the nerve, whether associated with an injury or not.

Nursing management of patients with peripheral nerve lesions

The nursing management of the patient with a lesion of the nerves is related to the amount of disability which it causes. This disability ranges from anaesthesia and temperature changes in a small area of skin to complete loss of the use of one or more limbs. Management of the patient is also related to the probability of complete recovery from the lesion or the possibility that no recovery will occur when the patient must be trained to accept disability for the remainder of his life.

Physiotherapy and peripheral nerve lesions. A major part of the management of the patient is by the physiotherapist and the occupational therapist. In the care of these patients, team-work is as necessary as in the care of any other orthopaedic patient. The physiotherapist contributes by keeping the joints mobile, i.e. preventing contractures at joints, maintaining the bulk and elasticity of muscles which have been temporarily deprived of a nerve supply and also by estimating the amount of recovery, if any, in the structure supplied by the affected nerve.

The occupational therapist aids the patient by providing activity to assist the work of the physiotherapist in preventing muscle wastage. When there is permanent residual disability, the occupational therapist helps the patient by re-training him to compensate for his disability and to manage his daily activities such as dressing, washing, shaving, feeding and transportation. She also collaborates with the Disablement Resettlement Officer in seeking new ways of managing his occupation or by changing his profession or trade.

Local management of the affected part. When skin is deprived of a sensory nerve supply the patient is unaware of pain or sensation; thus he has no knowledge of pressure, constriction, burning or any other injury: he is unaware that anything is wrong. He must therefore learn to protect the anaesthetic and paralysed limb and to avoid damage to it.

The anaesthetic skin must be kept clean, dry and free from local compressions such as crumbs in creases of skin, buttons and metal tags on clothing, stones in shoes or body pressure on it when lying or sitting. Such simple trauma as may be caused by a bad darn or a tight supporting strap or band on clothing can be serious.

The denervated area must also be protected from extremes of heat or cold. Hot water bottles, hot plates, lit cigarettes, hot water taps, radiators, and stoves are all hazards; in cold weather the hand or foot, if involved, must be covered by a loosely fitting glove or sock. Strong chemicals or washing detergents may also be a danger.

Manicure of the hands or pedicure of the feet should only be performed, on the paralysed side, by an expert. Trimming of corns and callosities must only be done by a trained chiropodist.

Involvement of the autonomic nervous supply reduces the efficiency of the venous return from the limb, thus, engorgement of the blood vessels with oedema and swelling will occur if the limb is allowed to hang down for a long time. For paralysis of the leg, the patient should sit with the affected limb raised so that the foot is level with the pelvis. When the arm or hand is paralysed the upper limb should rest on a table when the patient sits, so that the hand is level with the shoulder. Pillows or supports in the bed for the affected limb may also be necessary.

Splintage for peripheral nerve lesions

The splints supplied to patients with these conditions must be as unobtrusive and as light in weight as possible. They are supplied for a variety of reasons:

1　As 'lively' splints. These are spring loaded devices (Fig. 11.7) which oppose the action of unparalysed muscles. The patient contracts his unaffected muscles against the springs to exercise the muscles and prevent stiffness and deformity of the joints. They also act as partial functional substitutes for the paralysed muscles.

2　To maintain the limb in an acceptable and usable position. For example, if the patient has a dropped wrist, a 'cock-up' splint may be supplied to hold the hand in a position which will enable the patient to hold a writing or eating utensil (see Fig. 11.9).

3　To hold the limb in the 'optimum position of rest' so that the paralysed muscles are not stretched and the unparalysed muscles do not become contracted.

Splints for lesions of the upper limb

Abduction splint. This may be fashioned out of plaster of Paris or be a ready-made splint such as the Littler-Jones abduction splint (see p. 101). The nerve supply to the deltoid muscle which caps the shoulder, is the axillary (circumflex) nerve. This can be damaged in dislocations of the shoulder or in fractures of the surgical neck of the humerus. All fibres of the deltoid muscle abduct the shoulder; the anterior fibres also contribute to flexion; the posterior fibres to extension. The position of abduction at the shoulder ensures that no fibres of the muscle are unduly contracted and none are stretched.

Radial (musculo-spiral) nerve splintage. (i) The short cock-up splint. This is used to hold the wrist in an extended position to prevent contractures of the muscles on the anterior surface of the forearm, and to hold the hand and fingers in a functional position (see Fig. 11.9).

(ii) The radial 'lively' splint (Fig. 11.7). This consists of a series of springs attached to finger slings. Each finger and the thumb is supported in extension by the springs. Another spring extends the wrist. To flex the fingers, thumb or wrist it is necessary to oppose the pull of the springs; when the flexor muscles relax, the springs pull the wrist, hand and fingers back into the extended position. The patient exercises his functional muscles against the pull of the springs.

(iii) The ulnar 'lively' splint (Fig. 11.8). This splint opposes the actions of the extensors of the metacarpo-phalangeal joints.

Median nerve splintage (see Fig. 11.9). The median nerve enters the palm of the hand under the transverse carpal ligament at the front of the wrist. In the hand it supplies the short muscles which control the thumb, and the skin of the front of the thumb, index finger, middle finger and the lateral half of the ring finger and corresponding area of the palm. A lesion affecting the median nerve at the wrist causes paralysis of the muscles which flex, oppose and abduct the thumb. A median nerve lesion above the elbow causes also paralysis of the long flexors of the thumb, index and middle finger and of the pronator muscles of the forearm. The hand is then deformed with the fingers and thumb in an extended position with loss of ability to oppose the thumb to the fingers, as in holding a small object. This is described as the 'ape-like' hand because the thumb falls back to lie in the same plain as the fingers.

The median nerve splint is a wrist-band with a loop of material to pull the thumb across the palm of the hand. The thumb can then be opposed to the fingers.

The successful use of splints, particularly lively splints, for arm nerve lesions requires good co-operation from the patient. Carelessly applied splints do more harm than good.

Splintage for peripheral nerve lesions of the lower limb

Damage to the common peroneal (Lateral popliteal) nerve. In the lower limb this is the lesion most likely to require splintage. This nerve is the lateral half of the sciatic nerve: it first passes down in the posterior thigh. It then leaves the sciatic trunk to wind around the neck of the fibula where it can be rolled against the bone with one's finger. It then passes forwards to apply the muscles which lift the forefoot and extend (dorsiflex) the toes. When the nerve is damaged the forefoot hangs down, and the toes catch in the ground when walking. The following splints are available for use in the conservative treatment of the deformity:

Rizzoli splint (Fig. 11.10). This is a strong, flat spring which passes down the posterior surface of the leg to be inserted into the leather of the back of the patient's shoe. The upper end of the spring is attached to a metal band which passes round the calf. The splint is covered in flesh coloured material to make it as unobtrusive as possible. Once the spring is applied and the shoe is laced up, the foot is held in a corrected position and does not hang down in walking.

This splint is only for use on patients with paralysis of the anterior muscles of the leg. When the posterior muscles are paralysed, the spring and band would compress the back of the leg and cause a splint sore.

Drop foot springs (Fig. 11.11). These serve a similar function to the Rizzoli splint but are more obtrusive. The hinged bar of the splint passes down the side of the leg to be inserted into a socket in the heel of the shoe. The hinge is spring-loaded and the strength of the spring can be varied to meet the needs of the patient. It is functionally efficient but aesthetically unacceptable to girls.

Toe-raising springs (Fig. 11.12). These are easily seen on the patient. The spring forms a right-angled triangle with the foot and the leg. The upper end of the spring is attached to a band around the leg below the knee; the lower end is inserted into the upper surface of the toe end of the shoe. The

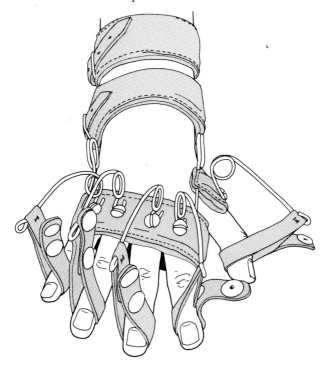

Fig. 11.7   The Radial 'Lively' splint.

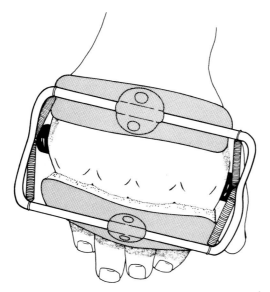

Fig. 11.8   The Ulnar 'Lively' splint.

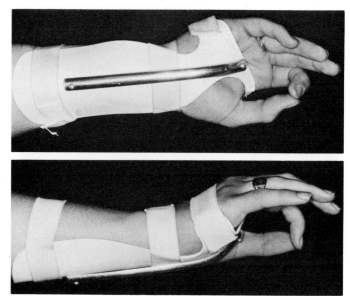

Fig. 11.9 (a) *Caption facing.*

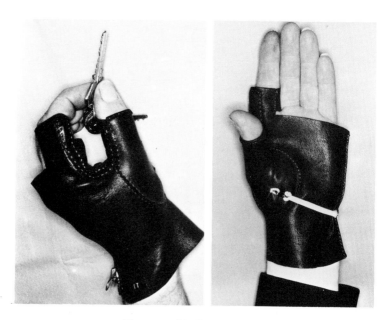

Fig. 11.9 (b) *Caption facing.*

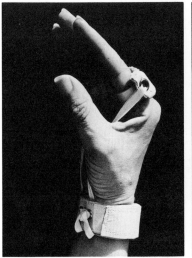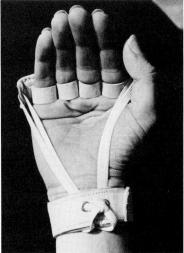

Fig. 11.9   (c) *Farnham Park Ulnar Nerve Splint*
To give the patient flexion at the metacarpo-phalangeal joints and allow
full function of the hand.

Fig. 11.9   (a) *Cock-up Splint*
Suitable for a radial nerve lesion or stabilization of the wrist joint. It is
moulded in rigid plastic. The palmar part of the splint should not prevent full
flexion of the metacarpo-phalangeal joints or opposition of the thumb.

The webbing straps are fastened with Velcro.

Where additional strength is required a reinforcement bar is shaped and
riveted to the splint.

Fig. 11.9   (b) *Farnham Park Median Nerve Splint*
The aim is to give abduction and opposition of the thumb, thus allowing
fine pinch.

To hold the thumb in abduction, a strip of spring steel is inserted in the
web of the thumb.

Opposition of the thumb is achieved by heavy shirring elastic attached at
the ulnar seam of the splint and hooked to the base of the thumb. It can be
unfastened when the patient requires maximum extension of the thumb.

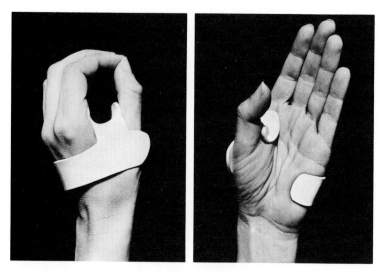

Fig. 11.9   (d) *Caption facing.*

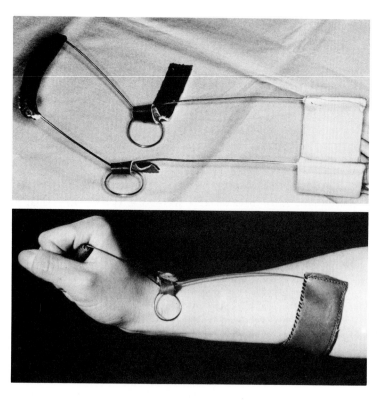

Fig. 11.9   (e) *Caption facing.*

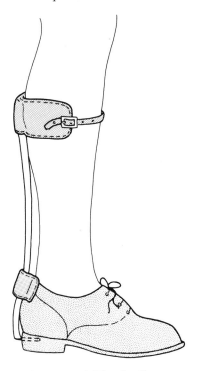

Fig. 11.10 A Rizzoli splint.

spring serves to lift the front end of the shoe and thus the foot. The band around the leg tends to slip down; if this happens the spring becomes ineffective. If the band is tightened to prevent it slipping, it may cause pain and oedema of the foot.

Fig. 11.9 (d) *Opponens Splint*
  Left: rigid plastic is moulded to the hand to maintain the thumb in abduction and opposition to allow pinch. Suitable for a median nerve lesion or functional retraining after opponens transplant.
  Right: palmar view of opponens splint.

Fig. 11.9 (e) *Oppenheimer Splint*
  Above: to show construction of Oppenheimer splint.
  Below: suitable for a radial nerve lesion, this splint allows full function of the hand. The piano wire construction draws the wrist into extension.

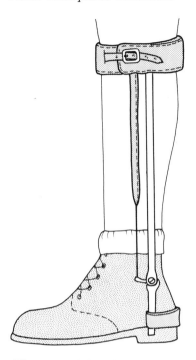

Fig. 11.11   A drop foot appliance.

Complete paralysis of the lower leg and foot

The leg below the knee is supplied by two main nerves; the common peroneal (lateral popliteal) and the medial popliteal nerves. If both are affected by a lesion, the leg and foot are flail; the foot is unstable when it is placed on the ground, for example, to support the body in standing or walking. The ankle and foot must therefore be stabilised so that the foot is 'plantigrade' and the leg is vertical—that is, so that it provides a stable platform upon which the patient can stand. In some instances this can be done surgically; if splintage is to be used, however, it must be functional rather than elegant; it must have sufficient strength to withstand a heavy work load.

Double below-knee irons (Fig. 11.13)

These are two parallel bars which pass down on either side of the lower leg. At the top of the splint they are attached to a supporting band which passes

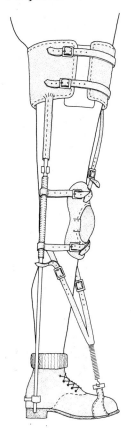

Fig. 11.12   A toe-raising spring appliance used with a caliper.

around the leg; at the lower end they are bent and inserted into rectangular sockets placed on either side of the heel of the patient's shoe. The shoe must be adapted when the splint is ordered. A strap passes from one bar to the other behind the leg at the level of the malleoli, to hold the bars in their sockets in the shoe. Whilst the patient is wearing this splint no dorsiflexion or plantarflexion of the ankle joint or foot is possible. Alternatively round sockets may be used with anterior and/or posterior stops which allow limited ankle motion.

Single below-knee iron with T-strap (Fig. 11.14). A single iron bar passes down on one side of the leg. It is attached at the upper end to a supporting band around the leg below the knee. At its lower end it is bent and inserted into a socket in the heel of the shoe. The shape of the socket may be:

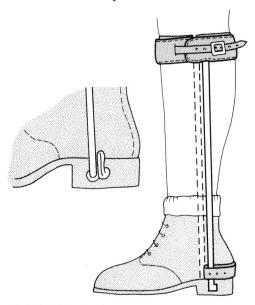

Fig. 11.13 (a) A double below-knee iron with square sockets and posterior strap. (Inset—drop-foot stops.)

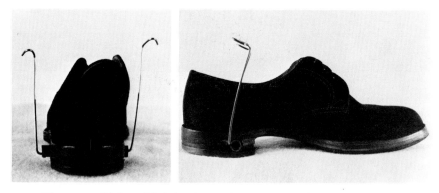

Fig. 11.13 (b) A modified shoe for a patient with a drop foot deformity. Heel sockets are for projections from below-knee iron.

1 *Rectangular* when the bar entering the socket is also rectangular. Thus no dorsiflexion or plantiflexion is possible whilst the splint is being worn, or
2 *Circular* with a cylindrical shape of bar to enter the socket. Thus plantarflexion or dorsiflexion are permitted when this splint is worn. However, a metal 'stop' on the shoe may be fitted. If this is in *front* of the bar dorsi-

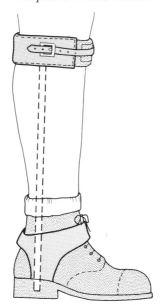

Fig. 11.14 A single below-knee iron with T-straps (an inside iron with outside straps).

flexion is prevented; should it be placed *behind* the bar plantarflexion is prevented.

T-straps (Fig. 11.14). These are straps which are attached to the gusset of the shoe. The crossbar of the T-shape fits around the ankle and over the below-knee iron. It is used to correct either an inversion or eversion deformity of the foot.

Correcting inversion of the foot
Inversion is a deformity which is present when the sole of the foot is turned inwards towards the median line. To avoid inversion, the patient is supplied with an inside iron and an outside T-strap.

Correcting eversion of the foot
Eversion exists when the foot is deformed with the sole of the foot turned away from the midline and facing towards the lateral surface. It may be looked on as an extreme example of flat foot.

An outside iron and an inside T-strap are used to counter excessive eversion.

12

Tendon Injuries

Relevant applied anatomy

The hand and foot are capable of performing many intricate movements. The fingers, thumb and carpal bones may be placed in many different positions. These positions may be used as means of expression or communication; or for delicate and fine movements such as are used in sewing, watch-making, or the assembly of computers or transistor radios. The fingers and hand must also be capable of grasping firmly as is required in gripping a hammer or any similar heavy object.

The foot must also be adaptable and capable of intricate movement. Most people do not make use of the full range of movements of which the foot is capable; it is sufficient for most of us to be able to put on footwear and transfer the body from one point to another by walking or running. The trained ballet dancer, however, makes use of most of the wide range of movements of which the foot is capable. Similarly in countries where people do not need to wear shoes, the local inhabitants have flexible feet which are able to perform very intricate movements.

A child who is born without upper limbs, or who develops paralysis of the arms during childhood, uses the feet as prehensile instruments, serving many of the functions of the hands. Thus writing, dressing, sewing, cutting, washing, management of the personal toilet, applying cosmetics and the use of cutlery for feeding are all possible using the feet to hold objects.

If all the muscles which are needed for the many complex movements of the hand and foot were placed on the hand or foot, these would be large, heavy and inelegant, with a limited range of movement. As a great many muscles are required for these movements they must be provided, but almost all of them must be situated at some distance from the hand or foot. Thus the muscles which provide the force for the powerful movements are placed in the forearm or calf. They act upon the hand and fingers, or foot and toes, by pulling upon long cords (tendons); these move the hand or foot in much the same way as a puppet-master works the limbs of his marionettes. Very fine intricate movements are actuated by small muscles situated in the hand or foot which have direct attachments to bone.

In order to close the fingers or make the toes curl down towards the sole of the foot, a set of muscles called flexors are required. These are in two layers—superficial (sublimis) and deep (profundus).

To cause the fingers to open, or the toes to elevate, a set of muscles called extensors are required.

These two sets of muscles operate in direct opposition to each other although they must collaborate to allow a harmonious movement. Thus the flexors relax so as to permit extension and the extensors relax to allow flexion.

It follows that if the tendons of the flexors are severed the digit will be pulled into an extension deformity and, if the tendons of the extensors are damaged the digit will be held in a flexion deformity.

To reach their point of insertion the tendons from the muscles must pass across the wrist or ankle; they must then continue on through the hand or foot until they are attached to bone. It is in these areas that the flexor and extensor tendons are most vulnerable. They are held in position by fibrous tendon sheaths and bands, inside which are the synovial sheaths which allow the tendons to glide freely with minimal friction.

Tendon injuries

Tendon injuries are common, especially in the hand; and are usually due to cuts with sharp objects such as knives, or injuries at work. But tendon injuries may also occur with crushing or blunt injuries even when the skin is not cut.

Tendon injuries of the hand

Extensor tendons. The most common tendon injury in the hand is a cut through the extensor tendons over the back of the knuckles. Fortunately, the prognosis after repair of the tendon is good. It is only necessary to sew up the tendon and immobilize the finger for some ten days, following which in the majority of cases an excellent result will occur.

Flexor tendons. Cuts of the flexor tendons are more complicated, but cuts of the flexor tendons in the palm recover quite well with direct suture. Cuts of the flexor tendons above the wrist are a little more complicated, as adhesions between the tendons are common, which is natural, considering that the tendons are closely related as they pass under the volar carpal ligament.

Therefore, if both sublimis and profundus tendons are cut, many surgeons believe the best treatment is to repair the profundus tendon and excise the sublimis completely. Certainly, as a general rule this leads to a better result than if any attempt is made to suture all the tendons, following which some adhesions between the different tendons and limitation of movement is extremely common. Naturally, if only one tendon is sutured, it is usual to repair this and the result is good.

Damage to the flexor tendons in the fingers is a far more complicated problem as in this situation adhesions between the tendon and the tendon sheath are almost inevitable. For this reason the majority of surgeons believe that direct suture of a cut flexor tendon in the finger is a mistake, and advocate simple repair of the skin in the early stages. Once the skin has healed, a second operation to replace the damaged tendon by a tendon graft is advised. The idea behind this procedure is that the tendon graft does not have any suture line in the dangerous interdigital portion, because it is attached distally to the distal phalanx and proximally it is attached to the appropriate tendon in the palm of the hand where adhesions are less likely to form, or more accurately, adhesions are more likely to be long and elastic and are less likely to limit movement. The donor tendon for the graft can be taken either from the palmaris longus of the same side, or from the peroneus longus muscle in the leg. Following a tendon graft it is usual to immobilize the wrist and fingers in the semi-flexed position for three weeks. This appears to be long enough to allow some union to occur between the graft and the donor tendon and yet not so long for dense adhesions to form.

Closed injuries of the tendons

Mallet finger

There are two common closed injuries of the tendons; one is the mallet finger. This characteristically occurs in middle-aged women and results from a relatively trivial injury to the tip of the finger when the tip of the extensor tendon is avulsed from its insertion into the base of the proximal phalanx (Fig. 12.1). As a result, the patient is unable to extend the distal phalanx actively. There is considerable controversy about the best treatment, but on the whole, results of the suture are poor for two reasons: firstly, the tendon is frayed and degenerate and secondly, it is so near the skin and therefore there is so little subcutaneous tissue that either infection or adhesions between the tendons and the overlying skin are inevitable. In addition, there is a certain risk of resultant damage to the nail bed which would ultimately cause permanent deformity of the nail.

Therefore, most surgeons advise that the distal phalanx should be hyper-extended for some four to six weeks. This can be achieved either by means of a plaster of Paris splint or a special splint, or by the surgical insertion of a fine wire through the distal phalanx into the head of the middle phalanx holding the joint in hyper-extension.

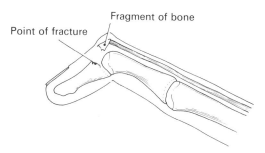

Fig. 12.1   (a) A mallet finger.

In general the results of treatment are only moderate, but in course of time a certain amount of spontaneous improvement occurs and the condition does not usually lead to severe disability, though it may lead to an ugly appearance of the finger.

Boutonnière injury

An analogous injury is the so-called Boutonnière injury affecting the proximal interphalangeal joint when the middle slip of the long extensor tendon is avulsed from the base of the middle phalanx. This injury also gives rise to considerable difficulties in treatment. As with a mallet finger, direct suture is difficult and usually gives a disappointing result. Some surgeons advocate prolonged hyper-extension of the proximal interphalangeal joint on the same lines as treatment for a mallet finger. Others believe that a mobilizing operation to replace the torn middle slip by suturing the lateral expansions

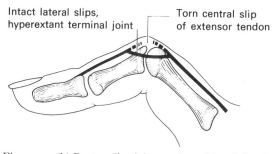

Fig. 12.1   (b) Boutonnière injury and resulting deformity.

together over the dorsum of the joint is the best treatment, but this in its turn may lead to limitation of flexion. The ultimate disability from this injury if left untreated can be severe, with permanent flexion of the interphalangeal joint and hyperextension of the distal interphalangeal joint.

Spontaneous rupture of tendons

Ruptured tendons—both flexor and extensor—also commonly occur in association with diseases such as rheumatoid arthritis. In particular, spontaneous rupture of the extensor tendons of the fingers at the back of the wrist frequently occur in rheumatoid arthritis. This may occur for two reasons; either the inflamed tendon sheath may strangulate the tendon and the rheumatoid granulation tissue eat into the tendon and weaken it or, alternatively, there may be a bony spike—e.g. at the dorsum of the lower end of the ulna, and the tendon may fray as it passes over the bony spike. Similarly, spontaneous rupture of the extensor pollicis longus tendon not uncommonly occurs following a malunited Colles' fracture. In the case of spontaneous rupture of tendons in rheumatoid arthritis, direct suture is usually the best treatment together with removal of the cause, whether this be a thickened tendon sheath or a spike of bone. In the case of spontaneous rupture of the extensor pollicis longus tendon, the best treatment is usually to employ the extensor indicis proprius tendon as a tendon transplant, detach it from its insertion and suture the transplant to the distal end of the extensor pollicis longus.

In the arm, rupture of the biceps tendon is not unusual. This commonly occurs in the older age group and is usually associated with osteoarthritis. The symptoms are pain and swelling plus momentary loss of use, but here the prognosis for spontaneous recovery is good, and operative interference is seldom—if ever—indicated.

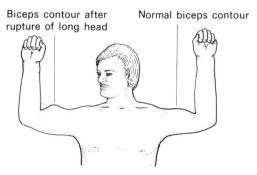

Fig. 12.2   Patient displaying abnormal biceps contour after rupture of long head.

Tendon injuries of the foot and leg

Tendo Achillis. In the foot and leg the most important tendon injury is spontaneous rupture of the Tendo Achillis. This commonly occurs in men of later middle age and is predisposed to by degeneration of the tendon. The patient usually gives a history of suddenly undertaking some unaccustomed exertion—for example, running in a parents' race in the school sports; the unexpected muscle action, together with perhaps a certain degree of inco-ordination causes a rupture of the weak tendon.

If left untreated this can give rise to considerable disability—inability to walk on the toes, impairment of normal gait, inability to run, and normally speaking it is wise to repair this tendon. However, it is a mistake to use unabsorbable material or chromic cat gut, as this area of the body is notoriously liable to develop infection which often becomes chronic. Following repair of the tendon the foot should be immobilised in a moderate equinus position for at least six weeks.

Quadriceps femoris. Spontaneous rupture of the quadriceps tendon also occurs. This may occur where the quadriceps is inserted into the upper pole of the patella or where the ligamentum patellae is inserted into the lower pole of the patella. The causes and symptoms are similar to those of the ruptured tendo Achillis, namely—unusual exertion in an elderly or middle-aged man, followed by sudden pain, haematoma formation and loss of ability to straighten the knee voluntarily. Again the treatment is by repair of the ruptured tendon, otherwise severe disability persists.

The peroneus longus has a definite but weak power of plantarflexion and its action may lead the examiner to underestimate the damage to the Tendo Calcaneus.

In both these instances, diagnosis may be difficult in so far as shortly after injury the gap in the tendon fills up with a blood clot and therefore cannot be felt, and to the inexperienced examiner the tendon appears to be in continuity.

Rupture of the quadriceps muscle in the middle of the thigh is also not uncommon. This usually occurs in younger people following a direct injury such as a kick at football. Here treatment is conservative and a short period of rest will lead to restoration of normal function, but if the condition is unwisely treated by vigorous massage, passive manipulation or excessive exercise, the haematoma may undergo ossification, leading to a persistent limp and limitation of flexion.

Tendon suture

As a general rule, a divided or torn tendon should be repaired by sewing the ends together (Fig. 12.3). Great ingenuity is needed to ensure that the suture is strong enough but not too bulky and that there is as little raw tendon surface as possible, as such raw surfaces encourage the formation of adhesions.

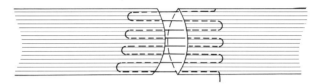

Fig. 12.3   Tendon suture.

Most surgeons prefer unabsorbable suture material such as silk, nylon or stainless steel. After suture the tendon must be held in a relaxed position usually for three weeks. The mature cells of a tendon are relatively inactive and play little part in the process of union. This means that in order that successful regeneration can occur, the two tendon ends must be put in to as close approximation as possible, and that the tendon repairing cells from the surrounding tissues must be able to reach the site of division. Unfortunately, this frequently leads to the formation of dense adhesions between the site of tendon injury and the surrounding tissues; surgical skill in repairing tendons tries to ensure that the tendon ends are held together until sufficient cells have grown into the tendon to allow repair to occur, but that the inevitable adhesions (i.e. the vascular tissue along which the cells travel) should not be allowed to become too strong.

Tendon repair

Many tendons, especially extensor tendons, can be successfully repaired by direct suture. This is not so with flexor tendons. Although in the hands of highly specialized technical surgeons the results of tendon grafting for damage have been good, in general there are still many indifferent results. This is chiefly because adhesions form between the tendon graft and the tunnel in which it glides. Attempts to prevent adhesions forming by wrapping materials round the tendon have been unsuccessful because the tendons must acquire a blood supply from the adjacent tissue and if the material is impermeable to granulation tissue the tendon lacks a blood supply and the ends do not unite. Alternatively, if the material is not impermeable adhesions still form.

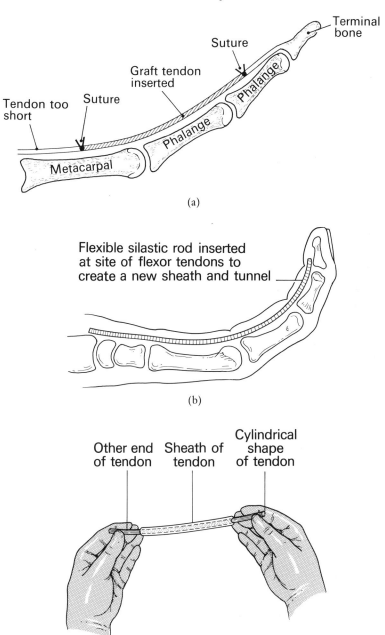

Fig. 12.4 (a) A tendon graft. (b) Silastic rod technique. (c) Tendon and sheath transplantation.

Therefore, it is inevitable that some adhesions must form. Ideally the aim is to make these as long and elastic as possible. With this need in view two developments in technique have been suggested:

1   One is that if the finger is badly scarred a silastic rod is inserted in the finger which is then vigorously moved passively for six to eight weeks. At the end of this time a smooth gliding sheath of connecting tissue will have formed around the silastic rod and provide a suitable bed in which the tendon graft can be placed. The rod is removed and a tendon graft threaded along the track in its position (Fig. 12.4b).

2   An alternative approach is to transplant, *in toto*, the fibrous and synovial tendon sheaths and both flexor tendons from a toe to the finger. In this case the blood vessels grow along the existing vinculae and there is little or no formation of tendon adhesions elsewhere. So far the results of this procedure have been excellent (Fig. 12.4c).

As with other tendon grafts the finger is splinted in semiflexion for three weeks.

Tendon grafts

In some situations, e.g. the fingers, direct suture usually fails as the suture line becomes adherent to the surrounding tendon sheath. By using a tendon graft to replace the divided tendon, a suture line inside the digital sheath is avoided (Fig. 12.4). It is customary to use either the palmaris or plantaris as a graft. The technique of suture and after-treatment are similar.

Tendon grafts are also used where there has been extensive destruction of tendons, for instance after burns.

Splintage for tendon injuries

The objective is to rest and relax the injured tendon and its attachment for the duration of healing. The position of the digit depends on which tendon is affected; if a flexor tendon has been divided, the finger should be immobilized in semi-flexion; if an extensor tendon has been cut, the almost extended position is required. The positioning of the digit will be arranged by the surgeon but extreme positions are usually inadvisable as they cause joint stiffness.

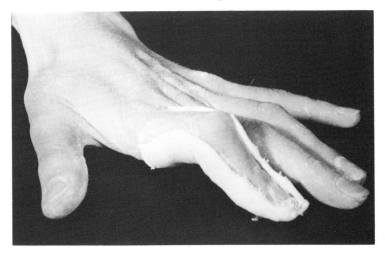

Fig. 12.5 A mallet finger splint.

Mallet finger splintage (Fig. 12.5)
This splint may be:
(a) commercially produced; these are made of polypropylene or other plastic material.
(b) improvised from aluminium sheeting and orthopaedic felt.
(c) made from plaster of Paris.
The position the finger is to be maintained in is: (i) complete hyperextension of the terminal interphalangeal joint; and (ii) right-angled flexion of the proximal interphalangeal joint.

Böhler's finger splint
This holds the affected finger in forward flexion and angulation. It extends from the tip of the finger, over the palm of the hand and five or six centimetres down the front of the wrist to end as a short crosspiece. It is held in position by bands of one centimetre wide zinc-oxide plaster.

Plaster of Paris splints for tendon injuries
A hand plaster is applied. This extends from the head of the radius, distal to the elbow, to just below the heads of the metacarpal bones. The wrist is fixed in a position of dorsiflexion (of about thirty degrees).
An extra slab is incorporated to include the finger; it should be about five centimetres wide and fourteen centimetres long. It is applied down the back of the finger and overlaps the posterior slab of the hand plaster by five centi-

metres. It encircles the affected finger without cutting into the webs on either side of the base of the finger. The tip of the finger is left exposed.

The encircling bandage of the hand plaster includes the base of the finger slab.

The thumb may be included in a hand plaster in the same way but the position of the thumb is more variable, related to the requirements of the surgeon.

Plaster of Paris splintage may also be required to support the foot and ankle in tendon injuries.

Long cock-up splint

This extends beyond the fingers and holds the wrist in extension. Only if all the extensor tendons are affected will this splint be used.

Nursing management for patients with tendon injuries

The patient with a tendon injury may also have had surgical repair of the tendon. It is therefore necessary:

1   To prevent haematoma formation by the use of a firm pad in the palm of the hand and the fingers and thumb curled around the pad; the affected finger is left clear. The bandage is also firmly applied but with the tips of the fingers and thumb exposed to ensure that there is no constriction of the hand and impairment of the blood supply. This pad and bandage is left on for twenty-four hours after operation.

2   To prevent swelling and oedema by elevating the hand above the shoulder in the immediate post-operative phase. A roller towel sling suspended from the hook of an intravenous infusion stand is suitable. The elbow, forearm and hand are suspended in the towel with safety pins through the roller towel, holding the limb in the desired position.

3   To prevent infection of the wound by adequate aseptic technique.

With any finger or toe splint there is a risk of occluding the circulation, therefore, the colour of the fingers or toes must be carefully observed.

When the surgeon decides that healing is adequate, physiotherapy and occupational therapy is commenced to accomplish as full a return of function of the limb as can be achieved.

Section C

Chronic Orthopaedic Conditions

13

Acute Infections of Bone, Joint and Hand

Relevant anatomy and physiology

All tissue must have a blood supply and bone is no exception; every long bone in the body has a blood vessel entering its shaft; the nutrient artery. In addition there are metaphyseal and epiphyseal vessels which supply the ends of the bone. The blood supply of flat bones and the carpal and tarsal bones is more variable. The blood vessels may be the routes of entry for micro-organisms; such a form of infection is known as 'haematogenous'. The micro-organism of haematogenous osteomyelitis, i.e. blood-borne infection of bone, is most commonly the staphylococcus aureus which is carried from a focus of infection elsewhere in the body; alternatively it may be a strepto-coccal infection or a complication of typhoid fever, diphtheria, pneumonia or abortus fever.

Bone is supplied with sensory nerves which carry nervous impulses (messages) to the central nervous system, signalling the occurrence of trauma or other lesions damaging the nerve; a kick on the shin is a painful experience! Infection is the successful invasion and multiplication in a tissue of micro-organisms; in osteomyelitis, the successful invasion and multiplication is in bone; there is, however, no room for increase in volume of the bone tissue—it is a hard, rigid tissue. An increase in the volume due to granulation tissue and pus (the products of infection) compresses the nerve endings and causes severe, excruciating pain which is not relieved by simple remedies; anti-biotics, surgical decompression and powerful analgesics may be the only relief possible.

Eventually relief of the pain may occur naturally when a SUBPERIOSTEAL ABSCESS forms. This is due to the products of the infection being carried through a track or sinus in the bone to the surface of the bone and beneath the periosteum—the membrane which surrounds the bone (see Fig. 13.2).

Pyogenic arthritis

Pyogenic means 'pus-forming'. Another title of the same condition is 'septic' arthritis and yet another, 'suppurative' arthritis.

A synovial joint also has an excellent blood supply and nerve supply. The haematogenous infection may be carried directly into the joint by the blood vessels entering it, or the infection may enter the joint from adjacent bone. The latter is unlikely to happen if a barrier of epiphyseal cartilage separates the infection in the bone from the nearest joint. Some joints, for instance the hip, have capsules which extend beyond the barrier of the epiphyseal line and the infection may enter the joint without having to cross the epiphyseal barrier.

Pain in joints

The nerve supply of the joint is both sensory and vasomotor. The sensory nerves supply the capsule and make the brain aware of pain or derangement of the joint. When infection occurs within the joint there is an increase of synovial fluid which, together with pus and tissue debris, distends the joint capsule. The stretching of the capsule is registered in the central nervous system as severe pain, as the peripheral nerve sensory endings are also stimulated.

Joint destruction

The surfaces of bone which meet at a synovial joint are especially suited to joint movement. The bone tissue is smooth and polished; it is additionally covered by a layer of smooth, slippery, glossy hyaline cartilage. The articular surfaces are also perfectly shaped to give optimum joint movement with little or no friction.

The presence of infection or loose bodies or crystals within the joint can be catastrophic. The joint surfaces may become roughened and eventually destroyed. When destruction has occurred, movement can only occur against considerable friction which impedes the movement and causes pain and a reduction in the normal range of movement. Eventually the roughened, uneven surfaces may unite and fuse together when the infection has gone; such a union is called *ankylosis*. This may be fibrous or bony.

Referred pain

The pain of a joint infection may not be felt as coming from the joint itself. Because of the irritation in the joint, reflex muscle contraction or 'muscle guarding' will occur. This phenomenon occurs when the muscles adjacent to a joint contract in a sustained spasm: the result is reduction of movement in the inflamed joint. The muscles become fatigued as the contraction in them continues, and then they relax which, in itself allows movement to occur when there is a recurrence of pain. The pain may be felt at the point of attachment of the muscle—namely, at a distance from the joint; for example, a patient with a hip infection may complain of a pain which is localized around the knee.

To pursue the subject a little further, the patient with an infection in a joint whose muscles are 'on guard' while he is awake may find that his muscles relax when he falls asleep. Any unexpected movement of the inflamed joint surfaces against each other may then result in sudden pain, causing the patient to scream or cry out. This phenomenon, known as 'night-cries', was well known to night nurses in orthopaedic units when treatment for tuberculosis was empirical, before the discovery of antibiotics. Efficient splintage, prevention of movement of the painful joint will overcome the need for 'muscle guarding' and also reduce the pain in the joint capsule.

Acute osteomyelitis

Acute infection of bone is known as acute osteomyelitis. It usually arises by a blood-borne spread from a focus elsewhere in the body, for example, a boil, tonsillitis, etc. It may occur as a sequel to a compound fracture or a badly treated wound. The clinical picture varies with the age of the patient.

Neonatal septicaemia
In the neonatal period septicaemia may result from infection of the umbilical cord (Fig. 13.1). The first sign is that the baby is ill, is listless, has a fever, cries, does not feed and may vomit. Detection of the local site of infection is often difficult but careful observation will reveal that the child does not move one limb as well as the other. The most common sites for acute infections in the new-born are in the upper end of the femur and the hip.

If the affected limb is examined carefully it will often be found that there is limitation of joint movement due to the reflex muscle spasm and that handling the affected limb makes the child cry. If the diagnosis is suspected it is wise to aspirate the affected joint and give antibiotics. If the child does not improve quickly with the treatment, open drainage of the joint is usually indicated.

In many instances the diagnosis is not made in the early stages and under

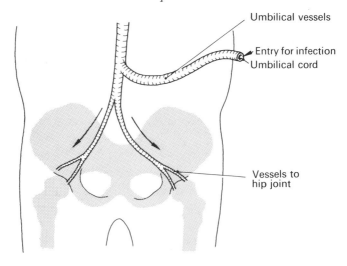

Fig. 13.1   Sepsis from umbilicus affecting a joint in an infant.

these circumstances extensive necrosis of bone may occur due to thrombosis of the blood vessels and cutting off of the blood supply.

Sometimes the first localizing evidence is the development of an abscess or even the spontaneous discharge of pus. In babies, acute osteomyelitis can lead to destruction of the growing end of the bone, leading to severe ultimate disability and marked shortening of the limb. Therefore, early diagnosis is of great importance.

Acute osteomyelitis in children

In older children acute osteomyelitis is common, especially in boys. The conditions may present in one of two forms. Commonly the child complains of acute pain near the end of a bone. There may be a small sympathetic effusion of the adjacent joint and the child will have some constitutional disturbance, raised temperature, loss of appetite, coated tongue, leucocytosis, etc. At this stage it may be difficult to distinguish the condition from acute septicaemia. It is nearly always the end of the bone (the metaphysis) which is affected. If untreated, an abscess may form which may burst either subperiosteally or ultimately subcutaneously, or it may burst into the adjacent joint. Again, there may be interference with the growth of the bone if the condition is untreated (Fig. 13.2).

Treatment is to give the usual measures for fever, to splint the limb, to take a sample of blood for blood culture and to give a wide spectrum antibiotic. If the condition does not improve within twenty-four hours, or if a

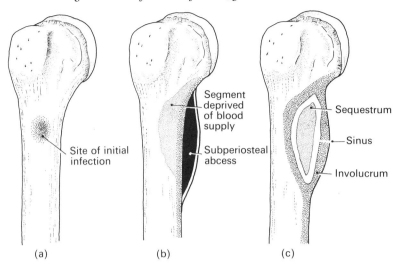

Fig. 13.2   Haematogenous osteomyelitis in bone. (a) Invasion. (b) Avascularization. (c) Necrosis and sequestrum formation.

subperiosteal or subcutaneous abscess can be felt, operation is indicated—namely, drainage of the abscess and sending a sample of pus for bacteriological examination and determination of sensitivity to antibiotics. Opinion differs about the advisability to operate on bones, but if there is an abscess inside the bone most surgeons consider that this should be drained by making a hole in the bone which will, among other things, relieve the pain. One of the advantages in operating is that it is possible to obtain a specimen of pus and determine the organism and its sensitivity even though the blood culture has been negative. On the other hand, operation may lead to a chronic sinus and is usually only advised if conservative treatment is not succeeding.

Alternatively, in children acute osteomyelitis may present in the form of a septicaemia with a high fever and temperature and occasional shock due to adrenal failure. As with small babies, localising the lesion may be difficult, and in this case it is usually wise to treat the condition conservatively in the first place, i.e. with massive doses of 'wide spectrum' antibiotics, blood transfusion and cortisone, and only operate when, and if, clear cut localisation in bone occurs.

Ideally the choice of an antibiotic should depend on isolating the organism and discovering its sensitivities and resistances. Unfortunately this takes time and even if a blood culture is taken as soon as a child reaches hospital it is likely to be 48 hours before much information is forthcoming—

and then it is too late and the fate of the bone has been settled. Therefore one must start chemotherapy at once on the 'best guess principle'. Everybody knows that certain agents penetrate bone better than others and that others act on a wider range of bacteria. In a serious condition like osteomyelitis most surgeons give two chemotherapeutic agents simultaneously.

If diagnosed and treated in the early stages, acute osteomyelitis will usually subside completely, but if it is either not diagnosed or not treated, the condition may become chronic (see Chapter 15). The common infecting organisms are staphylococci; streptococci and (less commonly) pneumococci.

Post-traumatic osteomyelitis

Following a compound fracture or following an operation on bone, acute osteomyelitis may develop. The symptoms and signs are similar but less dramatic. In adults also, acute osteomyelitis may arise as a new disease, but commonly acute osteomyelitis in adults is a recurrence of a previous osteomyelitis from which they suffered in childhood. Clinical features and treatment are similar.

Septic arthritis

Acute infection of the joints usually occurs following penetrating wounds. They also occur due to spreading of adjacent infection in bone or as part of septicaemia. In addition to the constitutional signs there will be swelling and pain with local heat in the joint with marked muscle spasm. In addition to giving the appropriate antibiotic, the treatment is immobilisation and aspiration of the joint.

If the condition does not improve with simple aspiration, open drainage is indicated. Following drainage of the joint it is usual to leave the capsule open but to suture the skin. Further aspiration and injection of antibiotics locally is often required. As already mentioned in new-born babies, spread from the upper end of the femur into the hip joint is a common and serious condition. Septic arthritis, as part of the septicaemia for example, secondary to pneumonia or a septic focus elsewhere, presents with similar clinical features and the treatment is the same.

After the acute infection has subsided specific orthopaedic treatment of the deformed and stiff joint, or, in the case of osteomyelitis, a weak bone, may be required.

Hand infections

Penetrating wounds to the hand are common, either from industrial accidents or in the course of domestic work. The most common injury is a penetrating wound of the pulp of the finger which will lead to pain, redness, swelling, loss of function and constitutional disturbance. These are usually treated by rest and the appropriate antibiotic, but if no improvement occurs within twenty-four hours, operation to drain an abscess is usually required.

Tendon sheath infections

These may occur as a result of direct penetration of the tendon sheath, e.g. by a thorn, splinter or other foreign body, or as a spread from a pulp infection. The whole finger is red and swollen, acutely tender and cannot be moved.

The treatment of tendon sheath infections is to drain the pus from the tendon sheath, send the pus for bacteriological examination to determine the organism and its sensitivity, then to immobilize the finger and give the appropriate antibiotics.

Following the tendon sheath infection, adhesions round the tendon and stiffness around the finger may occur, requiring a long course of physiotherapy.

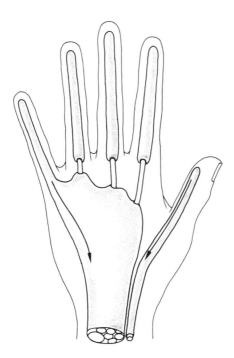

Fig. 13.3   The synovial tendon sheaths in the hand—to illustrate how an infection may track down to deeper tissues.

Deep palm infections (Fig. 13.3)

These may occur either following a tendon sheath infection if the tendon sheath erupts and discharges pus into the deep palmar space, or as the result of a deep penetrating wound. The whole hand is grossly swollen with a severe pain and constitutional disturbance.

The treatment is to drain the deep palmar space usually by a dorsal incision, apply the appropriate splint to the hand, and give the appropriate antibiotic. As in all infections, bacteriological examination of the pus and determination of antibiotic sensitivity is important.

Paronychia

Infections around the nail are fairly common, both due to penetrating wounds or superimposed on a chronic fungus infection. It is most important to diagnose the responsible organism and its antibiotic sensitivity but if the infection is fairly advanced it may be necessary to perform an operation, either lifting the skin round the base of the nail or, in extreme cases, removing the whole nail.

The principles of the nursing of patients with acute infections of bones and joints

The patient admitted with acute osteomyelitis or septic arthritis is often a bewildered, frightened young child with equally confused and worried parents. The onset may not have been sudden but the seriousness of the symptoms and signs often require emergency admission to hospital.

The condition may not be easy to diagnose. The history is often confused by a story of recent trauma; for example, reports such as 'fell in the playground', or, 'kicked by a brother or sister', may create difficulties in diagnosis; the pain may have originally been caused by a blow, but the general signs and symptoms of infection with fever and toxaemia usually clinch matters. A blow on a limb may, however, predispose the osteomyelitis. When a haematoma forms, stasis of the blood at that point may result in forming an ideal culture medium for any circulating pathogenic organisms.

On admission it is essential to warn the parents that an operation may be necessary and to gain their written authority for an anaesthetic and surgical intervention. The doctor must see the parents so as to help them to understand what is happening. The pain, fever and bewilderment of a child is hard to tolerate and sympathetic management of the parents is needed.

The patient is admitted to bed with a firm mattress and immobilization of the affected part is necessary. The form of the fixation depends upon the site of the lesion and the wishes of the surgeon; it may be simple temporary splintage such as traction, or more permanent immobilization. Examples of this are as follows:

1   *Foot, ankle, lower end of tibia and fibula:*
  (a) Club foot shoe.
  (b) Crab splint.
  (c) Plaster of Paris shell (Fig. 30.1, p. 512).
2   *Shaft and upper end of tibia and fibula, knee and femur:*
  (a) Thomas' splint.
  (b) Plaster cylinder with window at site of lesion.
  (c) Plaster cylinder converted into a back splint.
  (d) Aluminium gutter splinting.
  (e) Kramer wire splinting.
3   *Upper end of femur and hip:*
  (a) Pugh's traction.
  (b) Double abduction frame and saddle; this is not always satisfactory as it must be specially made for the patient; saddles particularly are not held in stock.
  (c) Double spica with window or bivalved with the anterior half removed. This is probably less satisfactory than:
  (d) A plaster bed with no foot pieces; extensor bows are incorporated instead for traction.
4   *Pelvis and spine:*
  Plaster bed (Chapter 30).
5   *The arm and hand:*
  Plaster shells.

The use of analgesic drugs to relieve the pain of the condition must be related to the diagnosis. Pain is, unfortunately, often the only indication of the seriousness of the condition. Heavy analgesic drugs may relieve the pain to the extent that it may be thought that the condition is improved and necessary definitive treatment may then be witheld. Explicit instructions of the doctor must be sought.

Preparation for operation
Drilling of the bone to release tension and evacuate pus or aspiration of an infected joint capsule will give relief from the pain, confirm the diagnosis and provide a specimen for a sensitivity test to the specific antibiotic needed for treatment. The patient is therefore prepared for operation but the timing of the operation, from the point of view of the operating theatre organization, may be difficult. The operation must be performed as soon as is possible, but

once the patient returns to the ward the operating theatre must be thoroughly cleaned and rendered aseptic before further operations can be performed there.

The patient is prepared as for any operation (Chapter 27, pp. 453, *et seq.*) with special consideration for the patient's pyrexial state.

Post-operative management

After the operation the following factors must be considered:

(a) Continued immobilization of the part until healing has occurred.

(b) Nursing management and observation of a patient with a severe pyrexia.

(c) Administration of:

(i) 'Wide-spectrum' antibiotics or chemotherapy until the micro-organism has been identified and (ii) the specific antibiotic for the micro-organism can be given.

(d) Care of the wound.

(e) Rehabilitation of the patient and the affected limb.

1 *Continued immobilization.* The immobilization of the part must continue but the wound must be visible for inspection and dressing; the splintage must be modified to meet this need. An infected joint must be kept at absolute rest until the acute phase of the infection has subsided and the antibiotic has taken effect.

Once the temperature of the patient has returned to normal and the signs of the infection have passed, radiographic examination of the joint will be made to assess possible damage to the articular surfaces. The surgeon must decide upon the optimum time for removal of splintage and mobilization of the limb. Until then, no movement is permitted without the direct supervision of the surgeon.

2 *Nursing and observation of the pyrexial patient.* Careful recording of the temperature, pulse and respiration is necessary to indicate the progress of the patient. Another indication of progress may be the erythrocyte sedimentation rate, and of course, return of appetite and liveliness are signs of recovery in a child!

A fluid balance chart is highly important in the management of any patient who has an infection; the patient with either osteomyelitis or pyogenic arthritis is no exception. The fluid intake and urinary output of the patient must both be maintained at a high level. The patient must be constantly encouraged to drink small quantities of fluids so that at the end of the day when the balance is estimated, large quantities have been drunk. In addition to replacing the fluid lost in perspiration as a result of the fever, dilution of the toxins from the micro-organisms and their excretion from the body by a large interchange of fluid will increase the rate of improvement in the patient. It will also prevent constipation.

As for any patient who is perspiring greatly, frequent blanket bathing and replacement of clothing will make the patient more comfortable. The mouth and teeth of the patient must also receive extra attention during the pyrexial stage. The diet can only be fluid, or very light.

Analgesic drugs will be ordered and the relief of pain will help the patient to sleep.

3 *Antibiotic therapy.* Occasionally antibiotics are introduced directly into the lesion in either a joint or a bone. This may be done either intermittently, by injecting the solution through a plastic cannula entering the capsule or bone cavity, or continuously, using an intravenous infusion outfit attached to the cannula. The solution used, the duration of the infusion and the rate of introduction will depend upon the wishes of the surgeon and the rate of improvement. In chronic osteomyelitis many surgeons advise irrigation of the cavity with saline before injecting antibiotics.

Antibiotics will also be given systematically by either the oral or parenteral route. The antibiotics must be recorded on the treatment chart of the patient.

In osteomyelitis, chemotherapy is usually necessary for six weeks if recurrence is to be avoided.

4 *Care of the wound.* (i) Drainage. The wound of the patient with acute osteomyelitis will often require to be drained. The form of drain will depend upon the consistency of the material found. Either corrugated rubber or a short length of rubber tubing may be used. A thick layer of surgical wool will be required over the dressing during the first days after the drilling operation. If serum is the only product found on drilling, drainage through a fine polythene tube connected to a drainage bottle with a negative vacuum pressure may be the method of choice to prevent haematoma formation. In either case the surgeon will give instructions about the length of time the drain should remain *in situ*.

(ii) Cosmetic effect. The appearance of the healed wound is important to the patient. An unsightly scar on the thigh or leg of a patient—particularly if a girl—can seriously affect her future career and leisure pursuits. The surgeon will take this into consideration but it is often difficult to avoid creating a prominent scar when wound drainage is necessary. Plastic surgery may be necessary later.

5 *Rehabilitation.* Once the pyrexial stage has passed, physiotherapy on the affected limb may commence. In the case of infective arthritis, movement must be restricted to muscle contraction only in the affected limb during the stage when the tissues are healing. A joint with soft, inflamed or healing tissues must not be moved except under the direct supervision of the surgeon in charge. The splintage must be left in position until clinical, serological and radiological signs indicate that movement is advisable.

In the management of a patient with osteomyelitis, however, when the joint is not infected, the physiotherapist will work to prevent the adjacent joints from becoming stiff as soon as the acute phase has passed.

The nursing management of suction irrigation systems

This is a system which is used in the presence of deep wound infection; for example infection of arthroplasty and implant surgery. It is also of value in some cases of chronic osteomyelitis.

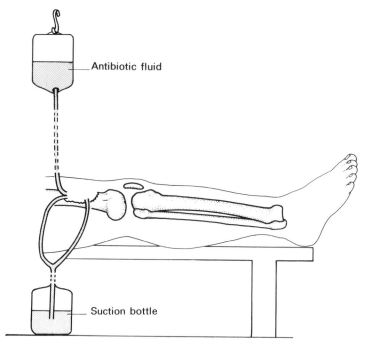

Fig. 13.4 Irrigation-drainage for chronic infection. The rate of suction must at least equal the rate of flow of the irrigation fluid.

Apparatus. Fluid is irrigated into the infected tissues, via suspended bottles and polythene tubing and is removed from the infected area by electrically driven suction apparatus via alternative polythene tubing.

The skin adjacent to the infected tissues is penetrated by four tubes, two entering and two leaving. These are 6·4 mm in diameter and multiperforated.

Suction is applied, at 90 to 120 mm of mercury, to the efferent tubes.

The Solution. This consists of a sterile detergent antibiotic solution. For example:
20% Alevaire
80% Normal saline
plus the antibiotic of choice.
(Alevaire is a wetting agent which is also mucolytic.)

The Antibiotic. The antibiotic used is related to the sensitivity tests. For example:
Cloxacillin ⎫
plus   ⎬ 1 gram to the litre
Ampicillin ⎭
may be used supplemented by parenteral antibiotics.

Nursing. Special nursing management is required. The maintenance of the regime is essential if the infection is to be overcome and the operative procedure saved.

The patient will be returned to the nursing unit, after the operation, with a bulky dressing over the wound. Balanced traction may be used to support the limb.

The dressing is replaced whenever it becomes wet. If a tube becomes clogged patency can be restored by moving it slightly.

Cultures are taken from the outflow tubes every 48–72 hours. (Cultures are usually negative by the third to the sixth day.)

A Typical Irrigation Regime.
1   Six litres of solution per day for the first two days.
2   Three litres per day, after the first two days, until further instructions from the surgeon.
3   If the clinical course is satisfactory the solution is changed to normal saline 12–14 days after operation.
4   After 48 hours three separate cultures are taken from the outflow tubes

at twelve-hourly intervals. If satisfactory the two input tubes are removed and the wounds closed by suturing. One day later the two suction catheters are removed.

General Nursing Care. Additionally the full regime of nursing care for any patient with a severe infection must be given. This includes careful charting of the temperature, pulse and respiration and an increased fluid intake by the patient which is recorded on a fluid balance chart.

14

Chronic Joint Diseases

Relevant anatomy and physiology

Healthy synovial joints move easily and freely; articular surfaces are smooth and the coefficient of friction is very low (approximately that of a skate on ice); the position of the joint and speed of movement are the only sensations noted by the central nervous system as normally there is no pain on movement. Engineers have put much thought into the design of efficient movable joints in machinery; few man-made joints can serve for the same span of trouble-free time as most human joints do and none have such a low coefficient of friction.

The animal synovial joint is efficient because it has built in features which are expensive and hard to produce in the manufactured product. These are:

1 *Completely congruous surfaces* at points of movement. The bony surfaces at the ends of bones are covered with a layer of hyaline cartilage; this is shiny, smooth, slippery and slightly elastic. In all joint movement, therefore, two glossy surfaces are in direct contact.

2 *Lubrication by synovial fluid.* The synovial membrane which lines the joint capsule is secretory. It constantly produces a fluid which serves to coat all the moving surfaces of the joint. Additionally, any structure within the joint not covered by hyaline cartilage is covered by synovial membrane and is therefore moist and slippery.

As the efficiency of any joint depends upon these features, it follows that any irregularity of the surfaces or interference with their lubrication will reduce the function of the joint. Lesions of the joint, such as those caused by inflammation or trauma, will damage either the moving surfaces of the joint which may then become roughened, or interfere with the lubrication of these surfaces either by under-secretion of synovial fluid or alteration in its physico-chemical properties. Deformity of adjacent bones may also affect the function of a joint.

The blood supply to joints

The joints, like all other tissues, require an adequate blood supply. This is supplied by adjacent main arteries and veins. The blood vessels normally form a network, or anastomosis, which surrounds the joint. These blood vessels enter the capsule and supply structures within the joint, they also provide a number of nutrient arteries which supply the ends of the bones which constitute the joint; an examination of disarticulated bones will reveal the presence of a number of small holes penetrating the joint near the articular margin; these are nutrient foraminae. Haematogenous or blood-borne infection may enter the joint and adjacent bone through these blood vessels.

The nerve supply to joints

Every joint is supplied by nerves which have two main functions:

1 *Efferent*. These control the blood supply of the synovial membrane and also the secretion of synovial fluid.

2 *Afferent*. These carry impulses which produce sensations of pain, position and movement. They also carry afferent impulses which initiate reflex contraction of the appropriate muscles without necessarily producing conscious awareness.

It follows that impairment of the nerve supply to the joint may affect the joint in two ways; (1) Reduction of the secretion of synovial fluid and (2) blocking of the 'reporting back' mechanisms so that the patient is unaware of pain producing a joint lesion and muscular control is deranged. This can lead to disorganization of the joint; such a joint is called a *neuropathic* joint.

The movement of synovial joints

The synovial joint cannot initiate movement on its own; it is made to function by the muscles which are arranged in the optimum position to be able to move the joint in a particular direction. The efficient function of muscles is dependent on their being exercised; therefore, if movement is reduced or lost, the muscles have little or no work to perform and as a result become thin, wasted and atrophic.

These same muscles, however, serve as a natural form of splintage if a lesion affects the joint; when the joint is deranged (e.g. inflamed or injured) the surrounding muscles contract, i.e. they go into spasm, a feature known as *muscle guarding*.

Tuberculosis

In the past the most common chronic joint disease was tuberculosis and this is still a common condition in many countries. Tuberculosis of joints is always secondary to a focus elsewhere in the body—in the lungs, cervical or mediastinal. The clinical features are insidious—loss of weight and general malaise with gradual development of pain, muscle spasm, restricted movement and deformity in the affected joint. The classical joint symptom is night pain.

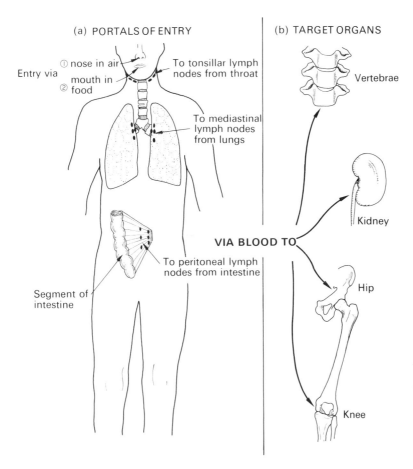

Fig. 14.1   The spread of tuberculosis in the body.

On examining the joint there is marked wasting of the adjacent muscles; marked limitation of movement and ultimately the development of a fixed deformity. It is important that this condition be diagnosed at an early stage. If tuberculosis of a joint is suspected in addition to clinical examination and radiological examination of the joint, it is important to take a radiograph of the lungs, to determine the erythrocyte sedimentation rate and to perform a Mantoux test. If the diagnosis is still in doubt, direct biopsy of the synovial membrane of the joint is usually wise.

Treatment in the first place is by resting the joint. Streptomycin, isonicotinic hydrazid (I.N.A.H.) and paraminosalicylic acid (P.A.S.) will be ordered. In the early stages, apart from the diagnostic measures, operation plays a relatively small part, but if there is chronic thickening of the synovial membrane this should be excised. If there is extensive destruction of bone and joint cartilage it may be necessary to perform an arthrodesis of the joint or, if the joint has assumed a position of fixed deformity, a corrective osteotomy may be required (see Chapter 6).

Nursing management of the patient with tuberculous infection of the skeletal system

General principles

Antibiotics and chemotherapy have completely altered the pattern of infectious disease. This is probably most obvious in the treatment of tuberculous infections. These drugs have reduced a problem that was once the scourge of mankind to reasonable proportions today. Only in countries where poverty abounds and there are inadequate public health and preventive medicine services is tuberculosis a major disease which has not been controlled.

Prophylactic inoculation with B.C.G. is widely practised in most countries nowadays. This, together with improved hygiene, better nutrition and the use of chemotherapy have much reduced the incidence of T.B. Nevertheless some patients still contract the disease.

Although streptomycin, I.N.A.H. and P.A.S. have altered the treatment of tuberculosis, certain principles in the care of tuberculous patients are still relevant and must be observed.

(a) *Prevention of spread*

1 *Pulmonary.* Although the patient with a skeletal infection has most probably gained his infection via the alimentary tract in food, the possibility of a lung focus must not be ruled out. For the protection of the nursing staff, other patients and the patient's relatives, all patients with tuberculous joints must be investigated for a possible pulminary lesion by clinical examination and radiography. If the patient has a cough, the sputum must be sent for

pathological examination. If such an infection is discovered the patient must be isolated and full precautions against droplet cross-infection taken.

   2   *Skeletal.* The cause of the spread of tuberculosis from any lesion of bone and joint is through the pus from the lesion. Dressings, exudate from sinuses or abscesses, or the debris obtained from the site at operation must be treated with the same care as any infected dressings in a well-organized hospital.

   3   *Staff.* Hospital staff must be protected. If their Mantoux reaction is negative, they should be given B.C.G. vaccination (Bacille Calmette Guerin).

(b) *Adequate sunlight, fresh air and ventilation.* Before the introduction of specific anti-tuberculous drugs the only treatment available was empirical; e.g. exposure to ultra-violet light by either natural or artificial sunlight, complete rest and a generous dietary regime. Although the need for such a regime has been reduced, the principles which underly it are still applicable and such patients should ideally still be nursed in such conditions.

(c) *A high protein diet.* The tuberculous patient may have suffered loss of appetite (anorexia) for some months before the condition was diagnosed; alternatively, he may have come from an environment where there was insufficient food. Good nutrition must be part of the regime and a diet with extra protein in the form of meat, fish and dairy produce is essential. With a poor appetite, encouragement to eat by the provision of frequent small and attractive meals may be necessary. Tuberculin tested milk is an important item in the diet.

(d) *Complete rest*
   1   *General.* The patient is given a regime of disciplined rest, particularly during the early acute stages of the infection. This must not be accompanied by extreme boredom, however, and the provision of diversional therapy is important. When it is noted that the anti-tuberculin drugs are effective and the patient's condition is improving, the rest regime need not be so restrictive.

   2   *Local.* The site of the lesion, particularly when it is a joint, must be put completely at rest until radiological and clinical examination shows that movement can be permitted. This means the skilful use of the correct splintage for the part. If the progress of the infection is arrested in time and splintage is correctly applied and used, the prognosis for the restoration of joint function is good.

(e) *Drug therapy.* The essential part of the anti-tubercular regime is the administration of drugs:

1 *Analgesics and sedatives.* If the patient has suffered prolonged un-relieved pain the use of suitable drugs to relieve the pain will improve his morale. Additionally, fear of nights disturbed by spasm and night-cries will be allayed.

2 *Streptomycin.* This is an antibiotic which can destroy the micro-organism of tuberculosis; it is given intramuscularly. The usual dose is one gram daily for adults. It has the possible side-effect of impairment of the function of the cranial nerves, resulting in deafness and dizziness, particu-cularly in elderly people if given over a prolonged period.

Some tubercular lesions have little or no blood supply entering them and the quantity of the drug reaching the micro-organisms may be inadequate. In such cases the orthopaedic surgeon may operate on the lesion to remove the avascular tissue and thus permit an increased entry of streptomycin via the new blood supply which ensues.

3 *Para-amino-salicylic acid (P.A.S.).* When streptomycin is given alone the micro-organisms soon develop a resistance to it. The administration of P.A.S. with it retards this effect. The usual dose for an adult is 15 g daily; it is given orally in cachets.

4 *Iso-nicotinic-acid-hydrazide (I.N.A.H.).* This drug is also active in destroying the micro-organism of tuberculosis but it is not so effective as streptomycin. Used in combination with streptomycin and P.A.S. it serves to provide a complete answer in the therapeutic management of tuberculosis. It is usually given as a daily 200 mg dose in the adult.

5 *Ethambutol and Rifampicin* are two relatively new drugs which are often used, particularly where there is evidence of the bacteria being resistant to streptomycin or I.N.A.H. These drugs are, however, potentially toxic and liver tests should be performed at intervals during treatment.

The dosage of all anti-tubercular drugs is, of course, reduced for child patients; the dose for a child is related to his age and body weight.

The main feature in the administration of these drugs is that they are maintained at a constant level in the body during the whole period of treat-ment. They must not be withheld or the micro-organisms may develop a resistance to them. They are usually given in the first instance for a period of six months; P.A.S. and I.N.A.H. may be continued beyond this time. In resistant or chronic infection the course of treatment with streptomycin may be repeated after an interval.

6 *Vitamins.* If the diet is adequate in fresh foods, particularly dairy pro-duce, green salads and fish of an oily nature, the vitamin intake of the patient will be sufficient. If there is any doubt about the vitamin content of the diet,

however, it must be augmented by the administration of synthetic vitamins, particularly A and D which are fat soluble.

These are the usual drugs which are administered to tuberculous patients; others are required to meet particular needs; for instance, iron for anaemia (in severe anaemia, blood transfusion will be required).

(f) *Fluid intake.* As a part of the therapeutic regime of the patient the fluid intake must be much higher than in normal circumstances. Extra fluid is essential when antibiotic and chemotherapeutic drugs are given so as to assist the excretion of the drugs and diminish the risk of their producing toxic effects. Another reason is to increase the interchange of fluids in discarding the toxins from infection and yet another is to prevent stasis and crystal deposition in the tubules of the kidney. If this occurs it may lead to stone formation.

Relevant nursing management in tuberculosis of the hip joint
This is a relatively common site for a tuberculous lesion. It may affect either the synovial membrane or the bone ends. At first the patient complains of a limp and pain in the hip; there is often pain referred to the inner side of the knee, as the obturator nerve supplies both the hip joint and the inner side of the knee. The patient walks with an abduction gait at first but as muscle spasm occurs the hip is then held in flexion and adduction, which gives the appearance of shortening of the limb.

Treatment. General—As already described in this chapter.
  Local—Aspiration of the joint cavity will be performed. This serves to provide material for culture and pathological examination. Splintage is also applied; this may be:

1 A Jones double abduction frame.
2 A plaster bed with extension bows.
3 A Hip spica, single or double.
  The hip is splinted and immobilised until healing occurs and the surgeon decides that movement is possible after radiological examination.
  Open operation and biopsy of the synovial membrane may be required to establish the diagnosis.

Relevant nursing management for patients with a tuberculous lesion of the knee
This is usually diagnosed early as swelling of the knee joint is easily seen.

The knee is often swollen but relatively painless; there is limitation of the range of movement. The patient holds the knee flexed and does not apply his weight to the leg.

It must be distinguished from other causes of chronic synovitis, e.g. rheumatoid arthritis, villous synovitis and synovial chondrominkosis.

Treatment. General—As already described in this chapter.

Local—(a) *For a synovial lesion*: Intra-articular injection of streptomycin and rest to the knee without rigid fixation; (b) *For a bony lesion*: Fixation of the leg in a Thomas bed-knee splint or a plaster of Paris hip spica.

For a bony lesion when the hyaline cartilage and articular bone have been eroded, full recovery of movement is unlikely. Surgical treatment is then usually necessary to fix (arthrodese) the joint in a good functional position.

Tuberculous lesions of other joints
This follows similar lines to those described for the hip joint and knee joint.

The complications of tuberculosis of the skeletal system
1 *Cold abscess formation.* This is a painless collection of pus and debris which may be present at the site of the lesion or may track to appear some distance from it, e.g. from the spine a tuberculous abscess may form in the psoas sheath and 'point' in the groin.

2 *Sinus formation.* If any abscess, tubercular or otherwise, is not surgically aspirated, the phagocytes of the blood will create their own pathway or channel to the surface of the body.

3 *Pott's paraplegia.* Tuberculosis of the vertebral column may result in the formation of an abscess which impinges upon the neural canal and compresses and constricts the spinal cord. This interrupts the nerve supply to the lower parts of the body, causing paralysis.

If a patient with Pott's paraplegia does not improve fairly quickly with rest and chemotherapy, operative decompression is usually needed.

The tuberculosis focus—pus, granulation tissue and necrotic material—which is pressing on the cord is removed either by an extra pleural route (anterolateral decompression) or transpleurally. After removal of affected tissue the spine may need stabilization by a bone graft.

4 *Amyloid disease.* The presence of a chronic tubercular lesion can result in deposits of wax-like materials in the visceral organs of the body. It is associated with deficiency of vitamins and proteins in the diet. It is rarely seen nowadays in countries where the tubercular problem has been overcome.

Amyloid disease primarily affects the kidneys, liver, intestines and (rarely) the peripheral nerves.

The main complications of skeletal tubercular lesions are deformities occurring at joints, in bone and in the spine. If the infection is diagnosed early enough and the treatment is adequate, deformities or shortening of limbs will be rare.

Rheumatoid arthritis

Rheumatoid arthritis is a disease of unknown aetiology characterized by the involvement of many joints which become painful and swollen. In addition there is a considerable constitutional disturbance. The patient feels unwell, is anaemic, has a raised erythrocyte sedimentation rate, and other organs such as the heart, lungs and kidneys may also be affected. The patient may also have chronic tenosynovitis and develop subcutaneous rheumatic nodules.

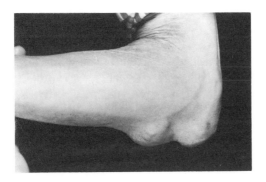

Fig. 14.2 Elbow of rheumatoid arthritis patient. Note rheumatic nodule.

In the classical syndrome the diagnosis is relatively easy but sometimes rheumatoid arthritis remains confined to one joint, even for a considerable period, and in that case the differentiation from chronic tuberculous arthritis is difficult. In addition to general care and pain relieving measures, rest of the joint in the acute stage is most important. If extensive synovial swelling persists, excision of the synovial membrane is usually advisable. If there is destruction of the joint it may be necessary either to perform some type of arthroplasty or occasionally to arthrodese the weak and painful joint.

A rather similar type of arthritis occurs in association with psoriasis. The treatment is on similar lines.

Relevant nursing management of patients
with rheumatoid arthritis

Patients have different manifestations of rheumatoid arthritis so that the nursing care and treatment of each patient varies. Some have only mild lesions affecting only a few joints, without much obvious deformity; others are very ill with gross deformities of most of the joints of the body.

This is also a condition which is the subject of much research at the present time. Although treatment is still largely empirical, progress in research and pharmacology may bring forth specific measures in the foreseeable future.

The present empirical approach to treatment has the following aims:

1 To retard or arrest the progression of the disease.

2 As the result of item (1) to prevent the joint deformity which is severely crippling and reduces the functional capacity of the patient.

3 To improve any deformity which has occurred and so increase the abilities of the patient.

4 To relieve the pain of the disease.

The cause is unknown but it is probably a multifactorial disease with heredity, virus and other infections, plus auto-immunity all playing their part.

Drug therapy

Salicylates. Aspirin is effective in relieving pain and in allaying inflammation in the joints. As much as four grams per day may need to be given in order to be effective and such a large dose can result in the following side-effects on the patient:

1 Slow bleeding from the gastric mucosa.

2 Haematemesis and malaena.

3 Iron deficiency anaemia.

4 Nausea, vomiting and dyspepsia.

5 Tinnitus aureus (ringing in the ears).

6 Deafness.

7 Dizziness and vertigo.

8 Asthma or urticaria in allergic patients.

Prolonged dosage may also result in damage to the tubules of the kidneys.

Selection of the type of aspirin to be given is important. Soluble calcium aspirin is preferred to the insoluble; enteric coated tablets pass through the stomach before dissolving in the small intestine; a long-acting tablet will reduce the number of tablets and times to be given; an advantage for night therapy to permit the patient to sleep.

Paracetamol. This is a safe and valuable analgesic as it does not cause any of the side-effects of aspirin and phenacetin when given in large amounts for a long time.

Phenylbutazone. This is an analgesic drug given with excellent anti-inflammatory results. It is often effective when aspirin cannot be tolerated by the patient or has no value in relieving pain. As the drug has serious side-effects it is usual to give a prolonged and careful trial of aspirin before prescribing phenylbutazone for patients with rheumatoid arthritis. These side-effects include:

1 Serious gastric disturbance including nausea and peptic ulceration.
2 Dermatitis.
3 Urticaria.
4 Oedema due to fluid retention.
5 Destruction of phagocytes in the blood stream with severe loss of resistance to infection (agranulocytosis).

Indomethacin. This is another anti-inflammatory drug which is used in the treatment of rheumatoid arthritis and osteoarthritis. It is a relatively new and potent analgesic. It may cause side-effects in some patients and these are avoided by giving small doses of the drug (25 mg 3 times daily, for example). The side-effects may be:

1 Gastric distress.
2 Urticaria.
3 Headache and vertigo.
4 Anxiety, restlessness and confusion.

Other 'anti-inflammatory drugs' are brufen and tanderil, it is often difficult to predict which drug will relieve a given patient with the minimum of side-effects. Penicillinase is also used to control the symptoms in otherwise intractable patients.

Gold salts. This method of treating patients with rheumatoid arthritis has been in use for many years but it is only recently that the drug has been proven to give definite improvement to some patients. Test doses are given initially and the drug is not given as a therapeutic regime until the other drugs have all been tried. It is only of value in the treatment of an active disease.

It has serious side-effects and the doctor will usually explain these to the patient before prescribing the drug: the side-effects are:

1 A severe exfoliative dermatitis preceded by itching.
2 Agranulocytosis due to damage to the bone marrow.
3 Hepatic damage causing jaundice.
4 Damage to the kidney tubules.

Patients on gold salts must have regular urine tests for the presence of albumen in the urine.

Chloroquine. This is a drug normally used for the treatment of malaria and amoebic inflammation of the liver, but it is occasionally found to be useful in the acute phase of rheumatoid arthritis.

It has the serious side-effect of damaging the retina of the eye and possible blindness if taken over a long period. There is a constant need for re-assessment of the drug regime of the patient. All drugs have potential toxic dangers however.

Corticosteroid drugs

Used pharmacologically the corticosteroid drugs modify or completely suppress the inflammatory reaction of the body so that there is little or no response to disease. These drugs will therefore *inhibit the signs* of activity of rheumatoid arthritis; they do not cure the disease.

If it is at all possible these drugs are *not* given to rheumatoid arthritic patients. The exceptional circumstances when they will be prescribed by the doctor are:

(a) As a 'last resort' treatment for the patient who is deteriorating.

(b) When the patient is severely disabled and an attempt is made to regain some independence.

(c) To restore wage earning capacity in special circumstances.

The possible side effects of these drugs are profound:

1 Excessive obesity.
2 Rashes on the skin, particularly on the face.
3 Hypertension.
4 Diabetes mellitus.
5 Lowered resistance to infection.
6 Peptic ulcers.
7 Osteoporosis of bone.
8 Mental changes.
9 Increased vulnerability to stress and trauma.

Some nursing observations of patients who commence treatment with corticosteroid drugs

1 Daily urine testing for glucose.
2 Daily blood pressure recording.
3 Weekly weight recording.
4 Temperature, pulse and respiration recording.

Additionally, careful visual observation of the patient is essential. Any change in the patient—no matter how slight—must be reported. Such signs as loss of appetite, increased pallor or other colour change, anxiety or loss of interest may be significant.

Patients on corticosteroid drugs who are to undergo a surgical operation will require increased dosage for the duration of the 'surgical phase' so as to avoid a sudden, severe (possibly fatal) reduction in blood pressure during or after the operation.

Rest

(a) *General.* A balance between rest and exercise must be achieved; too much of either is bad for the patient. If he rests for too great a part of his days, his joints become increasingly stiff, osteoporosis of bones and wasting of muscles occurs. However, some of his time of each day must be used as complete rest periods.

(b) *Local.* The inflamed joints must be rested and supported, particularly when the patient is at rest or asleep. Night splints made of plaster of Paris shells, plastazote or other plastic materials are made to fit each of the inflamed joints. These are applied and removed as necessary and may be easily replaced by new ones if the shape or range of movement should alter. The joints must always be handled gently and with extreme care.

Physiotherapy

The physiotherapist has an important role to play in the management of rheumatoid arthritis patients. From the onset of the disease through to rehabilitation it is necessary to maintain the widest range of movements possible in all the affected joints. This means that when the joints are inflamed and painful to move, short wave diathermy and hot packs are used to give relief from pain; this may enable the physiotherapist to move the joints of the patient and thus maintain function and prevent stiffness in the joint. As the disease becomes quiescent the movements become more active. Hydrotherapy, wax baths and faradic baths all have their uses.

Surgical treatment

The main approach to the treatment of the rheumatoid patient is by the use of a regime of drug therapy. Surgical help is used as follows:

1 Synovectomy of joints to retard the activity of the disease in a particular joint.

2 Repair of ruptured tendons.

3 Arthroplasty—replacement of stiff and painful joints by metal or plastic prosthetic devices.

4 Correction of deformity in joints and bones.

5 Arthrodesis—complete removal of a joint and the fusion of the bones involved in the joint.

6 Removal of thickened tendon sheaths.

7 Amputation of grossly deformed and useless, painful toes.

Psychological approach

The patient must be helped to adjust to his condition and made to feel involved in the management of the disease. He must know what is to be achieved and how. This means that an accurate statement of his prognosis is necessary and how, by his co-operation, he can improve his prospects.

The ideal arrangement for the management of the patient is in a rheumatoid arthritis unit staffed by a team who are experienced in creating the right atmosphere of cautious optimism.

The medical social worker is a necessary member of the team; she can do much to relieve the mental stress of the patient who is troubled by financial, family or other worries.

Rehabilitation

Dependency is the most severe problem for any patient. The patient with severe rheumatoid arthritis is more likely to be dependent on others if the condition progresses to involve many joints, causing them to be fixed and useless. Even matters such as transferring food from plate to mouth can become a serious problem, requiring extreme thought and effort. Toilet, the use of the lavatory and dressing may all become problems requiring complete assistance from relatives or attendants after discharge from hospital unless efforts are made to teach him how to live with his disability.

The occupational therapist has the important task of training the disabled patient to manage the activities of daily living, using devices and gadgets which will reduce the dependency of the patient on others. A comprehensive catalogue of such devices is maintained by the National Fund for Research into Crippling Diseases.

General health of patients

The standard of general health of the patient must be maintained. In the light of disabilities it is essential to see that the patient has a good diet, is free of treatable infections, has a high standard of personal hygiene, has no constipation or other bowel problems. He also requires interests and occupations so as to avoid boredom. When in hospital these problems are solved in the day to day management of the patient by the nursing and medical staff. After discharge it is essential that such supervision as is necessary is maintained by the patient's doctor and the visiting nurse.

Osteoarthritis

Osteoarthritis is the name given to conditions in which the articular cartilage becomes thinned and the adjacent bone develops outgrowths known as osteophytes. In addition there may be some thickening of the synovial membrane and an effusion into the joint may occur.

Primary osteoarthritis occurs in joints which were previously normal and usually several joints are affected. This condition may present in a fairly acute form and there may be repeated periods of pain and swelling, and periods of relative freedom from pain.

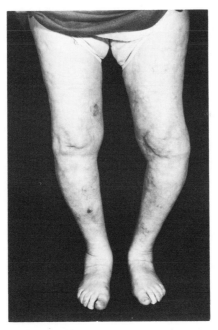

Fig. 14.3   Osteoarthritis of knee with genu varum. Note varicosed veins, which are often present in patients with osteoarthritis.

In the past it has often been confused with rheumatoid arthritis but it is important to make the differentiation as both prognosis and treatment are entirely different.

Secondary osteoarthritis has a similar clinical and pathological picture except that it is usually confined to one joint which is the site of previous disease. For example, in the hip conditions such as Perthes' disease, slipping upper femoral epiphysis, previous infection, trauma, congenital subluxation and congenital dislocation, are all likely to lead to secondary arthritis.

In the earlier stages osteoarthritis is best treated by weight reduction, mild analgesic drugs and physiotherapy. In the more established cases it may be necessary to perform an operation. Three main types of operation have been employed:

1   Arthrodesis (Fig. 14.4).
2   Replacement arthroplasty (see Fig. 19.21b).
3   Osteotomy (see Fig. 19.22).

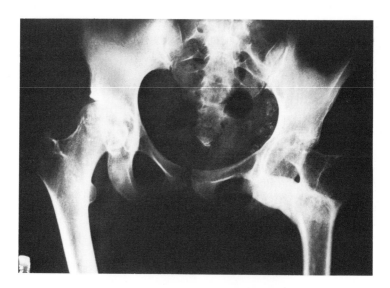

Fig. 14.4   Ischio-femoral arthrodesis of hip.

For an unknown reason, division of the bone adjacent to an osteoarthritic joint (osteotomy) relieves the symptoms and appears to favour repair of articular cartilage. In addition, if there has been fixed deformity of the joint —e.g. adduction deformity, or a fixed deformity of the knee joint, osteotomy will improve the mechanical stability of the joint and on these grounds alone it is a help.

Relevant nursing management for patients with osteoarthritis
Weight reduction. Often the initial treatment of a patient with osteoarthritis of either the hip or knee is to reduce the obesity of the patient; when the affected joints must bear excessive weight and possibly out of the normal alignment of the joint, with excessive pressure on a localized articular area, improvement is less likely to occur. It is futile to send the patient away with instructions to 'lose weight', without positive help in achieving this aim. Such patients are often 'compulsive eaters' who have long been aware of their excess fat but unable to apply the discipline to lose it. Medical supervision of an effective diet is needed with a diet sheet showing the patient that which can be eaten and which must be avoided (see Chapter 27). The patient must be weighed at each visit to the clinic and his current weight charted on a graph which he can see; this shows progress or otherwise and is an incentive to the patient to reduce weight.

Drug regime. The drugs used in the treatment of osteoarthritis are similar to those used in the treatment of rheumatoid arthritis and these are discussed in this chapter on pp. 223, 224, 225.

Physiotherapy. This is also similar to that for rheumatoid arthritis and this is discussed in this chapter on p. 225.

Osteoarthritis of the hip
See Chapter 19, p. 332.

Osteoarthritis of the knee
See Chapter 22, p. 376.

Gout

This is a disorder of purine metabolism of familial origin but an acute attack is usually precipitated by over-indulgence in food or drink, or physical or mental shock. It is characterized by a raised blood uric acid and the deposition of urate crystals, especially sodium biurate, near or in joints causing acute inflammatory changes. Repeated attacks lead to chronic synovitis and degeneration of the articular cartilage. The treatment is medical but inflamed irritable joints may need splinting for relief of pain in the acute phase.

Pseudo-Gout

In this condition, crystals of calcium pyrophosphate are deposited in the joint (usually they knee). The diagnosis is made by aspirating the joint and detecting the crystals with polarized light.

Connective tissue disorders

There are a number of congenital hereditary disorders of connective tissue characterized by joint laxity which ultimately lead to degenerative changes. In Marfans syndrome there are also scoliosis, dislocation of the lenses of the eyes and weakness of the wall of the aorta.

Villous synovitis

This is a condition in which there is thickening, reddening and hyper-vascularity of the synovial membrane. It is most common in the knee joint but may occur in the hip and ankle. The thickened synovial membrane may ultimately erode the adjacent bone and articular surface. The aetiology is unknown. If the condition does not settle down with rest it is usually wise to perform a subtotal excision of the synovial membrane (synovectomy).

Neuropathic joints

In certain neuropathic disorders, especially tabes dorsalis and syringo-myelia, there is disturbance of the afferent nerve fibres coming from the articular capsule and ligaments. These will lead to a loss of the normal protective reflexes and will ultimately lead to disorganization of the joint. In the early stages the joint will be the site of a chronic effusion and it may be painful.

Later on the pain disappears, the joint becomes a disorganized joint which is relatively painless; in addition there are signs of disease of the spinal cord such as absent reflexes. As far as the joint is concerned the main treatment is to provide some supporting appliance such as a walking caliper; occasionally the affected joint may be fixed (arthrodesed).

15

Chronic Bone Diseases

There are a large number of congenital abnormalities of the bone; some of the more common ones are described here:

1 Achondroplasia

In this condition there is general failure of longitudinal growth of the bones leading to a particular type of dwarf in whom the limbs, and especially the

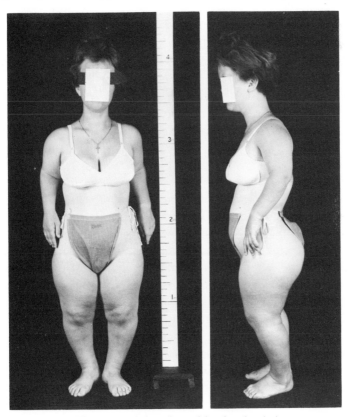

Fig. 15.1 (a) A patient with achondroplasia.

proximal segments of the limbs, are very much shorter than usual. The trunk, though shorter than average, is long in comparison with the limbs. The parietal bones of the skull are of normal size but the base of the skull is small, giving rise to the characteristic appearance as seen in Fig. 15.1.

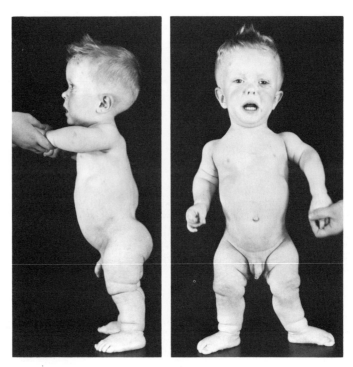

Fig. 15.1 (b) Inherited achondroplasia in an infant.

This condition may be inherited and may also arise as a spontaneous mutation. No specific treatment is known, but occasionally correction of growth deformities—e.g. genu varum, may be required. The patient's mental powers are nearly always normal. Narrowing of the spinal canal may lead to paraplegia. The short arms make management of a wheel chair very difficult.

2 Fragilitis ossium

In this condition the bones are excessively weak and fracture easily. Again, the condition may be inherited or may arise spontaneously as a mutation. Two main varieties are known, with different biochemical abnormalities— the severe form with multiple fractures from an early age and ultimately

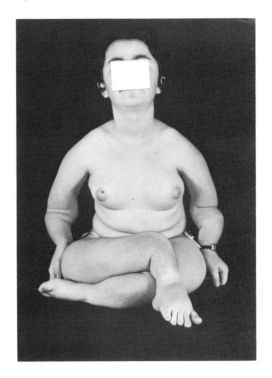

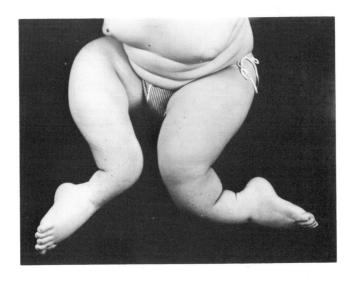

Fig. 15.2 (a) and (b) Patient with fragilitis ossium.

very severe deformities, and the milder type, which is associated with blue sclerotics, here, although fractures occur there are seldom severe deformities and the patient remains ambulant. There are varying degrees of severity—for example, the baby may suffer many intrauterine fractures and will often be stillborn. In addition to the weak bones, the child may have the characteristic blueness of sclerotics and may suffer from deafness during the course of growth. Deformities are likely to occur and in severe examples there will also be marked muscular weakness (Fig. 15.2a, b).

If a child has multiple fractures and deformed bones, the surgeon will perform a corrective osteotomy to correct the bone and will insert an intramedullary pin to hold the bone in the corrected position. When the child reaches puberty the bones will become stronger and the tendency to fracture will become less, though it may recur again in old age. In addition to deformity of the bones there may be deformity of the spine—for example, kyphosis or scoliosis, which require treatment on their merits.

3 Multiple exostoses (Fig. 15.3)

This is a hereditary condition in which osteo-cartilaginous lumps appear at the ends of several long bones. These may be associated with disturbance of growth and deformity of the limbs. Usually this condition is symptomless but occasionally exostoses press on adjacent structures such as nerves or blood vessels, or may interfere with joint movement, or they may become painful.

The exostosis may be fractured by injury, in which case it is painful. In general no special treatment is indicated for this condition, but occasionally operative removal is required due to pain or pressure on important structures. In addition, exostoses of the iliac bones or scapulae may undergo malignant changes.

4 Multiple chondromatosis

A superficially similar condition also occurs in which there are multiple cartilaginous tumours in the limb bones. This is commonly associated with gross disturbance of growth so that a typical case may have one leg several inches shorter than the other. In addition, multiple cartilaginous tumours may occur in both the hand and foot.

Chrondromatous tumours of the pelvis and scapula are liable to become malignant and, if they become painful or start to grow, they should be radically removed. In addition, conditions such as knock knee, bow leg, or spontaneous fractures may occur.

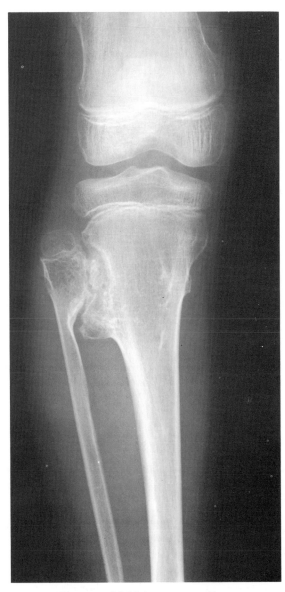

Fig. 15.3   Multiple exostoses of bone.

5 Osteochondrodysplasia

This is a relatively rare condition which is also hereditary, though it may occur as a mutation. It is characterized by enlargement of the ends of the long bones with consequent distortion of the joints, limitation of movement and the development of secondary osteoarthritis. No specific treatment is known, but the painful joints or deformity may require treatment in the usual way.

6 Cleido cranial Dysostosis

This hereditary condition is characterized by absence of the clavicles and failure of union of the symphysis pubis. The disability is slight, no treatment is known or required.

7 Paget's disease

This commonly occurs in the later half of life. It is characterized by pain and increase in volume and vascularity of bone. Degenerative changes often occur in the adjacent joint. It may lead to severe deformity and, in the case of the skull, may lead to interference in sight and hearing. The patient with Paget's disease is especially liable to three other complications:
(a) Spontaneous fracture.
(b) The development of sarcomatous changes.
(c) Hypertension.

Primary tumours of bone

Primary tumours of bone may be simple or malignant. Simple tumours of bone are the exostoses, chondromatoma, fibromatoma, osteoid osteomata, aneurysmal bone cysts and chondro blastomata. The usual surgical treatment is to excise the affected area and pack the resulting space with autogenous bone. Osteoclastoma, also called benign giant cell tumours, are locally agressive and destructive. Although they seldom metastasise they are likely to recur locally after simple curettage. If they do recur they should be treated by radical resection of the affected bone otherwise amputation may be required.

Primary malignant tumours of bone are the osteogenic sarcomata, the fibrosarcomata and the chondrosarcomata. In general, the prognosis in osteogenic sarcoma is extremely grave, especially in children. The normal features are pain and swelling, but secondary deposits in the lungs rapidly occur. The best treatment is still in dispute, but probably the surgeon will advise amputation followed by cytotoxic drugs.

The prognosis in chondrosarcoma is slightly better and here the best treatment is to perform an immediate amputation. Similarly, with fibro-

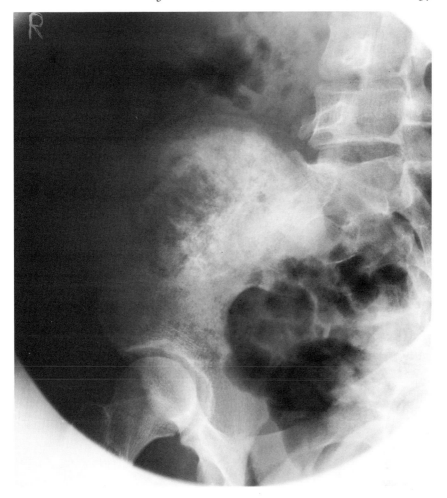

Fig. 15.4   Chondrosarcoma of pelvis.

sarcoma, the prognosis is much better than with osteogenic sarcoma. These can be treated either by radical local excision or by amputation. In general, if the tumour re-occurs after radical local excision, the surgeon will probably decide to amputate.

Secondary tumours of bone from malignant tumours elsewhere in the body are extremely common. They may present either in the form of pain or as a pathological fracture, or, in the case of the vertebrae, pain, collapse of the vertebrae and secondary involvement of the spinal cord may occur. The

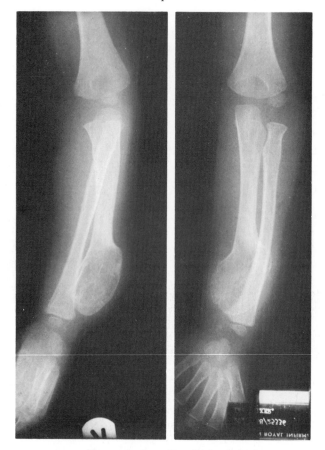

Fig. 15.5   Osteochondrodysplasia.

common primary sites are the breasts, prostate, lungs, thyroid, kidney and the gastro-intestinal tract.

The first two are hormone sensitive and will be treated by the appropriate hormone therapy. In addition, radiotherapy and cytotoxic drugs relieve the pain of secondary deposits in bone tumours.

In the case of actual or threatened pathological fractures of the long bones, intramedullary nail fixation is usually indicated as, even though it may not prolong the patient's life, he will be much more comfortable following such surgery.

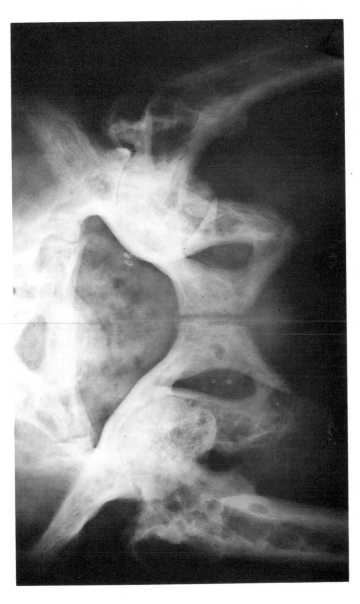

Fig. 15.6 Paget's disease.

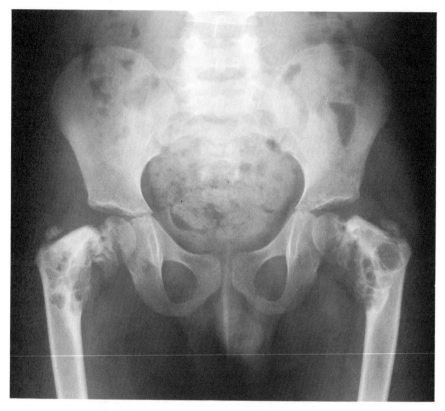

Fig. 15.7   (a) Multiple enchondromata of bone.

Other chronic diseases of bone include osseous manifestations of various blood disorders such as leukaemia, lymphadenoma and the ill-understood tumour known as Ewing's tumour which is often a secondary deposit in bone from the adrenals, though it may also arise from certain cells in the bone marrow. They are all lytic lesions which cause pain and ultimately fracture.

Neurofibromatosis
This is a hereditary condition in which multiple tumours occur on nerve sheaths. These may be deep or superficial, associated with these are areas of brown skin pigmentation and occasional lytic lesions of the tibia leading to spontaneous fracture and pseudarthrosis. Scoliosis is also a common complication, intraspinal neurofibromata may lead to paraplegia. Occasionally one of the tumours may become malignant causing severe pain.

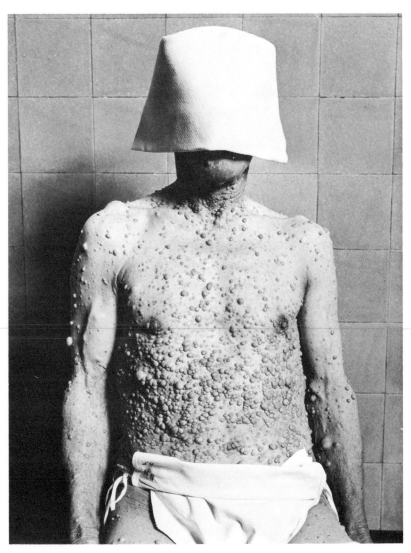

Fig. 15.7   (b) Neurofibromatosis of skin associated with bone lesions.

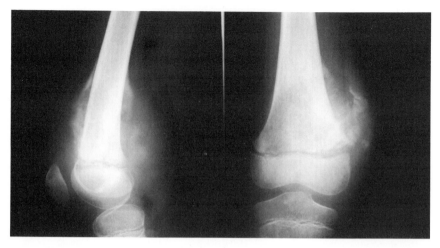

Fig. 15.8 Osteosarcoma of the knee.

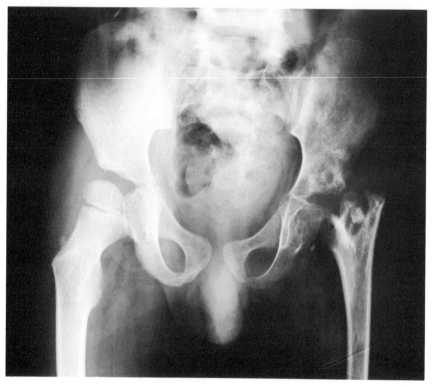

Fig. 15.9 (a) Osteomyelitis of femur, with destruction of femoral head, subluxation of hip and sequestrum formation.

We have already referred elsewhere to chronic diseases of bone—namely, osteoporosis, osteomalacia, chronic osteomyelitis due to specific infections such as syphilis, tuberculosis or yaws, and chronic osteomyelitis secondary to

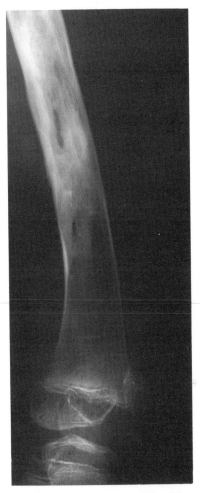

Fig. 15.9   (b) Chronic osteomyelitis of femur.

acute osteomyelitis. One of the complications of acute osteomyelitis is the formation of a chronic abscess known as a Brodie's abscess. This is characterized by pain and swelling of the affected bone, and an abscess cavity surrounded by sclerotic bone can be seen on the X-ray (Fig. 15.9). Treatment is to remove the dense wall of the abscess, remove the contents—e.g. sequestra, and give the patient the appropriate antibiotics.

Chronic bone infections

Chronic bone infections may arise as a sequel to acute osteomyelitis, as a complication of operative interference or as a complication of an open fracture. Once a bone infection has become chronic it is extremely difficult to eradicate it. Even the most penetrating of broad spectrum antibiotics probably do not reach 'buried' organisms at a sufficient concentration. One technique which has proved extremely useful is the continuous installation of an antibacterial solution by an irrigation tube combined with continuous suction to remove debris and excess fluid (see p. 210).

16

Affections of the Brain and Spinal Cord

Relevant applied anatomy and physiology

The control of most activities in the body is by the central nervous system; a general title for the brain and spinal cord. This is composed entirely of delicate nervous tissue and supporting connective tissue and blood vessels; without protection the central nervous system would be vulnerable to injury and it is therefore entirely surrounded by bone in the form of the cranium and vertebral column. Inside the cavity which encloses the central nervous system, i.e. the cranial cavity and neural canal, is a protective membrane called the theca.

The terms *upper motor neurone lesion* and *lower motor neurone lesion* will be used in this chapter. It is now necessary to define these terms.

Upper motor neurones

Refer to Fig. 16.1 as you read this section. The motor neurones in the central nervous system have the main function of transferring the impulses, which arise on the cortex, or surface, of the cerebrum, to other parts of the central nervous system. They form nervous tracts or pathways along which the impulses pass. Thus there are pathways between the cerebrum and cerebellum; others between the cerebellum and mid-brain and medulla oblongata; there are also pathways from the brain stem down the spinal cord and in the reverse direction. Every part of the healthy central nervous system has a communication via such pathways with other parts of the brain and spinal cord; these pathways are normally clear and free of obstruction.

Any pathological condition which impedes the passage of nervous impulses along these pathways between the cortex of the brain and the relevant segment of the spinal cord is known as an *upper motor neurone lesion*.

There are also nerve tracts which convey sensory or afferent impulses from the different levels of the spinal cord to the brain.

Lower motor neurones

Refer to Fig. 16.2 as you read this section (see also Fig. 17.1). As the central nervous system is protected within its bony cavity there must be a connecting

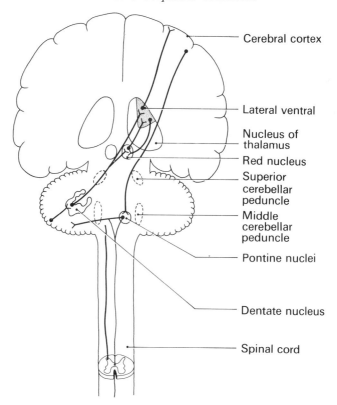

Fig. 16.1 Diagram of the motor pathways of the central nervous system, related to upper motor neurone lesions.

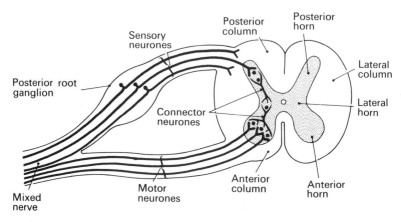

Fig. 16.2 Diagram of the roots of a spinal nerve within the spinal cord, related to lower notor neurone lesions.

nervous tract or pathway between the spinal cord and all of the bodily structures which are external to the theca. This communicating pathway is usually a spinal nerve which may also be called a peripheral nerve (see Chapter 11).

The spinal nerve arises from one side of a segment of the spinal cord by two roots which join before passing out of the neural canal to that part of the body which it supplies. Any pathological condition which damages, breaks or obstructs the nervous pathway from its origin within the spinal cord segment passing out along the spinal nerve to its destination in a peripheral organ (such as muscles or other structures) is referred to as a *lower motor neurone lesion*.

THE EFFECTS OF MOTOR NEURONE LESIONS

Upper motor neurone lesions	*Lower motor neurone lesions*
1 Spastic paralysis of the affected limbs.	1 Flaccid paralysis of the affected limbs.
2 Little or no muscle wasting.	2 Severe wasting of muscles.
3 Exaggerated reflexes.	3 Absence of reflexes.
4 Local temperature and colour changes absent; generalized effects on the skin may be present.	4 Local temperature and colour changes of the skin of the affected part.
5 Babinski's sign positive.	5 Babinski's sign negative.
6 Absent abdominal responses.	

Disorders of the brain and spinal cord

All skeletal muscle is innervated by a peripheral motor nerve arising from anterior horn cell and supplying a number of muscle fibres; the whole is known as the lower motor neurone complex. The exact control of the muscles of the limbs and trunk in standing and moving is a complex procedure based on what is known as the stretch reflex, i.e. the reflex contraction of muscle fibres when the muscle is stretched. The stretch reflex itself is subjected to a complex control by fibres originating in the brain known as upper motor neurone fibres.

Disorders of muscle action and muscle imbalance are divided into two main types—namely, upper motor neurone lesions and lower motor neurone lesions. Muscle imbalance leads to deformed posture, an abnormal gait, abnormal movements and ultimately to fixed deformities.

Lower motor neurone lesions

The causes of lower motor neurone lesions include anterior poliomyelitis and other virus infections, peripheral nerve lesions—traumatic, toxic and infective (e.g. leprosy)—and diseases of the motor end plate and muscle.

It is fairly easy to understand that if, for instance, the muscles which dorsiflex the foot are paralysed, the normally-acting plantar flexors are liable to produce a fixed equinus deformity.

The treatment of lower motor neurone lesions—that is if the lesion itself is untreatable—is to prevent deformity arising by suitable splints and exercises or, if deformity arises, to correct it by lengthening the tendons of contracted muscles and preventing recurrence of the deformity—for example, by tendon transplant (see Chapter 11). For example, if the anterior tibial muscles are paralysed, transferring the tibialis posterior muscle through the interosseous membrane to the dorsum of the foot. In certain circumstances fusion operations to fix or arthrodese flail joints are necessary.

Upper motor neurone lesions

In the case of upper motor neurone lesions the position is considerably more complicated as many different varieties of impairment of upper motor neurone control can occur. For instance, disorders of the spinal cord may, if they affect the posterior roots or columns (as in tabes dorsalis) give rise to loss of reflexes, diminution of muscle tone and disorder of joints known as neuropathic joints (Fig. 16.3). At a slightly higher level interruption of all upper motor neurones as, for example in traumatic paraplegia or certain spinal tumours, will give rise to increased muscle tone of the flexor reflexes, diminution of the extensor reflexes which are inhibited, and the characteristic posture with flexed and adducted hips, flexed knees and equinus deformity of the feet may develop if the condition is not treated.

Other diseases of the spinal cord such as Friedreich's ataxia, disseminated sclerosis, and syringomyelia may give rise to similar disorders.

At a higher level, disorders of the brain stem and cerebellum may give rise to disorders of posture, spontaneous increased rigidity, and spontaneous fine rhythmical tremor as in Parkinson's disease, intentional tremor as in diseases of the cerebellum due either to a tumour or disseminated sclerosis, or spontaneous writhing movements—athetosis.

At a still higher level, lesions of the motor cortex of the cerebellum may give rise to complete loss of voluntary movement or partial weakness and the increased loss of muscle tone. According to the extent of the paralysis, it is classified as:

Monoplegia   One limb.

Hemiplegia The arm and leg on the same side.
Paraplegia Both legs
Tetraplegia All four limbs.

According to the exact situation of the lesion the limbs may be spastic, ataxic or hypertonic, or there may be spontaneous movements, e.g. athetoid

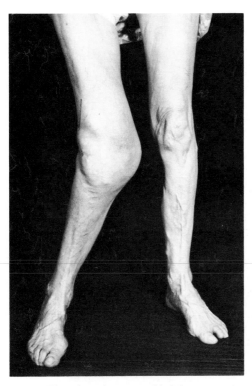

Fig. 16.3 A neuropathic joint.

movements or coarse or fine tremor. In addition, in all diseases of the brain there may be a varying degree of mental impairment, epileptic fits, deafness, impairment of sight or eye control, difficulty in co-ordinating swallowing and breathing, or in articulating.

From the orthopaedic surgeon's point of view the main essential is to avoid the development of fixed deformities and, in particular, pathological dislocation due to unequal muscle pull. A careful assessment must be made therefore of all muscles which are too active; these can be balanced either by tenotomy, myotomy, neurectomy or muscle transfer. In the case of the upper limbs where function is dependent on good voluntary control, good tactile and kinaesthetic sensation and good power of recognition, peripheral surgery to control muscle balance may correct deformity and improve appearance, but has less effect on improving function than do similar procedures performed in the lower limbs where the function is less dependent on voluntary control and is to a certain extent reflex and automatic. Myelomeningocele is discussed in Chapter 18.

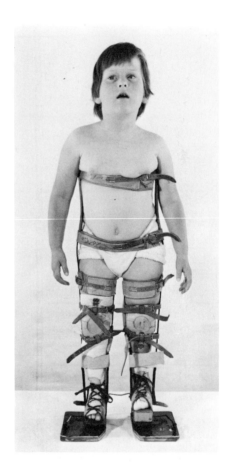

Fig. 16.4   Splintage on child with myelomeningocoele. This is a device for the use of children who are paralysed from the effects of spina bifida and other conditions. The child gains mobility by swivelling on each footplate in turn.

Notes about the splint may be obtained from the Department of Health and Social Security, DSB4A, Government Buildings, Warbreck Hill Road, Blackpool FY2, OU2, United Kingdom.

Having briefly indicated the general principles which govern the development of deformities and their treatment it is appropriate to consider a few of the more common neurological disorders which may require orthopaedic treatment.

Cerebral palsy
This condition which occurs in early life may be due to adverse antenatal influences, trauma at birth, rhesus incompatability or disorders of the neonatal period. There may be associated deafness and mental retardation. One

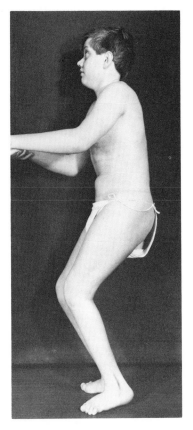

Fig. 16.5   Cerebral palsy.

limb (monoplegia), both legs (paraplegia), one arm and leg (hemiplegia) or all four limbs (tetraplegia) may be affected. At first the limbs are 'floppy' and the child moves his limbs less than normal and normal co-ordination of movement fails to develop. Later it may be possible to distinguish four different functional types:

1   Spasticity or hypertonicity—common.
2   Rigidity—uncommon.
3   Ataxia—loss of position sense—fairly common and often combined with spasticity.
4   Athetosis. In this condition the child's limbs perform involuntary, spontaneous writhing movements. The condition is usually caused by a lesion in the mid-brain secondary to rhesus incompatibility.

In general, orthopaedic measures do not improve athetosis and play only a limited role in ataxia, but correction of deformity and reducing the activity of hypertonic muscles in spasticity can be very useful. The most commonly employed measures are tenotomy (tendon division or lengthening), tendon transfer, myectomy (partial excision of muscles), neurotomy (division of nerves) and neurectomy (excision of part of a nerve). These measures should rarely be used under the age of five years; before this, physiotherapy—muscle stretching, muscle re-education and splinting are most useful.

There is some evidence that excision of the right amount of muscle by both reducing total muscle strength and removing some of the muscle spindles which initiate stretch reflexes, is the most controllable way of reducing muscle tone.

In adults, brain damage due either to injury, haemorrhage, infection, tumour or thrombosis usually produces hemiplegia. The patient is often left with a 'drop foot', flexed knee and hip and flexed wrist and fingers.

For a drop foot the following measures are available:

1   Wearing an appliance—e.g. a Rizzoli splint or below-knee iron and toe spring (see Fig. 16.4).
2   Lengthening the tendo Achillis.
3   Transferring the tibialis posterior tendon to the dorsum of the foot.

If there is a varus deformity of the foot this can be overcome by splitting the tibialis anterior and attaching the outer half to the base of the fifth metatarsal.

Flexion deformity of the fingers and wrist can be corrected by transferring selected flexor tendons, e.g. the flexor sublimus tendons to the back of the wrist, but if the 'body image' is defective, this will not lead to much improvement in function even though the deformity is corrected.

In all hypertonic disorders it is difficult to judge accurately the relative strength of muscles and their opponents and it is often wise to proceed slowly by graduated steps.

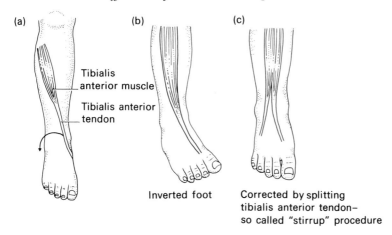

Fig. 16.6 (a) Tibialis anterior action.
          (b) Inversion due to tibialis anterior.
          (c) Corrected by splitting tendon.

Naturally in all cerebral lesion there may be other disabilities—mental retardation, fits, emotional lability, grimacing disturbances of swallowing, defects of hearing, sight and proprioception—all of which must be taken into account before advising orthopaedic treatment.

Proper control of the limbs depends on an adequate supply of information from the skin, joints, muscles and tendons of the limbs. Impulses from the periphery are normally interpreted in the brain creating what is often called a body image.

If in cerebral palsy, the damage to the brain dates from a very early age and is extensive the child never develops a proper body image of the defective limb and surgery can never restore good function. On the other hand if the brain damage is less extensive or only occurs after the child has already developed an integrated picture of the position and movement of the limb then surgery to correct deformities and reduce muscle tone can result in considerable improvement in function.

In the case of the lower limb certain surgical procedures are well established.

In the case of the upper limb there has been less certainty of the value of such surgery, but in selected patients procedures to correct fixed flexion deformity of the wrist and fixed flexion deformity of the fingers can be of considerable value. It should be borne in mind that when a joint is fixed in an abnormal position tendons may become displaced and have a new and harmful effect. For instance, in flexion deformities to the wrist the extensor carpi ulnaris tendon may subluxate to the front of the wrist and act as a flexor. Transplantation of the flexor tendons of the wrist into the extensor tendons of the fingers can produce a considerable improvement both in appearance and function.

Similarly, if the fingers are tightly pressed into the palm and the patient cannot extend them himself, transplantation of the superficial flexor tendons into the extensor tendon of the fingers can enable the patient to bend the fingers himself and greatly increase his range of function.

Finally, if there is inability to supinate the forearm, transplantation of the flexor carpal ulnaris tendon to the back of the radius, combined if necessary with division of the pronator muscles, can restore the power of supination.

In selected patients operation on the basal ganglia of the brain can reduce excessive muscle tone.

Parkinsonism

This disorder, due to a mid-brain lesion, is characterized by rigidity and fine tremor, there is poverty of movement and difficulty in initiating movement. Grotesque deformities—especially of the trunk—may occur. In general, orthopaedic measures do not help and may do harm. Splinting and attempted fixation of joints usually make the patient worse.

Disseminated sclerosis

This condition may manifest itself in several ways: in the cerebellar form there will be ataxia, inco-ordination of movement, intention tremor, dysarthria, and nystagmus. Specific orthopaedic treatment does not help cerebellar lesions, though measures such as Frankel's exercises and walking in front of a mirror may give the patient confidence.

In the spinal form with spasticity, measures to prevent or correct deformity and reduce excessive muscle tone as for cerebral palsy may help the patient. Occasionally supporting splints—e.g. below-knee irons—help a patient to walk. The disease runs a chronic, intermittent, fluctuating course, and every effort should be made to keep the patient ambulant.

Tabes dorsalis

Nowadays this condition is rare. It is characterized by ataxia, loss of joint sense, hypotonicity and areflexia. It may lead to the important complication of a swollen flail joint (neuropathic arthropathy or Charcot joint). Such a joint requires external support—e.g. by a caliper. Occasionally fixation (arthrodesis) is used, but this is not normally advisable.

Friedreich's ataxia

Like disseminated sclerosis, this may affect the cerebellum and the spinal cord. It develops in childhood, is progressive and may cause severe deformities, especially of the spine. The prognosis for life is poor as the heart muscle is usually weak.

Occasionally treatment of the scoliotic spine may be necessary either by external or internal supports, to enable the child to sit upright.

Syringomyelia

This is a slowly progressive disorder of the spinal cord which affects young adults. It may lead to spasticity of the legs, scoliosis, wasting of the small muscles of the hands, neuropathic joints and trophic lesions of the skin.

Orthopaedic measures may be required for the spinal deformity and for the spastic legs.

Lower motor neurone lesions

The most common causes of lower motor neurone lesions are (1) injuries, (2) poliomyelitis, (3) leprosy and (4) toxic or infective neuropathy. The principles of orthopaedic treatment are to prevent deformity and, where indicated, transplant tendons and arthrodese flail joints in order to prevent recurrence of deformity and obviate the need for wearing an appliance.

Acute anterior poliomyelitis

Poliomyelitis is an infection caused by one of three types of virus. This micro-organism usually gains entry to the body via the gastro-intestinal tract. After a period of incubation the virus attacks the central nervous system at any level of the spinal cord. As a result of this infection the spinal cord will undergo the inflammatory changes much as any other tissue of the body.

At first there is an increase in the blood supply in the area of infection; then the nervous tissue becomes inflamed, oedematous, and swollen. As a result, certain neurones lose their function and paralysis of the muscles served by that segment of the spinal cord will result. The amount of paralysis suffered by the patient is directly related to the quantity of nervous tissue affected. It varies from a disastrous complete paralysis affecting the whole trunk and all the limbs, to a minor weakness of individual muscles or no paralysis at all.

Later, this inflammation resolves. There may be no after-effects of the inflammation, that is complete healing of the nervous tissue, in which case there will be no permanent residual paralysis; or the neurones may be destroyed or scarred with permanent disability. *It must be emphasized however that only one-fifth of all patients affected by acute anterior poliomyelitis have paralysis.*

Most nations now have a vaccination programme against this disease which immunizes whole populations in childhood so that the major epidemics which were common in the past no longer occur. As there are still nations without an immunization scheme, however, poliomyelitis must still be considered a hazard to health. Epidemics nowadays are more likely to occur in areas where public health standards are low or where, due to parental carelessness, immunization of children is neglected.

The pattern of acute anterior poliomyelitis
The disease may be considered as having five distinct stages:

1   incubation,
2   onset,
3   greatest paralysis,
4   recovery,
5   residual paralysis.

1   *The stage of incubation.* This lasts approximately fourteen days. It is the time when the virus has entered the body and is multiplying; the nervous tissue provides a good culture medium for this type of virus. The patient will have no symptoms or signs. It is considered by some that the amount of destruction of nervous tissue is related to the activity of the patient in this stage; the more sedentary person will suffer less disability than the active athletic individual.

2   *The stage of onset.* Lasting forty-eight hours, this stage gives symptoms and signs which are similar to an attack of influenza. These may be mild, a coryza with headache and malaise, or more severe including pains in muscles with stiffness of the neck, spine or limbs.

One problem during an epidemic of acute anterior poliomyelitis is to know which disease is affecting the patient—influenza or poliomyelitis? As many patients with poliomyelitis recover at this stage and possibly have not called for medical help, it is difficult to know. We know that many adults have had subclinical attacks of poliomyelitis. The danger is that the patient remains a carrier for a long period after a subclinical attack and may provide a reservoir of micro-organisms to maintain the epidemic in a community.

The majority of patients with mild infections recover after this stage. During the latter part of this phase the patient may have symptoms and signs of meningeal irritation and the condition may be mistaken for meningitis.

3   *The stage of greatest paralysis.* During this eight week period the patient has paralysis directly related to the amount of nervous tissue involved. The anterior horn cells of the spinal cord are swollen and oedematous and unable to function in the affected area. If a large segment of the cord is affected, there will be major paralysis affecting a large number of muscles, on occasions the whole body from the neck downwards and including the respiratory mechanism may be paralysed. If only a small number of neurones are affected, the patient may have a paralysis of one or a few skeletal muscles.

An important principle of the management at this stage is to realize that it is the nervous tissue and not the muscular system which is infected.

In the care of the patient's muscular system there are four objectives:

(a) prevention of contraction of muscles,
(b) prevention of stretching of muscles,
(c) maintenance of a full range of movements in all the joints,
(d) prevention of deformities.

If the thoracic muscles are affected, the maintenance of adequate ventilation of the lungs is another requirement.

4   *The stage of recovery.* This can extend for a period of up to two years. There is a slow resolution of the inflammatory changes in the spinal cord. Motor neurones (anterior horn cells) which have been temporarily affected but not destroyed recover their function. As the nerve pathways which serve the affected skeletal muscles regain their function, so do the muscles.

The degree of recovery is variable from one patient to another. Some gain a great amount of function in their affected limbs and muscles; some hardly any, or none at all.

An important attitude in this stage of management is to avoid over-optimism in the patient. There is hope that complete recovery will occur, but it is best that the patient learns to adapt to his existing disability and lead as full a life as he can. If full recovery does happen this is a reason for rejoicing but foolish optimism must not retard progression to useful and happy living with the disability.

At first recovery is rapid; later the rate of improvement becomes less. After one year a big change is unlikely; after two years the condition is static.

5 *The stage of residual paralysis.* After the two years, it must be accepted that any paralysis remaining is permanent. The surgeon may decide to aid the limited function of the patient by the transplantation of muscles, elongation of tendons, tenotomies, arthrodesis of joints, neurectomy and any other form of surgical intervention which will assist the locomotion, posture or usage of the patient's limbs or body.

As a patient suffering from the effects of anterior poliomyelitis becomes older there may be deterioration in their muscle strength and their functional disability increases, e.g. a patient who can just walk at 20 may end up in a wheelchair at 55.

The management of the patient with acute anterior poliomyelitis

At all stages this requires a comprehensive team of workers representing most facets of patient care.

During the stages of onset and maximum paralysis the patient may require intensive care, particularly if the respiratory mechanism is affected. Intermittent-positive-pressure-ventilation, parenteral nutrition or tube feeding, a consistent two hourly turning routine and special bladder and bowel management may be needed for the survival of the patient. Such care is carried out in special hospital units and is beyond the scope of this book.

Up to six weeks from the start of the illness the patient's faeces contain the micro-organism of poliomyelitis and he is therefore infectious to others. His attendants must be adequately immunized against the infection and the patient nursed in isolation.

Relevant orthopaedic nursing

The orthopaedic team must have access to the patient at the commencement of his illness, particularly if there is paralysis present. The orthopaedic management of the patient may be classified into the following phases:

(a) Ensuring that during the stage of greatest paralysis deformity is avoided and that muscles and joints are maintained in the optimum condition for later rehabilitation.

(b) Later careful assessment of the degree of paralysis present in particular muscles, classification of the strength of the affected muscle and prevention of the deterioration of that function until recovery.

(c) Providing planned and logical rehabilitation during the stage of recovery to give the patient optimum improvement of function.

(d) Supplying adequate means for the patient to cope with any residual paralysis. This may mean surgical intervention, such as muscle transplantation, or the provision of appliances such as calipers and wheelchairs.

(e) Retraining the patient for daily living and earning a means of livelihood when a disability is permanent.

All of this requires adequate communication between each member of the team *and the patient*. The most effective course of action to aid the recovery of any patient can only be decided upon at a conference of all the health workers involved. Thus a meeting of the surgeon, physical medicine consultant, nurse, physiotherapist, occupational therapist, medical social workers and the disablement resettlement officer must be convened at relevant stages in the progression of the patient towards recovery. An ideal would be to involve the patient in the meeting, but if this is not possible he must be made aware of the decisions taken at the meeting and his co-operation sought.

Prevention of deformity during the acute stage
The whole body of the patient is nursed in the optimum position of rest. This means that the patient is supported in a posture which ensures that no joint is held constantly in a position which will overstretch any muscle or group of muscles.

The nursing positions used are similar to those used for the care of patients who have spinal injuries or paraplegia or tetraplegia. The principles of positioning are:
1   The head and spine are supported in the normal anatomical position, without distortion.
2   The shoulders are arranged with the arms either in abduction or flexion, depending upon the position in which the patient has been placed.
3   The elbows are adjusted into about 90 degrees of flexion.
4   The wrists are supported in slight dorsiflexion with the hands arranged around cylinders which are about 10 cm in diameter.
5   The hips are arranged in partial abduction and partial flexion. Extreme lateral rotation is prevented by the use of supporting pillows.
6   The knees are slightly flexed.
7   The feet are maintained at right angles by the use of firm pads.

It is most important that no part of the patient is maintained constantly and relentlessly in one fixed position so that a contraction requiring attention develops. The patient's position is altered at two-hourly intervals and on turning, the position of the shoulders, elbows, hips and knees is passively varied for him.

If a muscle group has weakness or paralysis there is a danger that the opposing muscle group will force the joint or limb into deformity. For example, the action of the posterior muscles of the forearm, supplied by the radial nerve, is to pull the wrist and fingers backwards into extension; if the lesion in the spinal cord affects the radial nerve, the posterior muscles of the forearm will be paralysed and the powerful anterior muscles will tend to pull the wrist forwards into a flexed position—this is known as a 'drop wrist'.

It may be necessary in these circumstances, to supply a plaster shell or splint to prevent deformity and to maintain the joint in an over-corrected position. This shell is removed at regular intervals so as to move the joint passively through its full range of movement before the splint is reapplied. The objective is that when and if recovery of the nerve occurs, the muscles and joints will have normal function. The splints supplied must be light in weight and should support, not fix, the affected part. Nor should they interfere with the function of normally working parts of the body, e.g. a wrist splint should allow normal use of the fingers and thumb.

Relative management during the stage of recovery

As part of progression towards the stage of recovery, the physiotherapist makes an estimate of the power of function of individual muscles. Various tests are used; some of these tests can accurately assess the function of a muscle so that its power can be recorded and improvement indicated at successive testings. Electromyography is used to indicate muscle activity; when a muscle tissue contracts, electrical potentials develop, the electro-myograph amplifies these potentials and records them graphically. Muscle power in a muscle is recorded by a figure between nought and five; nought indicates that there is no power and five indicates full power.

When it is established that power has returned to an affected muscle, or that a weak muscle is gaining strength, the physiotherapist commences re-education of the muscle until maximum recovery has been reached.

It is essential to know which muscles are functioning and which are not before deciding when the patient may progress from the horizontal position first to sitting and then to standing. For example, if the muscles which normally support the vertebral column are weak on one side (muscle imbalance) sitting upright without adequate support to the spinal column could result in a postural deformity such as scoliosis.

Relevant management for the stage of residual paralysis

If sufficient time has elapsed and no recovery has occurred in certain muscles or muscle groups, it must be accepted that the patient is left with a permanent disability. The patient must learn to enjoy as full a life as he can within the range of that disability. Chapter 11 (Peripheral Nerve Lesions), Chapter 31

(The Paraplegic Patient) and Chapter 27 (Comprehensive Patient Care) are relevant to this.

The management of patients with affections of the brain and spinal cord

(See also Chapter 27: Comprehensive Patient Care; Chapter 31: The Paraplegic Patient.)

Recent progress in neurology and neurosurgery offers much hope to the patient with disorders of the brain and spinal cord, as there are many advances in drug therapy and surgery. Often these patients must modify their way of life so as to adjust to their permanent residual disability. They come from the whole range of age groups, but those who require most help from nursing and physiotherapy staff may be classified as (1) the very young who have a congenital condition, (2) young adults who suffer from a neurological disorder and (3) elderly adults usually with cerebro-vascular disorders. All groups present different management problems.

The young patient

The child who has a disorder such as cerebral palsy must receive an amount of formal education comparable to the general schooling which is given to a normal child. The interruption of the pathways from brain to muscles may mean that the child does not develop the normal mechanisms of speech, seeing, hearing, limb and body control in walking, standing, running, writing, chewing and swallowing, or other daily vital activities. Training must be given by a team of specialists. This training will last throughout the formative years and the specialist team are best centred in one building so that schools for the complete education of the child from nursery to high school are usually the best answer. These may be resident or non-resident, according to local needs. Such schools may be paid for and organized by local authorities but voluntary organizations are often the most vigorous in initiating and maintaining such schools. The staff of such specialist schools represent a synthesis of many diverse interests. There are doctors of various specialities, nurses, physiotherapists, speech therapists, occupational therapists, social workers, teachers with special training for the education of the handicapped and many other staff who form a large team with the main objective of giving the optimum education and medical care to the patient.

Many children with brain damage also suffer from epilepsy. While sufficient anti-convulsive drugs must be given to control the attacks, it is important not to oversedate as this may make the child incapable of learning or co-operating in re-education.

The adult patient

The young adult. Once basic education has been achieved the problems for a person who acquires a neurological disorder are those of modification of daily living activities according to his disability and re-training for a new occupation, if this is possible. These are often patients who have brain destruction, perhaps as the result of a disease, head injury or cerebro-vascular accident; this will slow down their rate of comprehension and ability to remember as well as affecting speech, sight, hearing, locomotion and limb control.

The elderly patient. A large proportion of the patients with neurological disorders are those who are old. In this group are patients who suffer recurrent cerebro-vascular catastrophes or Parkinsonism. The prognosis is obviously not good in this group of patients, but optimism and a desire to achieve a return to normal living must be the keynote. Under some circumstances arterial anastomoses to short circuit obstruction in arteries supplying the brain may prevent permanent neurological damage or limit its spread. The term *geriatric* which is applied to the study of elderly patients, should engender the spirit of recovery and rehabilitation; it should not imply retirement to bed for a death. The geriatric team is composed of a group actively interested in this form of work—the rehabilitation of aged patients. The team consists of doctors, nurses, physiotherapists, occupational therapists, social workers, speech therapists, the ophthalmologist, chiropodist and many others. A similarity to the team who care for the young neurological patient will be noted.

Special aspects of care of patients with brain and spinal cord lesions

1 *Acceptance by relatives.* The neurological patient often has a gait, mannerisms and peculiarities which are symptoms of his condition; these may make him unattractive to his family and in the community. It is not easy to accept a person who may be chair-bound, mentally subnormal, socially unacceptable and requiring a great deal of repetitive intimate care for the remainder of life. Such a low state is found only in a small proportion of these patients however, and many require little assistance, and certainly less than these notes indicate. When possible, it is better for the patient to return to his own environment; he can experience loneliness and isolation just as a

healthy patient and no institution can replace the warmth of acceptance in the family circle.

The nursing staff should work towards the preparation of his relatives for the return of the patient to his home whilst he is still under treatment in hospital. Graduated return may be possible—encouraging the family to take the patient home in the knowledge that if the problems are too great, return to hospital is easily achieved for further rehabilitation. If this fails, admission to an institution which is properly staffed and equipped is a better proposition than when the health of a spouse or parent is affected by the attempt to manage an impossible situation.

2   *Training to achieve standing and walking.* When the patient can manage to stand and possibly walk—no matter how badly—a degree of independence has been achieved which gives optimism to both the patient and his relatives. He who can walk can reach the bathroom! The ability to progress to the bathroom means release for both patient and attendant, from the misery of soiled beds, bed-pans, urinals and commodes which must be emptied and cleaned. The physiotherapy staff work to this end from the day of admission of the patient to hospital. Muscles which are not paralysed must be preventing from wasting; methods of rising from a bed or chair must be taught; the best possible gait in the light of the disability is learnt. Tripods and stands, walking machines, splints and crutches all have their place in the process of achieving some form of locomotion (see Fig. 27.2)—no matter how slow and ungainly.

3   *Independence in feeding and the personal toilet.* Probably the most time-consuming aspect of patient care is that of feeding the helpless person. In hospitals it is a worry for an administrator to find sufficient people who have the time to sit by the bedside of helpless patients feeding them with small portions of food until the meal is consumed. It is often a greater problem in a family circle where the members must go to work or school or where patient care depends upon a single individual with limited time for many chores.

If the patient can learn to transfer food from crockery to mouth—even

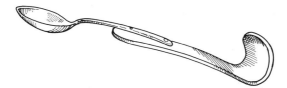

Fig. 16.7   Modification of a spoon for use by a patient with inability to grasp.

crudely and slowly—it relieves the hard-pressed family and makes the patient feel a degree less useless and futile. The same applies to washing, shaving, using the lavatory and dressing.

There are many aids which have been devised to assist the patient (Fig. 16.7, see also Chapter 27) in achieving a return of independence in these habitual tasks. The occupational therapy staff and social workers can advise on the method of obtaining such aids, which are often 'custom-made' to suit the individual patient.

4 *Re-training for employment.* It is not an easy matter to find employment for a person with a severe disability. Legislation exists in many countries which ensures that the large firms employ a small percentage of the physically handicapped population on their staff. If an employer has any choice in the matter (and he always has), he is more likely to employ a lightly disabled person to fill his quota rather than one who is slow and requires special concessions and considerations. Legislation usually does not apply in this respect to small firms with a few employees.

There are some State-assisted factories and voluntary organizations which help to find employment for the physically handicapped. The social worker assists by introducing the patient to the Disablement Resettlement Officer whose task is to find suitable employment for disabled persons. Often some form of home-employment is all that is possible in the light of the disability.

5 *A positive approach to general health.* Even though the patient has a severe neurological disorder which is untreatable, much can be done to ensure that no secondary condition contributes to his problems. A full assessment of the patient is therefore made so that treatment can be arranged for any associated conditions. Upper respiratory tract infections and other septic foci are cleared with antibiotic therapy. The eyes are tested and spectacles supplied if necessary. If hearing can be improved with a hearing aid this is an asset.

Conclusion
Given that the correct approach to rehabilitation exists, in relation to the residual disability, much can be done to make the way of life for the patient and his relatives acceptable and tolerable.

17

Affections of Muscles

Relevant anatomy and physiology

The skeletal muscles have the following functions:

1   To support the trunk in any chosen position; thus standing or sitting requires muscles to hold the body in a stable posture.

2   To stabilize the synovial joints of the limbs so that the limbs may be placed and held in the position in which they are required.

3   To move the synovial joints, and thus the body. Movements such as walking, running and jumping are caused by muscles.

4   To contract and apply precise controlled and varying amounts of pressure. Thus small 'feint' movements or powerful thrusts or pressures are equally required from any given muscle.

5   To prevent stasis in the tissues; the muscles have 'tone'; they contribute to the firm 'feel' of the tissues and cause movement when they are under pressure; they apply intermittent pressure to the blood vessels and thus help venous return.

6   To contribute to the activities within the abdominal cavity by varying the pressures as they compress the contents.

7   To cause respiration by varying the volume of the thoracic cavity as the walls of the chest and the diaphragm are moved by muscle tissue.

8   To assist communication with others by varying facial expressions and hand gestures.

This list of functions may be developed *ad infinitum* as the muscles contribute to most of the functions of the body.

Nerves and muscles

The efficient function of muscles depends upon communication with the spinal cord and the brain. In the transmission of instructions from the brain to the muscles, efferent or motor nerves carry the impulses; thus every muscle, no matter how small, must be supplied with a motor nerve branch. For co-ordinated activity of the whole body, the brain and spinal cord must be fully informed of every change in position in a muscle; afferent or sensory

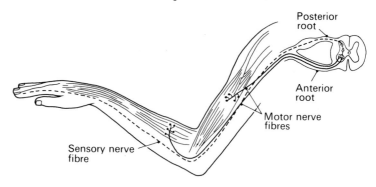

Fig. 17.1 The main features of sensory nerves from skin and motor nerve to skeletal muscle.

nerves constantly carry impulses (electrical messages) back to the central nervous system; every muscle must therefore also have afferent, sensory nerve fibres communicating from the muscle to the spinal cord and brain.

Any interruption in either the motor or sensory nerve supply of a muscle results in serious impairment of the function of the muscle. There must be communication for there to be proper control.

Blood vessels, blood and muscles

All the tissues of the body must have an adequate supply of circulating blood. The amount required by muscles is larger than that of many tissues; there is a direct relationship between the work performed and the quantity of blood needed by muscular tissue. When work is performed by a muscle there must be a corresponding supply of nutrient material such as glucose and oxygen; the greater the amount of work, the more blood with nutrition and oxygen the muscle will require. Every muscle has arteries, carrying oxygenated blood into the tissues, and veins carrying de-oxygenated blood away from the tissues.

Impairment or complete cessation of the blood supply to any tissue or organ is a serious matter; the function of the tissue will be reduced or the tissue will die. Ischaemia of muscles results in loss of function of the muscle, i.e. it is no longer elastic or contractile.

Diseases of muscle

Diseases of muscle may be either intrinsic or extrinsic.

Extrinsic causes. Extrinsic causes can be divided into neurogenic and vascular. In neurogenic diseases of muscle there is an affection of either an anterior horn cell of the spinal cord, or of a motor nerve; this leads to paralysis, wasting and finally, degeneration of the muscle fibres, with loss of electrical excitability so that the normal brisk response to an interrupted electric current (faradic current) is lost and the muscle will only respond sluggishly either at the start or at the end of a continuous (galvanic) stimulation (Fig. 17.2).

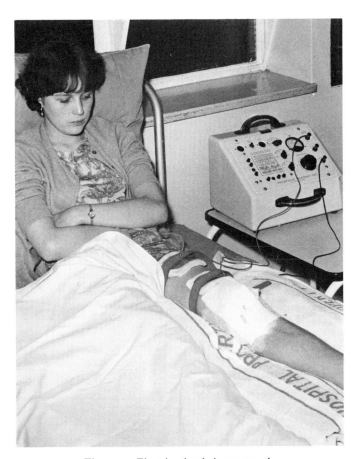

Fig. 17.2   Electric stimulation to muscles.

Vascular disorders of muscle are usually due to impairment of the arterial blood supply; this leads to death of the muscle cells, loss of contractility, replacement by scar tissue, fibrosis and contracture (Volkmann's ischaemic contracture, see Chapter 8). Such disorders usually occur in association with fractures, e.g. supracondylar fractures of the elbow in children, either as a sequel to spasm of the artery or to contusion of the wall of the artery and thrombosis with obliteration of the lumen (see Fig. 8.9b).

Similarly, the blood supply may be cut off by venous obstruction with back pressure on the capillaries and ultimately cessation of the circulation. It is very important that treatment e.g. plaster of Paris or bandages or a tourniquet should not cause or add to circulatory impairment.

Minor degrees of muscle ischaemia are probably very common in association with fractures, particularly fractures of the tibiae, and on occasions fractures of the femur may be associated with major damage to the femoral artery and ischaemia of the below knee muscles which may lead to deformities of the foot, such as an equinus deformity due to contracture of the calf muscle.

Intrinsic disease in muscle. A number of conditions loosely linked together under the title of 'myopathies' have been described. In general these occur in early childhood, e.g. about the age of five years, and become progressively worse during the growing period, ultimately leading to widespread weakness. A number of different clinical types have been described, the commonest is the so-called pseudohypertrophic type which particularly affects the calf, quadriceps and trunk muscles so that the patient has difficulty in standing and getting up from the lying position. He tends to have a characteristic

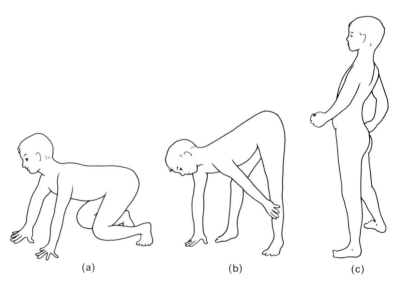

(a)   (b)   (c)

Fig. 17.3   Series of drawings to show muscular dystrophy patient rising from the ground (a) on all fours, (b) kneeling and (c) standing.

posture and a lurching, waddling gait, with an exaggerated lordosis (Fig. 17.3). The condition is more common in boys and is usually caused by a sex-linked dominant gene, i.e. it is inherited through the mother.

Other muscle dystrophies are the facio scapulo-humeral type (Dejerine) which primarily affects the face and shoulder girdle muscles. It commonly comes on somewhat later in life and has a rather better prognosis.

Another type is the Charcot-Marie-Tooth muscle dystrophy which primarily affects the dorsiflexor and evertor muscles of the leg and produces an equino-varo-cavus deformity of the feet. This also usually has an hereditary basis.

In addition, muscle wasting and weakness may occur in a wide variety of other conditions—e.g. in the presence of malignant disease and particularly in carcinoma of the bronchus; in association with diabetes, and with various forms of chronic arthritis; various endocrine disorders—e.g. thyroid and adrenal disorders, and in association with a number of rare disorders of carbohydrate metabolism.

The whole subject of primary muscle disease is a difficult and complex one, and in every case of marked muscle wasting it is important to institute a thorough investigation of the causes which may include electrical tests, electromyography and muscle biopsy. Often the primary disease cannot be treated, but orthopaedic treatment—physiotherapy, preventing and correcting deformities, supporting apparatus and stabilising operations, may help the patient to remain mobile.

Arthrogryposis. This is an uncommon congenital condition in which the child is born with multiple deformities, widespread replacement of muscle tissue by fibrous tissue, and a peculiar abnormality of the subcutaneous tissue and fascia so that the normal flexion creases in the skin are absent and the child's limbs have a curious smooth 'seal-like' appearance. It is common for such children to have club feet, flexed knees, dislocated hips; in some minor cases the condition occurs affecting only a few muscles. Basically the treatment is to correct deformities by lengthening contracted muscles and tendons and also joint capsules; if necessary, corrective osteotomies of bone are performed. There may be associated congenital anomalies of the skeleton.

Myositis ossificans. This condition occurs in two forms: a localized form may occur following injury—in particular the brachialis anticus muscle in front of the elbow and the quadriceps muscle in front of the thigh are the two commonest sites, but minor degrees may occur in other situations. It is believed that osteogenic cells grow into a haematoma and form bone there.

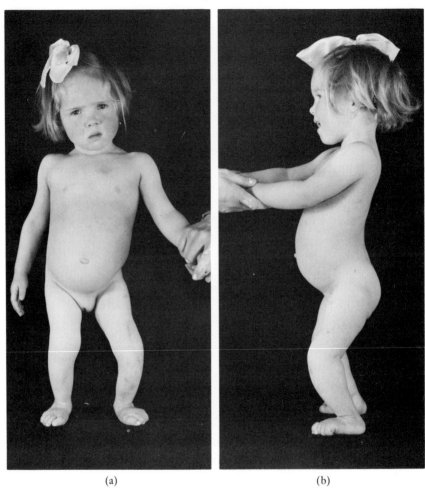

(a)   (b)

Fig. 17.4   Patient with arthrogryposis.

Basically the treatment is to rest the condition in the acute phase and, as the acute phase settles down, graduated exercises are commenced but massage and forced movements only aggravate the condition.

The generalized form of myositis ossificans is extremely rare; the cause is unknown but it is a progressive condition in which the skeletal muscles are gradually replaced by bone leading to progressive stiffness, deformity, and ultimately complete immobility usually leading to death from respiratory infection. No effective treatment is known.

Congenital absence of muscles. Certain muscles of which the commonest example is the pectoralis major may be congenitally absent. Usually there is relatively little functional disability and the main problem is the cosmetic blemish.

Progressive muscle fibrosis. Progressive fibrosis and shortening of muscle may occur as a sequal to multiple injections (e.g. of antibiotics in infancy). The most commonly affected muscle is the quadriceps, quadriceps fibrosis causes progressive restriction of knee flexion. The treatment is to lengthen the tendon of the affected muscle, or to separate the affected part from the normal part of the muscle.

18

Deformities of the Spine

Relevant applied anatomy and physiology

The normal vertebral column is not 'as straight as a poker'; if it were it would be deformed. The existence of curves in the spine make possible a variety of functions. For example:

1   The cervical curve holds the head vertically upright and makes possible a wide range of binocular vision.

2   The thoracic curve increases the volume of the thoracic cavity; it forms part of the thoracic cage.

3   The lumbar curve assists the positioning of the centre of gravity of the body over its base, the feet.

4   The sacral curve increases the volume of the pelvic cavity. This use of curves in functional anatomy is continued into the legs. The femora are also curved; this contributes to placing the centre of gravity of the body over its

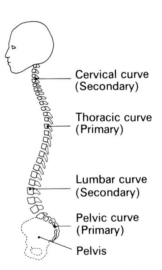

Fig. 18.1   A normal spine.

272

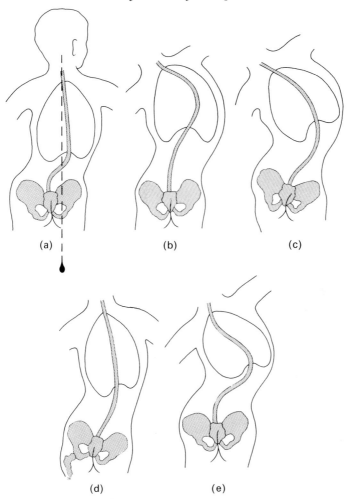

Fig. 18.2   Uncompensated curves: (a) lateral shift of trunk, (b) high thoracic
curve, (c) long C-curve without secondary curves, (d) long lumbar curve, (e)
severe curve with inadequate compensation.

base. Because the body is arranged so neatly over the base by the curves, the
minimal muscular effort is necessary to maintain the body in the erect posture.

Normal variations exist in the depth and length of the curves. These
variations are related to age, sex, race, height and weight. For example, the
lumbar and pelvic curves are more pronounced in the female than in the male
because of the depth of the pelvic basin from the anterior to the posterior
surfaces.

Slight variations may also exist from one person to another, such anomalies are acceptable as normal. For example, a slight lateral curve to the right in the cervical region may exist in right-handed people, and to the left in left-handed people.

The curves are also classified as primary and secondary. The primary curves—the thoracic and pelvic curves—are those which form when the infant is in the uterus; the normal fetal position produces these. If the fetus assumes an extended position there will be severe difficulties in parturition. The secondary curves first form when the infant lies supine on a flat surface, later either in lying prone or sitting, he learns control first of the head and later the trunk thus achieving the upright posture as part of normal development.

Spinal growth

(a) Man is the only animal who achieves a bipedal posture by a combination of lumbar lordosis and fully extended hips.

The new-born baby has flexed hips and flexed cervical and lumbar spine.

Growth therefore involves more than increase in size; there is also differentiation and change of shape.

Growth in the height of the body is cause by an increase in (1) the length of the long bones, (2) the depth of the skull and (3) the depth of each vertebral body.

Each vertebral body increases in depth at the epiphyseal plates. These are layers of growth cartilage which form a lid and a base, to each vertebral body, in the young person. At the junction of the bone and the cartilagenous growth plate new bone is deposited so that each vertebral body grows deeper and thus the total effect on the spinal column is an increase in height.

(b) The spinal canal increases in size by growth cartilages situated between the pedicles and the bodies.

The neural arches and articular, spinous and transverse processes also increase in size by growth cartilages.

Spinal musculature

Each vertebra interlocks into its adjacent neighbours. The whole vertebral structure is then secured together by a number of ligaments (eight to each pair of vertebrae). However, the upright position and the many variations in posture and movement of the vertebral column depends upon a large number of small muscles. The majority of these muscles are arranged down the paraspinal grooves on the posterior surface; they are thus directly attached to the projections of each of the vertebra—the two transverse processes and the spinous process. A number of muscles which are not attached to the vertebral column affect its movements however; these are the muscles of the neck, the pectoral muscles, the respiratory muscles, the muscles of the abdominal walls and the latissimus dorsi muscles. No matter what the situation of the muscles they are normally balanced so as to maintain the correct posture of the vertebral column. Imbalance of these muscles will lead to spinal deformity.

The nerve supply to the spinal muscles

The muscles directly attached to the vertebral column are supplied by a small branch from each spinal nerve, the posterior primary ramus. This leaves the neural canal on its lateral surface (see p. 246). As a corollary of spinal deformity these branches may be constricted; this nerve root pressure may impair the nerve supply to the posterior spinal musculature causing muscle wastage and paralysis which, in its turn, increases the postural problems of the patient.

The vertebral column as a boundary to the thorax and abdomen

The vertebral column gives support to the ribs and the abdominal muscles. It is also the posterior boundary of the thorax and abdomen.

Severe deformity of the vertebral column may encroach on the volume of these cavities, greatly reducing the space available for the lungs and heart and the organs and intestines in the abdominal cavity. The patient will sometimes have severe respiratory distress because of a reduced vital capacity and digestive disorders due to compression of the viscera of the abdomen.

Deformities of the spine

Spinal deformities are important because: (i) of the risk of pressure on the spinal cord and nerves leading to pain and paralysis; (ii) the cause of the deformity may, in its turn, produce pain; (iii) there may be interference with other organs, particularly the heart, lungs; (iv) spinal deformity is a serious cosmetic matter and secondary effects on the arms and legs may induce impairment of motion and excessive liability to fatigue.

Nomenclature. The normal spine is capable of four main movements, namely —forward flexion, extension, lateral flexion and rotation. Corresponding to these, though not necessarily identical with or caused by them, are the four main types of spinal deformity—namely, increased forward angulation (that is, posterior convexity or kyphosis), increased backward angulation (posterior concavity or lordosis), lateral flexion and rotation. The last three are usually

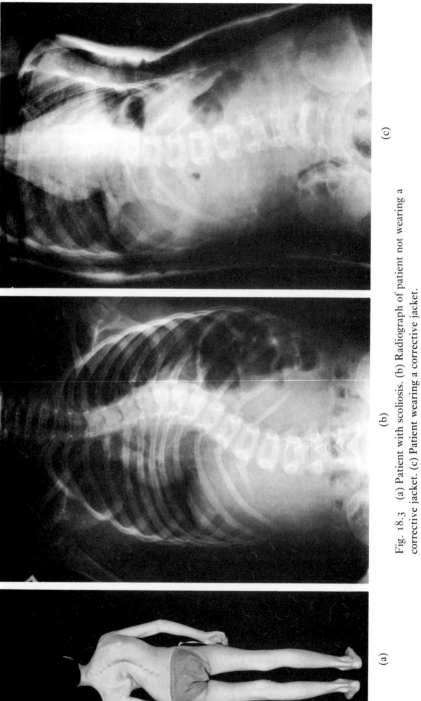

Fig. 18.3 (a) Patient with scoliosis. (b) Radiograph of patient not wearing a corrective jacket. (c) Patient wearing a corrective jacket.

combined and termed *scoliosis*. Causes of spinal deformity are the same as elsewhere in the body—namely, failure of growth; muscle imbalance and destruction of bones or joints by infection, injuries or tumours.

Kyphosis. Of these deformities, kyphosis is the most frequent and important and may lead to pressure on the spinal cord with paralysis of the limbs. The causes can be conveniently divided into disturbances of growth and destructive processes.

Congenital kyphosis. Disturbance of growth may be of congenital origin—for example, a congenital wedge-shaped vertebra or split of the vertebral body, or even absence of vertebral bodies. In extreme cases where there is also paralysis of the legs and sphincters, as in myelomeningocoele, excision of the affected vertebrae followed by prone nursing in a plaster shell may be required.

In all severe kyphoses whatever the cause there is a risk of paraplegia developing. Every effort should therefore be made to prevent progressive

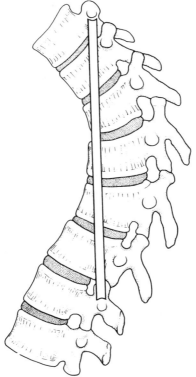

Fig. 18.4   Intertransverse strut graft for kyphosis—usually bilateral.

kyphosis becoming worse. One useful procedure is to insert bilateral inter-transverse struts (Fig. 18.4).

Other congenital abnormalities of the spine include a central spur of bone (diastematomyelia) and failure of fusion of the neural arches which may be associated with varying degrees of mal-development of the spinal cord and membranes (myelomeningocele) see Fig. 18.13.

Myelomeningocele. Intrauterine failure of development may lead to various degrees of failure of closure of the neural arch. This may be slight and only detectable on radiography, or severe with failure of development of the spinal cord and complete paralysis and sensory loss in the legs and lower part of the body.

Where there is also failure of skin closure and the spinal meninges and cord remnants are open to the exterior there is a high risk of meningitis unless a skin closure is performed. This however does not cure the paraplegia; in addition many of these babies develop hydrocephalus unless the cerebrospinal fluid (CSF) is drained into a vein or the peritoneum (see p. 297).

Severe spinal defects can be detected *in utero* in which case the parents are usually allowed to decide to have an abortion rather than bring a badly deformed, paralysed and probably mentally retarded child into the world.

The paraplegic myelomeningocele patient will require continuous medical and surgical care for urinary infections and incontinence, leg and spine deformities, ulceration and infection of anaesthetic areas, not to mention fits, clumsiness of hands and occasional blindness due to the hydrocephalus. The CSF drainage device may become blocked and infected and require repeated changing. Clearly such a child requires tremendous parental attention and other children in the family may suffer as a result. In making their decision parents should be aware of all these facts.

Adolescent kyphosis. During adolescence, failure of growth of the vertebral bodies may occur. This is usually an inherited condition and causes varying degrees of kyphosis, usually in the lower thoracic region which is called adolescent kyphosis or Scheuermann's disease. In old age, softening of the bones (osteoporosis) often leads to severe kyphosis.

Infections. Tuberculosis and other infections of the spine may cause severe deformity both by destruction of intervertebral discs and vertebral bodies and by interference with growth in children. This condition is usually associated with serious constitutional disorders, pressure on the spinal cord and the formation of abscesses either in the neck, chest, abdomen or groin.

Tumours. Tumours of the vertebral bodies may be either primary or secondary. Primary tumours may be benign or malignant. The most common primary malignant tumours are myelomatoma; the most common secondary deposits are from primary tumours in the lungs, breast, prostate, kidneys, thyroid or stomach.

The treatment of all these conditions is first of all the appropriate treatment of the causative condition, e.g. radiotherapy and cytotoxic drugs for tumours, antibiotics for tuberculosis. Purely orthopaedic measures include rest in recumbency in the acute phase and the wearing of a spinal support in the convalescent phase. Operations may be necessary to correct severe deformity, to remove dead and infected tissue or to remove a portion of tissue in order to establish the diagnosis (biopsy).

Lordosis. If the kyphosis is localized there will usually be compensatory lordosis above and below the affected area. Apart from compensatory lordosis, lordosis is rare. However, it may occur as a congenital lesion due to failure of development of the posterior vertebral elements, or it may occur in association with paralysis of the abdominal muscles and flexion deformity of the hips (see Fig. 3.5).

Scoliosis. The combination of lordosis, lateral flexion and rotation is usually known as scoliosis. This may be caused by congenital defects in the vertebrae in which case there are usually associated rib defects, e.g. absence or fusion, and often other congenital defects affecting the limbs, diaphragm, kidneys, etc. In addition, scoliosis may occur as a sequel to a variety of muscle disorders—e.g. muscular dystrophy, poliomyelitis and a number of brain and spinal cord diseases such as syringomyelia and Friedreich's ataxia, but in the majority of patients with scoliosis the cause is unknown. There are two main types of so-called idiopathic scoliosis: one type which is present at birth or which appears in early infancy and another type which occurs in early adolescence.

Of the infantile curves, approximately ninety per cent recover spontaneously but the remainder become relentlessly worse with growth, indicating that there is a disturbance of vertebral growth. The adolescent type of scoliosis tends to worsen progressively during the growing period and to become stationary when growth is complete.

Ideally the treatment of scoliosis is to treat the cause—e.g. growth disturbance or muscle imbalance. Unfortunately, it is often impossible to be sure of the cause: in this case treatment must be empirical; in milder cases the deformity can be controlled by stretching and the application of splints, of which the Milwaukee brace is the most effective (Fig. 18.7). More severe cases may require operations either to correct the deformity, correct muscle imbalance, or to fix the spine in its corrected position. The operations therefore include wedge resection, epiphysiodesis, release of muscles and ribs on the concave side, and instrumentation such as the insertion of a Harrington rod or a spinal plate (Fig. 18.9).

There is widespread recognition that scoliosis is due to a combination of muscle imbalance and impairment of normal spinal growth both of which factors interact on each other, and once a deformity is present it is likely to be progressive until it ultimately becomes severe and fixed. Therefore, it is desirable to try to correct scoliosis at the earliest possible moment. Both muscle imbalance and growth disturbance may be due to a wide variety of extra spinal causes which frequently cannot be diagnosed or treated.

In mild cases a plaster jacket, exercises and wearing a Milwaukee splint are extremely valuable. It is important to recognize that the real value of the Milwaukee splint is that it is a medium through which the patient can apply stretching exercises to her spine and its success depends on the splint fitting well and the patient performing the exercises assiduously in the splint (Fig. 18.7).

It is difficult to apply an effective Milwaukee splint in small children with prominent abdomens and small pelves. In such children the intermittent wearing of a corrective plaster cast will often carry them through till they are older, or have been cured. I recommend wearing a plaster jacket for six winter months and then free exercising for six summer months.

An alternative procedure is fusion of the laminae on the convex side, and fusion of the ribs to each other on the convex side. A 'costodesis' acts as an inhibitor of growth on the convex side of the spine.

In more severe curves fusion of the spine combined with grafting is often the most useful method of treatment but it is desirable to loosen up a curved spine as much as possible before operation. Although this can be done by means of plaster casts and direct pressure, the application of direct traction is useful in the more severe cases. The most effective way of applying the traction is by the use of a halo-splint which can be combined with either counter-traction on the legs, counter-pressure on the pelvis by a halo pelvic apparatus or more simply nursing the patient in a sitting posture with a weight and pulley lifting the patient off the bed (Fig. 18.5). This is certainly an effective method of applying traction in severe spinal deformities though if the spine is very rigid the method may have to be combined with operation interference to divide structures which prevent correction whether these are fibrous or bony. Halo-traction (Fig. 28.18c and d) may also be employed in the treatment of other deformities, for example kyphosis, or for severe neck deformities and dislocations. The method must be used with care or damage may occur to the cervical spine or intracranial structures.

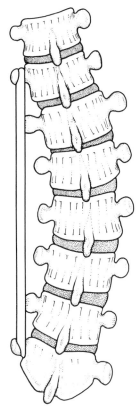

Fig. 18.5   Unilateral intertransverse graft for scoliosis, this may be combined with instrumentation.

The nursing management of patients with congenital and growth deformities of the spine

The child with a deformity of the spine requires prolonged observation in order to estimate the degree of curvature and to note whether it is static or progressive. It is important to take the necessary action before a slight curve which is unnoticeable under clothing becomes an obvious deformity which cannot be disguised even by the most skilled dressmaker. It is essential that the patient must attend clinics regularly for several years for clinical examinations and radiography so that the curve can be measured accurately and recorded in order that any necessary re-adjustment of corrective splintage can be carried out (Fig. 18.7). The frequency of the clinic attendances will depend upon the surgeon's estimate of the probable rate of deterioration, the age of the patient, the rate of change in the curve and other relevant factors; visits may be weekly, monthly or six-monthly. For the patient's sake the visits should not be prolonged, tedious, embarrassing or unpleasant experiences. It is desirable that patients with spinal deformities should be seen at a special clinic where the number of patients is reduced and there are staff and facilities available for measurement, radiography, clinical photography and splint adjustment.

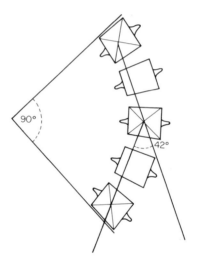

Fig. 18.6 Measurement of abnormal curvature of the spine. Two different methods of measuring a lateral flexion deformity are illustrated. Cobb's method (i.e. the angle between the upper surface of the highest and the lower surface of the lowest vertebra) gives a higher reading than Ferguson's (the angle formed by joining the centres of the highest lowest and apex vertebrae).

Examinations and tests

1   *Radiography.* The direction of the radiographic picture is in relation to the curve of the spine; if the curve is a scoliotic curve, from one side to the other, an antero-posterior film is used; if the curve is kyphotic, from the anterior to the posterior surface, a lateral radiographic film is taken; if kypho-scoliotic the radiographer may decide to make the angle of filming at some degree between antero-posterior and lateral. When the film is de-

veloped the curve is accurately measured on the film using a set-square to mark a line at right-angles to the upper and lower margin of the curve, towards its concavity. The degree of the angle formed where the two lines meet is recorded on the notes (see Fig. 18.6). Although accurate radiographic records are important, care must be taken not to over-irradiate the patient.

2 *Clinical photography.* A comprehensive set of photographs enable the surgeon to note any deterioration or improvement in the deformity by comparing the patient's present condition with that recorded on the photographs previously taken. A posterior aspect, lateral aspect and bending posture are required at each visit; exactly the same distances, lighting and enlargement of the photographs are used on each photograph.

3 *Vital capacity test.* When the thorax is deformed the amount of air taken in by the patient during a full inspiration after complete expiration of air is affected. As the curve increases and the spine becomes more fixed, the vital capacity becomes less. An estimation of the vital capacity at each visit is useful.

4 *General clinical examination.* The patient is examined clinically at each visit. Particular note is taken of:
   (1) Any neurological abnormalities
   (2) Any abnormalities elsewhere, e.g. asymmetry of limbs, head or ears, cafe-au-lait spots, joint laxity, etc.

As the patient will have prolonged treatment it is unkind and unnecessary to retain him in hospital. If multiple operations are required the patient should usually be sent home and to school during the period between surgical intervention. If instructions to the parents are adequate they can usually manage the care of a patient in a plaster jacket or other splint. If the patient is retained in hospital for any period, schooling must continue; special hospital schools exist for this purpose and collaboration between the patient's normal school and the special school will ensure that there is no interruption in the flow of education.

Conservative management

External splintage may be used to prevent deterioration of a deformity or as part of treatment in correcting it. It may also be necessary to use external splintage to immobilize the spine in a suitable position as part of surgical treatment by epiphyseodesis or spinal fusion.

Milwaukee brace (Fig. 18.7). This is a spinal brace which was first devised by Professors Blount and Schmidt with their splintmaker. The Milwaukee brace applies fixed traction (see Chapter 28) between the pelvis and the occiput of the patient. Lateral pressure is also applied by suitable pads. This is probably the most important element and the patient is taught to increase this pressure by deep breathing and pulling on the pad simultaneously. This serves to straighten abnormal curvature of the spine and maintain correction until full ossification of the spine is complete and regression unlikely. A positive cast of the patient's trunk from the level of the chin to the level of the great trochanter of the femora is made, with the patient standing and with head traction applied. The finished positive cast is the model upon which the splintmaker devises the appliance. A plumb line marking on the negative cast is transferred to the positive cast to guide the splintmaker; he must know if the patient has any lateral tilt when the negative cast is made. The main parts of the Milwaukee brace are:

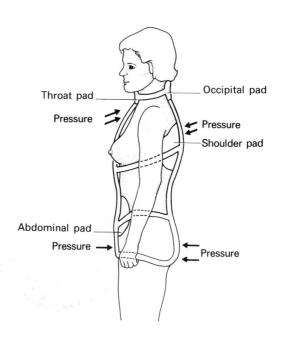

Fig. 18.7   Milwaukee brace showing pressure points.

(i) *A block leather pelvic belt.* This is broad and is modelled so that it rests on the crests of ilium on either side. It is carefully moulded into the waist and pelvis during manufacture; it is firmly fixed with a corset lace. The skiving of this is made of soft leather. Alternatively a moulded plastic belt can be used.

(ii) *Anterior (one) and Posterior (two) upright bars.* These are made of strong yet light-weight alloy. The length is adjustable to meet the increase in height of the patient as growth and improvement occur.

The lower end is set firmly on to a metal alloy inlay which is set into the layers of the block leather pelvic band; this must be a strong union as the downward thrust on the bars is great.

The upper ends support a head piece on the anterior surface and on the posterior surface. Thus when the bars are correctly adjusted an upward thrust against the head is maintained.

(iii) *Pressure pads.* Pads, supported by straps, are supplied to apply constant pressure on the apex of a projecting curve to increase correction.

To apply the splint. The brace is fitted to the patient and the pelvic band is fastened on. The length of the upright bars is adjusted with the patient lying supine. The chin piece and occipital piece fit firmly against the head. When the splint has been in position for a few days the upright bars will again need adjustment so that the chin piece and occipital piece support the head effectively but slight nodding movement is allowed; when some correction has been achieved the curves will straighten as the length of the spine increases. Sufficient room is permitted for the patient's head to be lifted off the head supports by stretching her spine upwards. The patient wears the brace constantly—night and day. The areas under pressure—the chin, the back of the head and the iliac crests—will require constant attention to avoid soreness.

Special clothing must be devised for wearing over the Milwaukee brace.

The success of the Milwaukee brace depends on the co-operation of the patient and her parents.

Wearing the brace for a long time may cause considerable psychological stress in a teenage girl. Other children, particularly boys, may make cruel and offensive remarks. The girl may lose her boyfriend. Some girls completely reject the brace.

Corrective jackets

Opinions vary as to the efficiency of plaster of Paris jackets, their application and function. A variety of jackets exist and personal modifications are frequently introduced. The jackets most commonly used in the management of scoliosis are:

1 The Abbott jacket
This was devised by E. G. Abbott, an American orthopaedic surgeon. It requires an Abbott frame which helps to extend the spine and cause de-rotation of rotational deformities by using slings which pull laterally in the relevant direction. When sufficient correction of the spine is achieved on the frame a plaster of Paris jacket is applied over a thick layer of felt over a stockinette vest, extending from the level of the suprasternal notch to the pubis; the patient's concavities are filled with padding under the jacket. Windows are cut in the jacket over the areas of the greater concavity and the excess padding is pulled out through the windows; the patient assists correction by performing breathing exercises, the greatest expansion of the thorax being into the spaces remaining in the jacket where the excess wadding has been removed.

2 Risser localizer jacket
This uses the same principles as the Abbott jacket but localizer pads are placed over the convexities of the curves of the deformity under the plaster jacket.

3 Risser turnbuckle jacket
This is a jacket which is divided at the level of the apex of the curve after application. On one side—the convex side—a hinge is inserted at the level of the break. On the other side—the concave side of the curve—an extending turnbuckle is inserted which widens the gap in the division as it is manipulated. Thus the curve is over-corrected.

4 Wedging jacket
This is the method preferred by R. Roaf. It is a comparatively simple method of correcting a scoliotic curve.

The method of application. A stockinette vest is put on to the patient and over this a thick layer of felt arranged as follows:
    Pelvic band. The piece of felt about 2 cm thick and as wide as the depth

of the pelvis to fit firmly around the pelvis is sewn to form a seam at the front. The following measurements are recorded: (i) The circumference of the greatest width of the trunk of the patient and (ii) the distance from the seventh cervical vertebra to the gluteal fold. These are used to measure the two pieces of felt that form the vest; each rectangle of felt is half the distance of measurement (i) in width and the whole of measurement (ii) in length. Two parallel cuts 5 cm apart and 17 cm deep are made in the centre of the upper edge; the narrow strip thus formed is the axillary strip; it is not cut off until the jacket is finally trimmed. Each piece of felt forms a lateral half to the vest; the upper edge is sewn for about 5 cm to form an armhole. With the lateral halves in position and the patient's arms through the armholes, the two halves are *not* sewn together. Trimming at the front and back may be necessary to make the vest fit snugly against the patient. Another stockinette vest is then applied over the felt. Extra circles of felt are positioned over bony prominences. The patient is now positioned supine on the shoulder box and pillows and hip prop, or else the orthopaedic operating table is used and the jacket applied as in Chapter 30, p. 525. The jacket is then extended either upwards to form a head piece, as in Chapter 30, p. 530, or downwards to incorporate the relevant hip and thigh over a thick layer of wool padding. This depends upon the level of the curve and the instructions of the surgeon; upper curves require that a head piece be fitted and lower curves a hip spica.

Some correction of the deformity can be obtained during the application of the jacket by applying it in two parts. A lower part to the apex of the curve; when the plaster is sufficiently set the position of the patient is altered to cause the relevant correction before the remainder of the jacket is applied.

The cast is allowed some days to dry and harden completely.

Wedging the jacket. A marker film is taken in the radiography department. This shows the apex of the existing curve of the deformity and the point at which the wedging cut must commence and finish. Using an electric plaster saw, a cut is made through the plaster from the level of the centre of the apex of the curve on the front to the waist, and then around to the level of the starting point on the back. A second parallel cut is made 15 cm from the first and a segment of plaster removed (Fig. 30.5).

The gap must now be forcibly increased by bending the uncut part of the jacket. This is done by arranging the patient over a sandbag and increasing the gap with forge tongs. When the underlying stockinette and felt are exposed they too are cut so that skin is showing. A short length of wood is used to keep the gap open; this is 2·5 cm wide, 4 mm thick and as long as necessary for the correction achieved at this time. A short length is used at first and the length increased at future wedging sessions.

The area adjacent to the wedging cut is greased with petroleum jelly and a plaster bandage used over the grease, to close the gap until further wedging is to be done and the bandage can easily be removed. Later when the maximum correction is achieved, the cast is fully strengthened with a thick layer of plaster bandage.

The nursing management of patients fixed in wedging jackets

It requires little imagination to know that any of the jackets and appliances described in this chapter are unpleasant to wear. The lining retains the heat of the body, they are heavy to support and sitting, lying down and walking are all difficult to manage. A great deal of tolerance is required from the patient and she deserves an explanation of what is being done and why. She will need much nursing help in all personal matters such as feeding, using the lavatory, and washing until she gains some form of independence.

Careful observation is necessary to see that the skin on the edges of the jacket does not become sore or that nerve pressure is not occurring; a reasonable margin of space for the arms is needed. When a hip spica is incorporated, the leg is placed in abduction to increase the space for the perineum to avoid soiling the lower end of the jacket with faeces or urine.

Encasement in plaster in this fashion may also affect the alimentary tract causing loss of appetite, poor digestion and constipation. Small, frequent and attractive meals may be preferred to three large meals at set times. A record of bowel actions is maintained and evacuant suppositories used to relieve any constipation or difficulty in defaecation.

Relevant nursing management of patients before and after surgical operations on the vertebral column

Spinal surgery takes many forms. Examples of such operations are:

1   Operations to close an opening into the neural canal, as in spina bifida occulta.

2   Epiphyseodesis, or growth arrest, in correcting congenital scoliosis or kypho-scoliosis.

3   The insertion of correcting jacks and hooks such as the Harrington rod to correct the curves of scoliosis or kypho-scoliosis, or the insertion of a corrective plate.

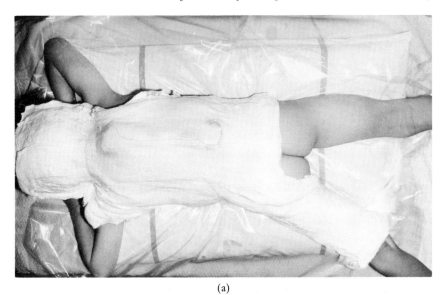

(a)

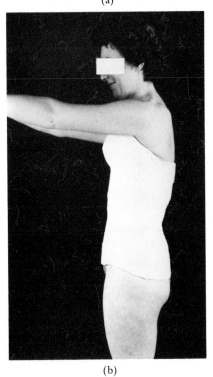

(b)

Fig. 18.8   (a) A plaster bed made on the patient, after an operation to correct scoliosis. (b) Patient wearing a plaster jacket.

4 Spinal fusion to fix a number of vertebrae together to maintain any correction gained by using wedging jackets.

5 Decompression of the neural canal to remove debris from an abscess compressing the spinal cord in the neural canal or a tumour or spur of bone.

6 Operations to relieve the pressure on a nerve root causing low back pain and sciatica.

7 Osteotomy to reduce the fixed deformities of ankylosing spondylitis.

There are other examples of spinal surgery. The management of patients for all of these operations has similarities and these are now discussed. Many patients who require spinal operations are 'elective' cases; that is, there is not the same urgency as in some other operations. The preparation can be comprehensive so that by the day of operation everything is planned and ready. Although some spinal deformities have serious consequences such as paraplegia and impaired vital capacity, most are more an aesthetic blemish than a physical disability. The physical, psychological and educational disadvantages of treatment must be weighed against the ultimate benefits.

Wearing a plaster jacket or Milwaukee splint for long periods is a great emotional hardship to an adolescent. Repeated X-rays may impair fertility; operations leave scars which may be ugly. Long periods in hospital can interrupt education and separate the patient from friends. Boredom during recumbency is another problem. Orthopaedic nursing includes a consideration of all these facts and helping the patient to face them.

Preparation of a plaster bed and turning case

The use of internal fixation during operations on the spine has reduced the need for these. Many patients who are mature enough to co-operate, are cared for either on a latex foam bed or a pillow bed on top of a firm mattress. In young patients, however, a plaster bed and turning case are necessary. Enquiry must be made to find out the wishes of the surgeon in the post-operative care of the patient.

A problem in preparing a plaster bed for a patient with a spinal deformity is that the deformity may have been reduced and the shape of the bed may be incorrect in the post-operative phase; as an inefficient bed is useless or harmful to the patient it may be necessary to make special arrangements for making the bed on the patient after the operation. This can mean making two plaster beds. The first one is heat dried for as long as it can be after removal from the patient's body; the second is properly dried, mounted on a stand, and lined with a thin layer of wool under stockinette as described in Chapter 30, p. 531, the patient is placed in the first bed for return to the ward and immediate post-operative care. When the second bed is ready the patient is

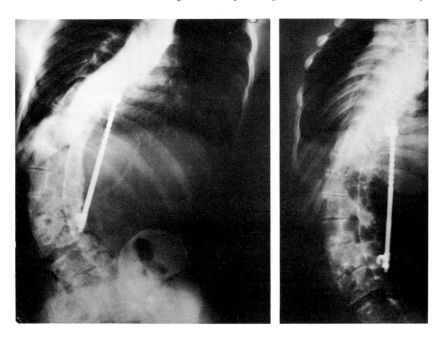

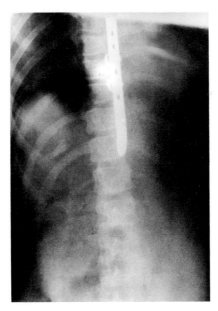

Fig. 18.9 (Above) Harrington rods and (below) spinal plate in place, after operation.

transferred to this three or four days after the operation. When there is no likelihood of a variation in the shape of the patient as a result of the operation the plaster bed and turning case are made as soon after admission as possible; thoroughly dried, mounted on a stand and lined as described in Chapter 30, p. 453.

The patient then uses the plaster bed intermittently during the days before operation to practise sleeping, eating, defaecation and micturition whilst lying in the bed. The plaster bed and turning case with turning straps are sent to the operating theatre when the patient is ready for operation.

If the patient has been nursed on her plaster bed constantly before operation she will require turning into her turning case for pre-operative preparation of the skin on the back of her body; this is the opportunity for completely cleaning and re-furbishing the bed; a new lining is made and fitted.

Clinical examination

The patient is given a full pre-operative examination and investigation as described in Chapter 27.

Physiotherapy

The physiotherapist is an important member of the team managing spinal operations. Physiotherapy commences as soon as the patient comes into the hospital and continues up to discharge home. Pre-operatively the patient must meet and know the physiotherapy staff. They will carry out the following procedures:

1 Estimation of the vital capacity, particularly if the thoracic volume is reduced by the deformity. This knowledge is important to the anaesthetist, to the surgeon and to the physiotherapist in the immediate post-operative phase.

2 Estimation of muscle power if any paralysis exists because of pressure affecting the function of the spinal cord. A record is made of the power and function of every relevant muscle; a scale of muscle power is used which indicates a power between 0 and 5. The nought represents paralysis and the five shows full muscle power and function. This knowledge is again useful to show any improvement in function as a result of the operation.

3 Training the patient to perform the exercises she must do after the operation. This serves to reduce some of the stress in the post-operative period.

Other pre-operative preparation. Apart from the relevant features already mentioned, this is the same as for any orthopaedic patient (see Chapter 27).

Relevant post-operative management of patients who have had surgical operations on the vertebral column

The general nursing management of the patient is the same as that for any post-operative patient who must be nursed in complete recumbency (see Chapter 27, p. 455, *et seq.*

Special features

Wound drainage. The site of operation is usually deep and extensive. Haemostasis is carried out as the surgeon works; despite this, oozing into the wound will continue for some time after operation and adequate vacuum drainage is necessary. A polythene tube drain is used; this passes out from the wound site through a stab wound at a point some distance from the operation wound. It is connected to a drainage bottle which has been prepared by creating a vacuum in it. The fluid content of the wound bed is therefore sucked out as soon as it forms, and haematoma formation is unlikely. This bottle must be scrutinised frequently; if it fills, the drainage tube is clamped off and the full drainage bottle is replaced with a new one, also with a vacuum in it. If the bottle does not fill and there is no increase in the quantity, this indicates either that the drainage tube is obstructed or that there is no more serum or blood to drain from the wound. Instructions must be obtained from the surgeon to ascertain when the drain is to be removed. This is done without uncovering the operation wound. As the patient is lying on the wound—perhaps on a plaster bed—the drain is drawn out in one action, not in stages as with non-vacuum wound drains.

Haematoma formation. If haematoma formation does occur it will be a source of discomfort to the patient. The presence of the haematoma may be indicated by pyrexia and restlessness. It will retard healing and may provide the material in which infection can best occur. If the presence of a haematoma is suspected it will be necessary to turn the patient on to the turning case, uncover the wound for examination and redressing; the haematoma fluid will probably exude during the dressing.

Infection. A prophylactic antibiotic cover will be given to the patient to prevent the serious complication of infection of the wound. The observation charts of the patient should indicate the presence of an infective lesion even though the wound is not visible. A rise in temperature, however, must be due to other causes—an infection of the tonsils for example, but if other reasons for the pyrexia have been eliminated, the wound must be examined. To do this, when the patient is in a plaster bed it is again necessary to turn her into the turning case, using turning straps (see Chapter 30, p. 540).

Thoracic problems. The vertebral column forms the posterior boundary to the thoracic cage. Many spinal operations, particularly those for correction of deformity in the thoracic region, are close to the pleural cavity; a complication of the operation may be that the pleura is penetrated and air or blood enters the cavity. As the pleural cavity contains a potential vacuum, the entry of air or blood breaks the vacuum and the part of the lung near the point of entry may collapse. The surgeon and anaesthetist are aware of this eventuality and are ready to cope with it should it arise.

The anaesthetist will maintain the lungs in an inflated state until the surgeon has taken action to close the pleural cavity and leave *in situ* a suitable apparatus for evacuating either air or blood from the cavity. This may be either an underwater seal drain or a patent one-way evacuant valve which permits air to leave the pleural cavity but prevents its re-entry.

(i) *Management of an underwater seal drain.* The patient returns to the recovery ward with a thoracic drain in position. This is connected by an air-tight connection to a bottle half filled with sterile water; the tube from the thorax opens underneath the surface of the water. A second tube permits the exit of air from the upper half of the bottle.

As the patient inhales, the water will be seen to rise a little way up the tube. The position of the bottle is important; it must be kept much lower than the level of the thorax; if it should be raised to the level of the thorax, or higher, the water will enter the thorax.

(ii) *Management of a thoracic one-way valve.* The main care required is to ensure that the valve is not compressed or the opening blocked. The wound of exit for the valve must, of course, be kept properly dressed and observed for bleeding.

The underwater seal drain or the one-way valve are removed by the surgeon and the opening sutured usually after a thoracic radiograph has been taken.

The nursing observation of a patient with pleural involvement includes careful assessment of respiratory function. Variations in the rate, volume and regularity of respiration, the colour of the patient's skin, the pulse and blood pressure or general distress in the patient may indicate that pneumothorax or haemothorax has occurred and emergency surgical action is necessary.

The total amount of fluid which enters the bottle and its haemoglobin content must be accurately measured as this indicates the amount of post-operative blood loss.

Antibiotic and chemotherapy. Prophylactic coverage against infection is usually standard practice for all major spinal operations. For patients who have had decompression of a tuberculous abscess of the vertebral column the drugs supplied for treating the tubercular infection—streptomycin, para-amino salicylic acid and izo-nicotinic hydrazid—must be given until the regime of drug therapy is completed.

Recovery after paralysis. When compression of the spinal cord or spinal nerves were present prior to operation, observation is needed to note improvement as a result of operation. The physiotherapist will make daily tests of relevant muscles when such recovery is anticipated.

Other discomforts. The post-spinal-operation patient will undergo the same problems as any patient; inability to micturate; pain, abdominal discomfort and paralytic ileus. These all require attention and are discussed in Chapter 27.

For plaster beds, divided plaster beds, turning cases and turning straps see Chapter 30.

Other spinal deformities

Sternomastoid 'tumour' and torticollis

The common syndrome which affects the neck in infancy is a swelling of the sternomastoid muscle—the so-called sternomastoid tumour. This always disappears in time but may lead later to failure of growth of the sterno-mastoid muscle which in itself causes torticollis. In this syndrome the head is turned to the opposite side but is tilted towards the affected side; the face and ear on the affected side are smaller; the eyes are asymmetrical. Treatment is to divide the tight muscles (Fig. 18.10). Following this, special exercises and/or a corrective collar are usually advised.

It is important that treatment be instituted at an early age. If correction is deferred, permanent changes in the face and skull will occur.

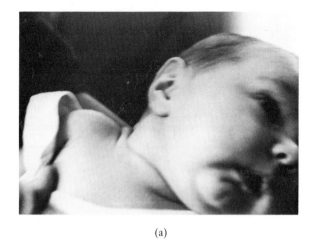

(a)

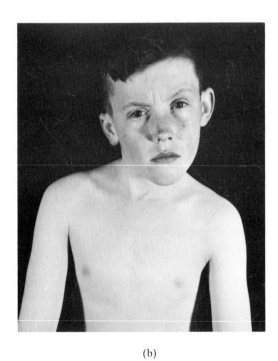

(b)

Fig. 18.10 (a) Patient with a sternomastoid tumour. (b) Patient with torticollis.

Klippel-Feil syndrome

Congenital fusion of the cervical vertebrae is not uncommon and is associated with a short, stiff neck. The characteristic feature is that the hairline goes right down to the upper part of the trunk (Fig. 18.11). There may also be torticollis and the condition must be distinguished from sternomastoid torticollis. This condition may be associated also with congenital elevation of the shoulder (Sprengel's shoulder, Fig. 18.12). In this condition the scapula is small, fixed and elevated; it is often attached to the spine by bony or fibrus tissue. Some cosmetic improvement can be obtained by excising the upper ribs on each side but the stiffness of the neck remains.

Sprengel's shoulder

In the early stages the best treatment is physiotherapy and later excision of the upper part of the scapula, together with division of the muscle fibres, fibrous bands and anomalous bone is the best treatment.

Lumbo-sacral region

There are many diseases which affect the lumbo-sacral region. Of these the most common is myelomeningocele. This is often associated with hydrocephalus, and if left untreated the child develops meningitis and dies. His life can be saved by excision of the meningocele, skin closures, and inserting a Spitz-Holter valve into the ventricles of the brain in order to prevent hydrocephalus. The child will have a varying degree of paralysis of the legs, bladder and bowels, and a severe spinal deformity such as kyphosis, which all require the appropriate treatment (Chapters 16 and 31).

Another common deformity in the lumbo-sacral region is spondylolisthesis with forward slipping of the fifth lumbar vertebra on the first sacral. In extreme cases this may give rise to pressure on nerves. If the symptoms are sufficiently severe the best treatment is a lumbo-sacral fusion; in many patients the most simple measure of wearing a supporting corset is sufficient.

Generalized degenerative disc disease is not uncommon and is known as osteoarthritis, which causes pain and stiffness. This can usually be successfully treated by physiotherapy, weight reduction, improving the abdominal muscles and the wearing of a supporting corset, but occasionally operation is necessary to remove the appropriate disc or fuse the affected area of the spine.

Ankylosing spondylitis

Spondylosis must not be confused with spondylitis which is a generalized

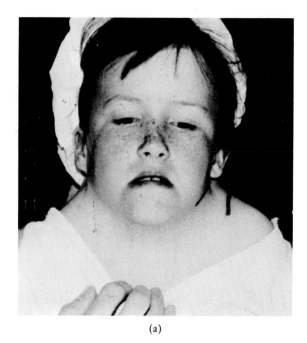

(a)

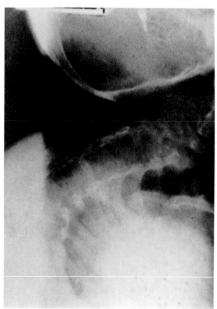

(b)

Fig. 18.11   Patient showing Klippel-Feil syndrome.

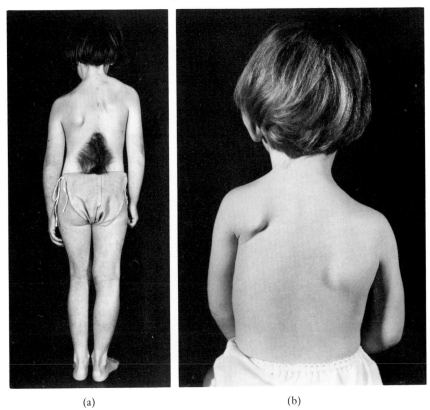

(a)   (b)

Fig. 18.12   (a) and (b) Patients showing congenital elevation of the shoulder
(Sprengel's shoulder).

inflammatory disease of the ligaments and discs, leading to pain, stiffness,
kyphosis and ossification of the ligaments of the spine. In the early stages it
should be treated by analgesics, physiotherapy and exercises.

   If the condition does not respond to this treatment, radiotherapy relieves
the pain but may cause undesirable complications such as leukaemia if it is
repeated. In advanced cases, correction of the deformity by lumbar osteotomy may be required. This disease also causes limitation of rib movements
with the risk of chest infection developing. The disease process may also
spread to the hips, causing stiffening and ultimately bony ankylosis of these
joints. Patients with ankylosing spondylitis are vulnerable to trauma and
even mild trauma can cause a fracture, with displacement and spinal cord
damage.

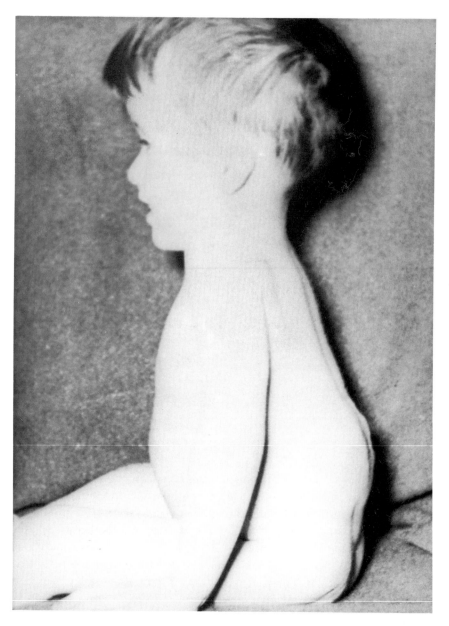

Fig. 18.13   Patient with myelomeningocele.

The nursing management of patients with ankylosing spondylitis

Patients with ankylosing spondylitis have amounts of disability which vary from one patient to another. Those with a mild affection may only have some limitation of bending and may not be aware that they have a lesion; others may be so severely disabled that the whole spine from head to sacrum is fused into an immobile mass; even worse, some patients also have involvement of the hips and shoulders.

The main approach to management is the prevention of extreme deformity and the maintenance of as active a life as is possible with the presence of the disability. All patients with lesser degrees of disability can continue with an occupation and employment and even those with the severest disability can manage some form of money-making activity. Provided the fixed residual deformity is tolerable, many skills can be achieved by the patient. This means that a straight spine with the head in a normal position is preferred to a curved spine with the head fixed horizontally and the line of vision pointing towards the floor. If the patient remains seated constantly in a slumped posture with rounded shoulders, as the condition progresses, this is the inevitable result. The earlier the condition is diagnosed and treated, the better his posture will be in the residual deformity.

The patient must be encouraged to maintain a balance between rest and activity, although normality of daily living is the aim.

1   Patients diagnosed with the earliest stages

The patient is advised to maintain a regime of daily exercises taught by the physiotherapist. In addition to muscle improvement, all the joints are put through their full range of movements, the chest is expanded to its full capacity and bending of the spine to its maximum before full extension and rotation movements are practised.

When sitting, the patient is encouraged to adopt—reflexly—a bolt-upright position without leaning the elbows on the arms of the chair; a high straight chair is better than a low bucket seat type of chair.

When lying down, a hard base to a firm mattress is essential; the habit of sleeping without a pillow, or using only a thin pillow, should be developed.

To prevent flexion deformity of the hips patients should lie prone for half an hour twice daily.

2   Correcting deformity in more advanced stages of the disease

A full plaster of Paris bed, including a head piece, is made as in Chapter 30, p. 306. When dry, it is reinforced with strips of malleable metal passing over the apex of the curve; these strips are bolted through the plaster and the plaster shell is then cut from side to side so that the metal strips serve as a crude stiff hinge. The head portion is weighted with a block of wood attached to it. The bed is then mounted on a stand with the upper portion free of the stand and unsupported. Blocks of wood of various depths are supplied to support the upper portion of the bed as the patient rests on it. The bed is lined as described in Chapter 30, p. 535.

Such a bed may be divided at any level or in more than one place. The objective is to reduce the degree of deformity before the patient's spine fuses into an unacceptable position. The patient spends much of his time on the bed but must be removed from it for some time of the day for physiotherapy.

3   Operative correction

Late treatment includes osteotomy of the spine to improve posture; this may be at the cervical or the lumbar level. The lumbar operation is used whenever possible as it is much safer. Other forms of surgery may be necessary, including arthroplasty of the hips.

Complications of ankylosing spondylitis

   (i)   Limitation of all movements and postures.

   (ii)   Reduction of respiratory volume and the vital vapacity.

   (iii)   Inability to carry out the normal evasive movements to protect the head and neck in falling, so that these are vulnerable to injury.

   (iv)   Difficulty in looking towards the front; vision is usually directed downwards.

   (v)   Severe muscle wasting mainly on the posterior aspects of the body; this may be caused either by disuse atrophy or nerve root compression.

   (vi)   The spine is very vulnerable to trauma.

   (vii)   Iritis is not uncommon.

   (viii)   The condition also affects the heart valves and the aorta.

   (ix)   Doubtless many other problems exist which only the patient with a rigid spine could enumerate.

Osteoporosis

Osteoporosis is very common in older women after the menopause, making them liable to fractures even with relatively slight trauma. There is some evidence that hormone treatment given in the very early stages decreases the osteoporosis. Calcium and vitamin D tablets are advised.

Deformities of the spine in systematic conditions

The bones of the spine are also subject to the same disease processes as bones elsewhere in the body, in particular, Paget's disease, rickets and fragilitis ossium may cause pain and deformity. In older patients, softening of the bones due to osteoporosis or osteomalacia may lead to kyphosis and pain. Also, secondary malignant tumours often develop in the spine.

19

Deformities of the Hip Joints

Relevant applied anatomy and physiology

The hips, like the knees, receive the total weight of the body above the level of the joint during locomotion. As one leg is used to propel the body forward onto the other leg, the whole body weight is accepted by the limb on the ground. In fact, in running, the thrust through the joint may reach four times the body weight. When standing on both legs the weight of the body is divided between the limbs. The heavier the weight of the body the greater the weight borne by the hip joints and knee joints.

The mechanical stresses applied to a ball and socket joint impinge from different directions according to the posture of the body. When the posture of the body is a good one the hip joint withstands the stresses easily throughout the life of the individual; most people have no hip joint problems. If the posture is bad, however, the stresses applied to the joint arrive repeatedly and constantly from an abnormal direction and the strain on the joint can affect its efficiency. Thus distortion or stiffness of the vertebral column, disorder of the joint on the opposite side, severe postural distortion of the trunk, or paralysis, can affect the efficiency of a joint of the lower limb. Serious obesity is a factor in applying abnormal stresses to the weight-bearing joints.

The structure of the hip joint

The hip joint is formed by the articulation of the pelvis with the femur. The pelvis presents a deep cavity (the acetabulum) which receives a ball-shaped head arranged on the neck of the femur.

The socket, the acetabulum, is further deepened by a lip of fibrocartilage called the labrum which fits snugly around the base of the head of the femur to improve the strength of the joint. There is a pad of fat in the floor of the socket.

A ligament connects the head of the femur to the acetabular rim, within

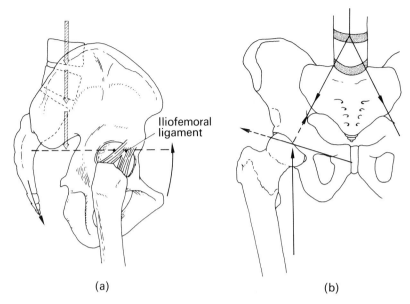

(a)   (b)

Fig. 19.1   (a) A normal hip. (b) Directions of the stresses operative during standing.

this ligament (ligamentum teres) an arterial supply and venous return serve the head of the femur; other blood vessels enter the neck of the femur at its base and pass up the neck towards the head.

The joint capsule

As the joint is an important weight-bearing joint the capsule must be strong. It is composed of a fibrous sheath, which arises around the margins of the acetabulum and then passes downwards to be inserted around the base of the neck of the femur. It is further supported by (a) a layer of extracapsular ligaments and (b) a cuff of muscles exterior to the extracapsular ligaments. The efficiency of the joint depends upon this cuff of muscles; if these are paralysed the hip is unstable and may be easily dislocated.

Trendelenburg's sign

If a normal person stands on one leg the fold of the buttock on the opposite side rises due to the gluteus medius muscle of the weight-bearing leg contracting and tilting the pelvis towards the side on which he stands (Fig. 19.2a). If there is instability of the hip—for example, with a dislocation, fracture of the neck of the femur, paralysis of the abductor muscles, coxa

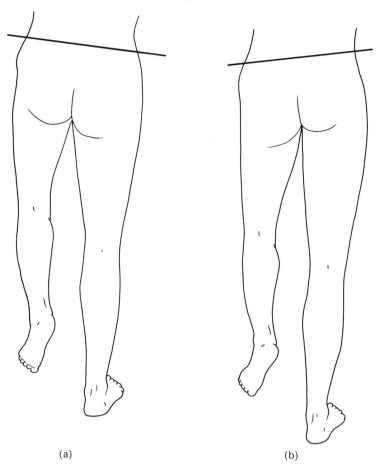

(a)   (b)

Fig. 19.2   Trendelenburg's sign (a) Negative: normal. (b) Positive: abnormal.

vara, or a fixed adduction deformity, then instead of the opposite buttock
rising it falls; this is known as a positive Trendelenburg sign (Fig. 19.2b).

Thomas' sign
If there is a fixed flexion deformity of the hip this may be masked by an
increased lumbar lordosis. Therefore, in testing for flexion deformity the
patient should lie flat on a firm couch; the opposite hip is then flexed until the
lumbar spine is straight—this is ascertained by the examiner feeling that the
whole of the lumbar spine is flat on the couch. Any residual flexion of the
affected hip is then easily seen and measured.

Congenital dislocation of the hip

Congenital dislocation of the hip is one of the most serious hip disorders and is more common in girls. It can usually be recognized in the neonatal period if the baby is carefully examined. Two different tests are used, as a preliminary screening test the hip is examined for laxity. In a lax hip the head of the femur can be felt and heard to slip over the rim of the acetabulum when the flexed hip is abducted and adducted.

Most lax hips become stable particularly if the abducted position is maintained by double nappies or an extra plastic nappy (Craig Splint). If, however, it is found that there is limitation of adduction then there is considerable risk of sublaxation and dislocation developing. In this case full plaster fixation in abduction is indicated.

A few years ago it was hoped that the neonatal diagnosis and treatment of all babies with lax hips would eliminate congenital dislocation of the hip. Unfortunately, this has not been found to be completely effective, probably because there are two types of congenital dislocation of the hip: (1) the lax joint type, which can become normal especially if the neonatal hips are splinted in abduction, and (2) the dystrophic type in which there is failure of development of the acetabulum. This latter type does not usually reveal itself at birth but it becomes more marked as the child grows. If the diagnosis is made at an early age and treatment, i.e. fixation in abduction, is given, this may stimulate the acetabulum to grow normally, but if the child is already walking before the diagnosis is made conservative treatment is less effective and open reduction is often indicated. This takes two main forms; one by an approach from the medial aspect, the adductor muscles, psoas tendon and infero-medial capsule of the hip joint are divided, thus enabling the head of the femur to sink deeply into the acetabular socket without fixation.

Alternatively, some surgeons recommend a lateral approach and removal of the internal portion of the capsule known as the limbus, which they believe is a hindrance to normal development of the acetabulum. At a later age if the acetabulum is not developing properly reconstruction may be necessary. There are three main types of procedure:

1   An osteotomy of the pelvis which is above the acetabulum with the medial displacement of the inferior fragment which produces an effective deepening of the acetabulum (Chiari) (Fig. 19.3).

2   An osteotomy of the pelvis at the same level but with rotation of the lower fragment, the fragment being held in place by inserting a bone graft between the upper and lower parts of the pelvis and transversing the bone with Kuntscher wires (Salter).

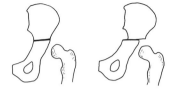

Fig. 19.3   Pelvic osteotomy of Chiari

3   The construction of an enlarged acetabular roof or shelf by partially dividing the ilium and turning down a flap of external cortex from the ilium over the femoral head.

All these procedures give considerable improvement both in appearance and function. It is not known for certain whether they delay the onset of osteoarthritis in later life nor is there any evidence at the moment which of them is the most effective.

The newly born

At this stage the hip is not truly dislocated but the capsule is lax and the hip can easily be subluxated. There is also usually some difficulty in fully abducting the hip. The test for subluxation is to flex the hip and then gently abduct the legs; if the joint capsule is lax the head of the femur subluxates posteriorly

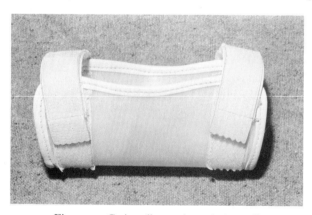

Fig. 19.4   Craig splint, or leg-splaying splint.

in flexion and adduction (Fig. 19.5a). As the flexed leg is abducted the head of the femur can be felt to slip over the posterior rim of the acetabulum as it enters the hip socket. If this sign is present the child should be kept with her legs fully abducted for at least three months; one of the most convenient methods is to apply the so-called Craig splint (Fig. 19.4) over the baby's nappies. Other splints have been devised with the same purpose but are slightly less convenient. If the instability of the hip is diagnosed early, the majority of cases become perfectly normal with this treatment, but occasionally either this does not happen, or the condition has not been diagnosed at birth. A valuable sign that all is not well is limitation of abduction. This is an indication for plaster fixation. Under these circumstances a limp will be noticed when the child first walks and in addition, the affected leg will be shorter and slightly externally rotated.

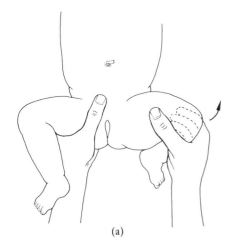

(a)

Fig. 19.5   (a) Barlow's test for abduction of flexed hip.

(b) Child in double hip-plaster (frog plaster).

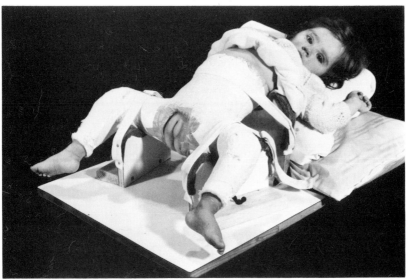

(b)

The toddler

It is not easy to detect a limp in a toddler as her gait is a little unstable anyway, but again, careful examination of the limbs will show if there is limitation of abduction and also that if the examiner presses on the leg when the knee and hip are flexed, an up and down movement of the leg in relation to the pelvis can be felt—this is known as telescoping. However, the diagnosis must be confirmed by X-ray.

In a nine month to two year old child the best treatment at this stage is to apply traction (see Chapter 28, p. 472) to the leg for some two or three weeks and then to reduce the hip by a closed reduction—i.e. by abducting the flexed hip. Reduction must be confirmed radiologically. The hip is then maintained in the abducted position by a double hip spica (Fig. 19.5b) for some nine months until the acetabulum has grown to a normal shape. Occasionally it is impossible to reduce the hip, or the acetabulum fails to develop and, under these circumstances open operation may be required. Operation is also usually required in the older child in whom the condition has not been diagnosed until she has been walking for some months.

The obstacles to reduction of a congenital dislocation of the hip are many; there may be tightness of the psoas muscle, tightness of the external rotator muscles of the hip, a large ligamentum teres, an ingrowth of fibro–fatty tissue into the floor of the acetabulum, or inturning of the cartilaginous labrum (a limbus) which normally forms the rim of the acetabulum. The acetabulum may be small and shallow and the head of the femur is too big to fit into it, or there may be a forward inclination of the femoral neck (anteversion) (Fig. 19.6b).

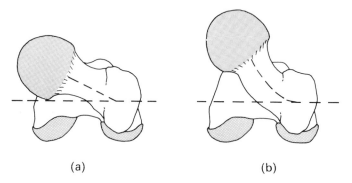

(a)   (b)

Fig. 19.6   Anteversion of femoral head and neck.
   (a) Normal; angle of plane through head, neck and great trochanter is 0–30 degrees to plane through condyles.
   (b) Anteversion; angle greater than 30 degrees.

If any of these conditions are present, closed reduction is unlikely to be successful and operative reduction will be necessary. The hip is exposed and the cause, or causes, of the persisting dislocation are established and treated. For example, tight muscles are divided, a thickened ligamentum teres is excised, and so on. It is then noticed whether there is any anteversion of the neck of the femur and the position in which the hip is most stable is ascertained. A double hip spica is then applied with the leg in this position. If there has been gross anteversion of the neck of the femur it may be necessary to perform a corrective osteotomy at a later date, but with the proper treatment anteversion usually corrects itself.

The older child and the adult
In older patients with unreduced dislocation of the hip (especially with a bilateral dislocation of the hip) operative intervention is more likely to do more harm than good and it is usually wise to leave the hips in the dislocated position. Indeed, many patients with bilateral dislocation of the hips have relatively few symptoms—at least until they are well past middle age. If the patient has bilateral dislocation of the hip and one is reduced, she is left with unequal legs—that is, she is worse off than if she had never been treated. Also, partial reduction of a dislocated hip is more likely to lead to painful arthritis at a comparatively young age than if the hip is left dislocated. However, if the hip has been reduced but the acetabulum fails to develop, then an operation to construct a deep acetabulum is necessary. There are many ways of achieving this but the best known and longest established method is by forming a bony shelf above the head of the femur. When and if pain becomes severe hip replacements by prostheses are advised.

The nursing management of infants with congenital dislocation of the hip

The newly born
If a dislocation of the hip is diagnosed in the infant soon after birth the results of treatment are better than if the condition is missed and treatment is not commenced until the child is older. Once the head of the femur is in its normal position, natural growth will occur.

The young infant is nursed with the thighs in complete abduction and external rotation on a suitable appliance; examples of these are:
1   Craig splint (Fig. 19.4, p. 308).
2   Fredjka splint (Fig. 19.7, p. 312).

3   Von Rosen splint (Fig. 19.8, p. 313).
4   Barlow splint (Fig. 19.9, p. 313).

The Craig splint and Fredjka splint. These are applied over the infant's diapers or napkins. They are removed for bathing and replacing soiled napkins and re-applied immediately afterwards.

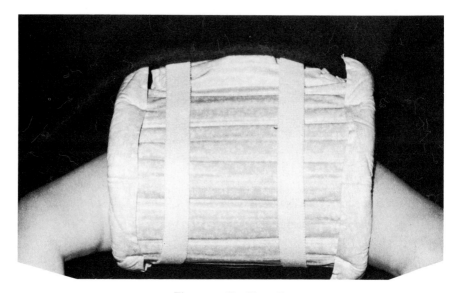

Fig. 19.7   Fredjka splint.

The Barlow splint and Von Rosen splint. These are malleable metal splints with a washable plastic covering, which hold the infant firmly and constantly with the hips in the abducted and externally rotated position. They are applied directly to the skin of the infant and are moulded to the circumference of the thighs and to the shoulders. They are applied in the hospital and the infant's mother can then take her baby home to care for her in the splint, and bring her back to a future clinic. The mother must be instructed as follows:
1   The splint is *not* removed from the infant. Bathing, washing, changing clothing are managed with the splint *in situ*.
2   To note the condition of the infant's skin. The splint must not cut into the flesh at any point. To check, when the Barlow splint is used, that there is no 'scissoring' effect behind the neck.
3   To note that the splint is serving its function. A fit and lively infant may wriggle out of the splint.

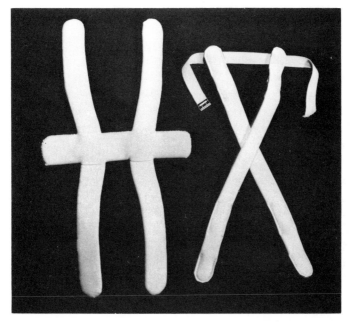

Fig. 19.8 Von Rosen splint.   Fig. 19.9 Barlow splint.

4 To note that the splint is large enough and that the infant has not grown too large for it.

5 To return the infant to the hospital if she has any doubts about the splintage.

If all is well the splint is discarded before the infant is three months old. This is considered to be the ideal way to deal with congenital dislocation of the hip; it depends, however, upon diagnosis of the condition within a day or so of the infant's birth. An obstetrical course for nurses should include instruction on the method of testing the hips of newly born infants.

The older infant
Once growth and ossification occurs around the hips with development of adjacent musculature, reduction of the dislocated hip is a more serious problem. Abduction and traction is first applied to reduce the dislocation to be followed by prolonged immobilisation.

Traction—(a) *Alvik traction.* This is a method of applying reduction traction to the hips without completely immobilising the infant on a frame (Fig. 28.17). The child has a greater range of mobility and can be turned laterally or prone without the traction force being affected. It is described in Chapter 28.

(b) *Traction on a double abduction frame with a (C) shaped cross-bar* (Fig. 28.3; also Chapter 28). The principles of this form of traction used to reduce the dislocation are:

1   To abduct the thighs by gradually increasing amounts, whilst maintaining traction longitudinally along both legs. Each thigh is abducted to 90 degrees.

2   To apply a cross pull on the affected hip, to pull the head of the femur into the acetabulum.

The double abduction frame (sometimes called a divaricator) consists of two longitudinal bars which extend from the nipple line to extension bows 150 cm beyond the feet of the patient; these bars are jointed at the level of the hips and each of the leg portions of the bars can be locked firmly into varying degrees of abduction. The frame also has:

(a) Nipple bars which are hinged to fit around the patient's thorax.

(b) Pelvic bars which are hinged to fit around the patient's pelvis.

(c) An abducting bar which is shaped into an arc of a circle on to which the leg bars can be locked.

(d) Knock knee bars to which the legs can be padded and bandaged to prevent a knock knee deformity.

(e) A saddle of soft leather filled with animal wool upon which the trunk and thighs of the patient rest. This is supplied with the leg pieces abducted to 45 degrees.

Preparation

The child is measured for the frame and saddle. Until these are supplied the traction is maintained by Pugh's method (Chapter 28, p. 479). The measurements required are:

For the frame:

(a) From the nipple line to the gluteal fold.

(b) From the gluteal fold to 4 cm above the external malleolus.

(c) Around the nipple line plus 5 cm to allow for the saddle depth.

For the saddle

(a) From the spinous process at the base of the back of the neck to the tip of the coccygeal vertebra.

(b) From the coccyx to the level of the tibial plateau.

(c) One third measurement (c) of the frame measurement.

Sometimes it is preferred to order two saddles; one with the leg pieces at 45 degrees and one with the leg pieces at 90 degrees to the mid-line. This makes the provision of saddles very costly as the infant is kept on the frame for a limited time only. If reduction by this method is not achieved within a reasonable time (four to six weeks) surgical reduction is usually undertaken.

Method of application

After bathing the child, extensions are applied to the legs as in Chapter 28 p. 472 if the Pugh's traction extensions need replacement. The infant is then lifted onto the saddle and this is checked for size and level of fixation. The upper margin of the saddle should be at the level of the base of the neck when the leg pieces terminate at the level of the ends of the femora. The saddle width should not extend beyond the sides of the infant's trunk.

The leg bars of the abduction frame are fixed at 20 degrees from the mid-line. It is often preferred to cover the metal of the abduction frame with 2·5 cm wide strips of old linen bandaging before use. The infant is lifted onto the frame; the level of the saddle and patient are correctly adjusted and the saddle is fixed to the frame by its tapes. The extensions are firmly tied to the extensions bows, and the nipple and pelvic bars (guarded with leather sheaths) are closed over the front of the patient's trunk. Manual traction on the legs is maintained for the whole duration of this manoeuvre.

The cross bar of the frame is now attached by traction cord to the foot of the cot; the lower legs of the cot are now elevated onto blocks. This is to provide counter-traction as the child's body now tends to slide away from the extension bows towards the bed head.

The legs are padded against the knock knee bars and the legs bandaged with calico bandages to the knock knee bars. The ankles and feet are left free for exercise.

Gradual increase in divarication now begins; a few degrees each day on each leg until each leg is about 40 degrees from the mid-line. Cross pull now commences to pull the head of the femur into the acetabulum on the affected side.

A small padded gutter splint is applied to the lateral surface of the affected thigh; this must not extend up too far towards the hip or down too far towards the knee. A strong piece of calico is now passed over the centre of this splint and is tied off onto the opposite side of the frame. Medial rotation of the femur is to be achieved as well as downwards pull on the femoral head.

After the cross pull has been applied the divarication is continued until each leg is abducted to 90 degrees or until the surgeon decides that it is adequate.

Nursing routine

The child must be maintained in a state of scrupulous cleanliness even though she is not habit trained. The saddle is liable to soiling and a diaper should be arranged to protect this.

As the latter stages of divarication are reached the child may become fretful; this should be reported, but the main essence of management is kindliness, sympathy, and mothering.

Maintenance of reduction

When the dislocation has been reduced—either by Alvik traction or traction on a double abduction frame, or surgically—the hips are held immobilized in the divaricated position by the use of splintage such as a Denis Browne dislocation of the hip splint or the Putti-Forrester-Browne splint (Fig. 19.10), or by the use of a frog plaster or a Batchelor plaster. Alternatively, the head of the femur can be pulled down by a Thomas' splint until it is opposite the acetabulum. Under anaesthesia the hip is then reduced by abducting the leg and after radiological confirmation, a double hip spica is applied.

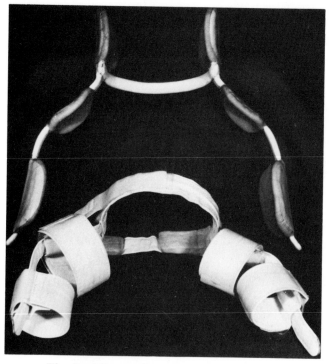

Fig. 19.10 The Putti-Forester-Browne splint (*top*) for older children, (*bottom*) for tiny infants.

Frog plaster. The use of a frog plaster (see Fig. 19.5) has the advantage that the patient's mother can manage the care of her own child at home. Given tolerance and the use of various devices such as the 'Plowden perch' (Fig. 19.11) (devised by Miss M. H. Plowden when she was Ward sister of the infants' ward at the Robert Jones and Agnes Hunt Orthopaedic Hospital, Oswestry, Shropshire, England) for supporting the infant either in the

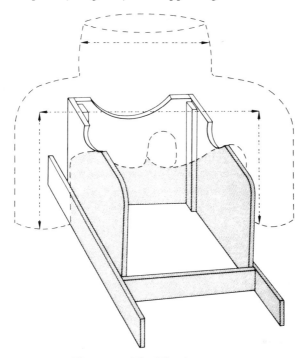

Fig. 19.11   The 'Plowden perch'.

upright position for defaecation, or when feeding, or when recumbent for sleeping. Other useful devices include carts with small castors for wheels to enable the child to propel herself around the floor. The mother can also carry her child when out of the home on visits or on public transport.

The frog plaster consists of a bilateral hip spica which extends from the nipple line to 4 cm above the malleoli of the ankles. The hips are held in the divaricated position and the knees are flexed. The hip spica is applied with the child supported on a hip prop and with the head and shoulders on pillows.

Wool roll is used to make a layer of wool over the skin of the area to be covered by plaster. The first bandages are applied in figure-of-eight patterns around the pelvis and thighs on both sides. These first layers are then extended up and down to cover the whole area of the frog plaster. These first layers are then reinforced by long slabs which strengthen the sides of the spica and the lateral surfaces of the leg pieces. The edges of the plaster are then trimmed and finished.

The genital area of the spica is vulnerable. It must be as narrow as possible to give strength to the area but this makes it liable to soiling, by faeces or urine, which is most unpleasant for the patient and her attendants. The area may be protected by incorporating a layer of polythene sheeting on the top surface of the plaster, or by the use of a fibre glass coating.

Batchelor plaster. This consists of full length leg plasters applied over wool roll with the knees partially flexed. The hips are held in the abducted and internally rotated position and the two leg plasters are connected to each other by a bar of wood which is incorporated into the plaster.

Rehabilitation
As the limbs of the child are immobilized for a long time (usually at least nine months), it is necessary to carry out a planned programme of physiotherapy to re-educate all the muscles of the hips and legs.

Coxa vara

Another congenital disorder of the hips is coxa vara. Normally the neck and shaft of the femur makes an angle of about 120 degrees, but if this is reduced it is called coxa vara (Fig. 19.12). The condition is characterized by

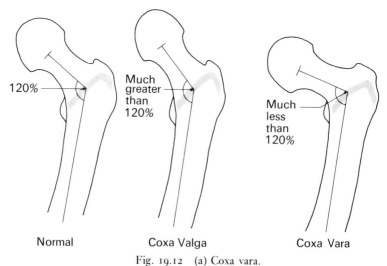

Fig. 19.12   (a) Coxa vara.

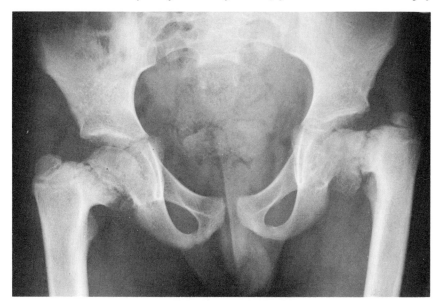

Fig. 19.12   (b) Radiograph of coxa vara.

limitation of abduction, instability of the hip and a positive Trendelenburg sign.

Coxa vara, if severe, should be treated by a cuneiform osteotomy (Fig. 6.1c), excising a segment of bone, after which the bones can be either fixed in position by a small nail-plate or the patient is treated on a double abduction frame. Mild degrees of coxa vara do not necessarily require any treatment and may be part of a more generalised musculo-skeletal syndrome. In addition, coxa vara may be associated with congenital shortening of the femur. This may be severe and lead to marked disability, but unfortunately for this type there is no known effective treatment (Fig. 19.13).

Osteochondritis (or Perthes' disease) (Fig. 19.14)

Between the ages of five and ten years it is not uncommon for changes to occur in the head of the femur leading to pain and limitation of hip movement. These changes are in the nature of an osteochondritis and are usually attributable to ischaemia of the head of the femur. They may also occur in a congenital dislocation of the hip following reduction. The clinical features are limping, muscle spasm and limitation of abduction and internal rotation.

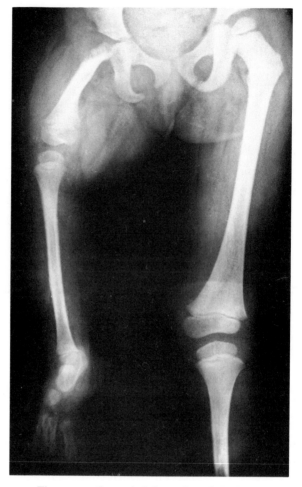

Fig. 19.13 Congenital shortening of the femur.

The earliest radiological sign is an increase in density of the head of the femur. This is followed by fragmentation, flattening of the head of the femur and changes in the metaphysis, namely, broadening of the metaphysis and the formation of cysts in the metaphysis. If untreated, the head of the femur becomes mushroom-shaped and deformed, there is permanent limitation of abduction and rotation and later degenerative changes occur in the articular cartilage.

Treatment usually consists of relieving the hip of weight-bearing until restoration of normal bony structure occurs. This may be achieved by putting

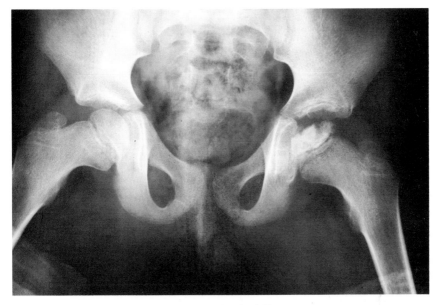

Fig. 19.14   (a) Perthes' disease.

the patient to bed with traction on the affected leg, by giving him a weight-relieving caliper with a patten on the opposite foot (Fig. 19.16), by giving him a pair of crutches and preventing him using the leg, by the application of a sling, or by applying a 'broomstick' plaster (Fig. 19.15).

In general, the prognosis for Perthes' disease in young children is good, but in the older child it is not so good. There is considerable disagreement among surgeons about how much treatment affects the ultimate result. Although a large number of operations have been suggested for the treatment of Perthes' disease so far none have been proved to be consistently sucessful.

The nursing management of children with Perthes' disease

As already stated the approach to treatment for these patients depends upon (a) the age of the patient, (b) the stage at which the condition is diagnosed and (c) the opinion of the surgeon. Some patients are managed in bed without traction, some are lightly fixed in bed on Pugh's traction or weight and pulley traction (see Chapter 28); some are firmly fixed on a double abduction frame, some with broomstick plasters, some are ambulant with a leg sling and crutches and some are ambulant with a weight-relieving patten-ended caliper.

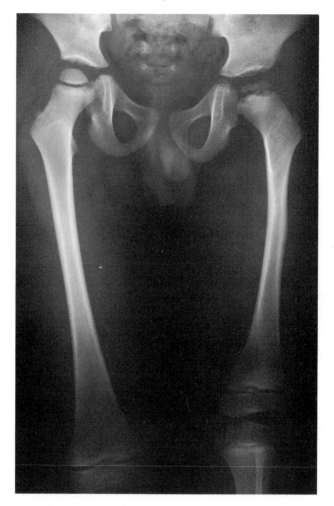

Fig. 19.14 (b) Short leg with osteochondritis of hip.

Traction using a Jones' double abduction frame. This has already been described on p. 314 of this chapter. The only variations from that description are that this frame is larger in size to suit an older patient, that the cross bar is straight with holes at 2·5 cm intervals to provide the increase in abduction, and that a groin strap is used to apply counter-traction to the extensions on the leg. The measurements are also the same as those stated on p. 314.

The patient is nursed on Pugh's traction until the frame and saddle are made and supplied. Once these are available, the patient is lifted carefully by a

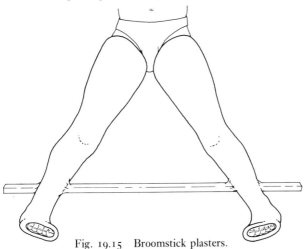

Fig. 19.15   Broomstick plasters.

team of nurses onto the saddle and then onto the frame. During this time the traction on the affected leg must be maintained; this is done by one helper supporting the axillae of the patient whilst another applies firm manual traction along the length of the affected leg with one hand behind the heel of the patient, along tendo calcaneum, and the other over the forefoot of the patient; the foot is held at right angles to the leg.

The manual traction must be maintained until the extensions are tied and the groin strap is applied to the *unaffected* hip. Thus the patient is on fixed traction with traction applied by the skin extensions and counter-traction by the groin strap.

Care of the groin strap and groin. The groin strap is moulded into an arc during manufacture and is composed of a tube of soft leather sewn with the seam away from the skin and filled with animal wool. It must be kept in the curved shape; to straighten it will crack the leather. The leather is kept soft with saddle soap which is applied regularly once weekly. The groin strap or skin extensions are not removed unless manual traction is first applied. A second groin strap is kept in reserve and this is used to replace the one to be cleaned and saddle soaped.

The groin is a delicate area of skin which requires special care when a groin strap (or the ring of a Thomas' splint) is in position. The skin under the groin strap is regularly washed with soap and water, rinsed, dried and rubbed with surgical spirit or a barrier cream to harden it, and lightly powdered with talc. Care is taken not to wet the groin strap with either water or methylated spirit and it is held up off the skin during this procedure.

Other comments. Although the nipple bars are fitted and fastened, some surgeons permit the release of the nipple bar so that the child can lift the thorax off the saddle.

Constant supervision of any patient on an abduction frame is essential. The position of the trunk, the alignment of the pelvis, the position of the legs, the feet, the saddle and the tension of the extension cords must be inspected at least twice daily. The bandages on the legs are removed and re-applied daily.

Thomas' patten-ended calipers. These may be used to relieve weight-bearing on the affected hip.

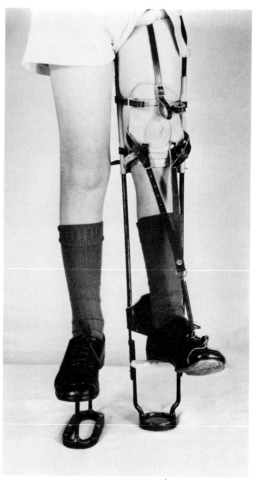

Fig. 19.16 Thomas' patten-ended caliper and raised shoe.

Broomstick plasters. Long leg plasters are applied over stockinette covered by wool roll, with the stockinette turned back over the ends of the plaster. If the feet are not to be included, the knees are flexed to 30 degrees. Should the feet be included, the knees are flexed to 5 degrees. A broomstick covered in plaster of Paris bandage is fixed to the calf of each leg plaster. The degree of abduction and rotation are adjusted on fixing the broomstick with plaster bandage.

The objective in applying broomstick plasters is to keep the child from applying weight to the hips whilst allowing a wide range of movement and activity. Often the child can go to his home instead of being confined to bed in hospital. He can often manage to get to school on special wheeled appliances, provided there is tolerance of this at the school.

Slipping upper femoral epiphysis (Fig. 19.17)

Following the pre-adolescent growth spurt, relative weakening of the periosteum occurs in relation to the speed of growth and increase of the patient's weight. This may give rise to the syndrome of slipping upper femoral epiphysis which is specially common either in very fat or very tall children and may be associated with endocrine disturbances. The condition presents in one of three ways.

First of all there may be chronic aching pain in the hip with a gradual development of a limp, adduction and external rotation of the leg, with limitation of abduction and internal rotation. Secondly, following a short period of such symptoms a minor injury such as a stumble, may precipitate severe pain in the leg with inability to walk. The patient is found to have a short adducted and externally rotated leg; this is the so-called acute-on-chronic syndrome (Fig. 19.17). Lastly, on rare occasions, a major injury may lead to fracture-separation of the femoral epiphysis. This is equivalent to a fracture of the neck of the femur in older patients.

Following an acute episode, an attempt may be made to reduce the displaced epiphysis, either by gentle traction or by gentle manipulation under an anaesthetic. If it is possible to reduce the epiphysis then it is usually fixed in place by the insertion of four pins up the neck of the femur (Fig. 19.17). Similarly if the displacement of the epiphysis is slight then it should be prevented from slipping further by fixing it with multiple small pins or nails. If, however, it is impossible to reduce the displaced epiphysis, either due to delay or because the onset has been slow and insidious, and the epiphysis has become fixed in its new position, the surgeon has two alternatives. Either he may proceed to reduce the displaced epiphysis by open reduction, or he may perform a corrective osteotomy in the intertrochanteric region. For most

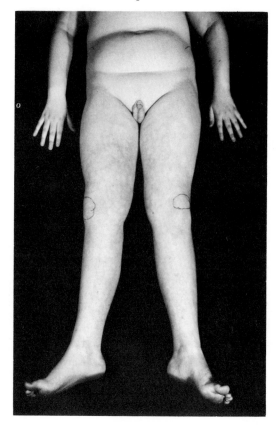

Fig. 19.17 (a) Patient with slipped upper femoral epiphysis.

surgeons the latter is the safer procedure and will give rise to a limb which is normal in appearance but slightly limited in movement, but in expert hands open reduction of the displaced epiphysis will yield an excellent result. All methods of treatment are associated with the danger of damage to the blood supply and of avascular necrosis leading to a stiff and painful hip and degenerative arthritis. Therefore, forcible manipulation or operations which may endanger the blood supply to the upper femoral epiphysis are to be avoided.

Acute infections of the hip joint

These are not uncommon in the neonatal period due to a septicaemia associated with sepsis of the umbilical cord. The child is 'off colour', pyrexial, loses appetite and weight, but often only the keen observer will

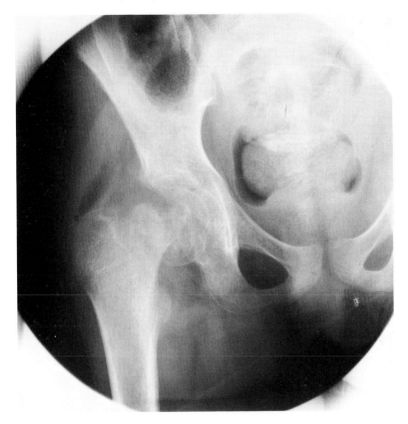

Fig. 19.17   (b) Radiograph of slipped upper femoral epiphysis.

detect that the hip is affected. Sometimes the first local sign is of redness and swelling and even of discharge of a small abscess from behind the greater trochanter. If, however, the condition is diagnosed before this because there is evidence of the hip joint being painful and the hip muscles are in spasm, then this condition should be treated by operation or open drainage of the hip joint and the institution of antibiotics. If diagnosed at this early stage, the prognosis is good, but if the diagnosis is delayed, serious consequences follow.

Sometimes, due to distention of the joint capsule, the hip dislocates, in which case it must be reduced and held in position—for example, by traction on a frame. If the infection is not recognised in time there will be extensive destruction of the head of the femur (Fig. 19.19) leading to permanent shortening, adduction and instability of the hip joint. As delay is so serious it

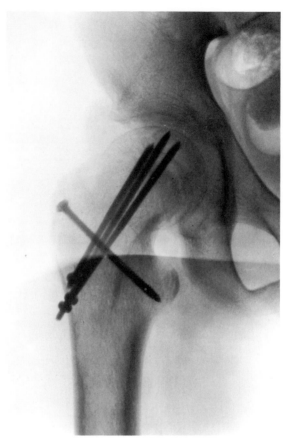

Fig. 19.17   (c) Radiograph of slipped upper femoral epiphysis, with four pins
in neck femur.

is wiser in a suspected hip infection to 'look and see' rather than 'wait and
see'.

Infections of the hip joint may occur in older patients as part of a septicaemia but, as the patient complains of pain in the hip and can draw his
parents' attention to it, diagnosis is easier: the condition should be treated
as for septic infection of any other joint (see Chapter 13).

Chronic infection of the hip joint

The most common chronic infection is tuberculosis (Fig. 19.20). This is
insidious in onset, causing pain—especially at night, a limp and ultimately

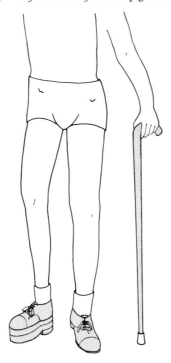

Fig. 19.18   Externally rotated leg in patient with osteo-arthritis.

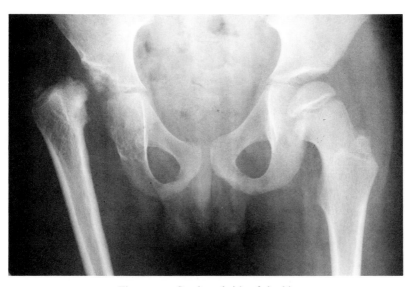

Fig. 19.19   Septic arthritis of the hip.

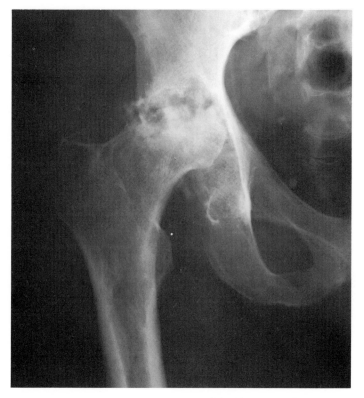

Fig. 19.20 Destructive arthritis of the hip (tuberculosis).

limitation of abduction and extension. If untreated, the limb will become shortened, adducted, flexed and internally rotated. In the early stages the treatment is by antibiotics, chemotherapy and, if necessary, synovectomy. Indeed, in order to establish the diagnosis at an early stage, biopsy of the synovial membrane is often necessary.

At a later stage if there has been destruction of the joint treatment will either be by arthrodesis of the joint or, in younger children, by corrective osteotomy to correct any deformity (see Chapter 14).

Rheumatoid arthritis of the hip joint

Rheumatoid arthritis of the hip may present in a very similar way. Usually there will be signs of other joints being affected, but occasionally rheumatoid arthritis of the hip is monarticular for a considerable period when the

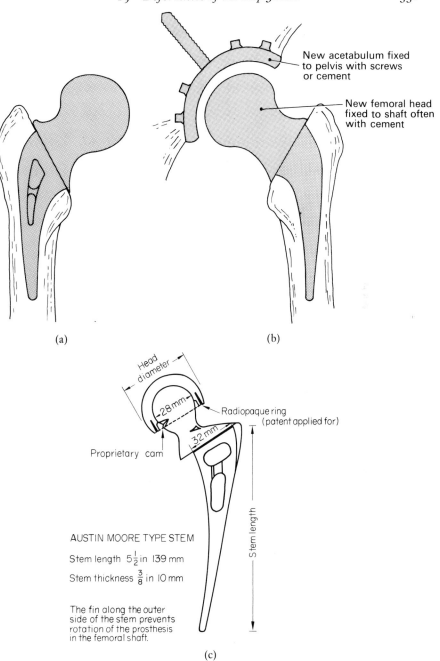

Fig. 19.21   (a) An Austin-Moore prosthesis. (b) Principles of total hip replacement.

differential diagnosis from tuberculosis may be very difficult. Monarticular 'rheumatic' involvement of the hip is not uncommon in children. Apart from the systematic treatment for the rheumatoid arthritis, it may be necessary on occasions to restore movement to a stiff hip. This can best be achieved either by excision of the head and neck of the femur—the so-called Girdlestone operation—or by replacement arthroplasty (Fig. 19.21a). (See also Chapter 14.)

Ankylosing spondylitis of the hip joint

Ankylosing spondylitis is primarily a disease which causes stiffness of the spine and ossification of the spinal ligaments: the exact aetiology is unknown, but the ankylosing process may spread to the hips, ultimately causing stiffness of the hips and bony ankylosis. If this is a serious disability to the patient, movement can be restored as in rheumatoid arthritis—that is, either by excision of the head and neck of femur or by a replacement arthroplasty (see also Chapter 14.

Chronic degenerative arthrosis or osteoarthritis of the hip joint

Two forms are recognized: the first, or primary form, is when there has been no preceding disease or abnormality of the hip. This appears to be a genetic condition. It may be associated with osteoarthritis in other joints. There is also the secondary form where it is known that the patient has had previous disease—for example, congenital subluxation, Perthes' disease, slipping upper femoral epiphysis, dislocation of the hip, or infection. The dominant symptom is, of course, pain, but here there are two main syndromes: there is the pain-at-night syndrome and the pain-on-activity syndrome. It is not understood why there should be two different syndromes or the exact underlying pathological causes.

In addition there will be restriction of movement—particularly of abduction, internal rotation and extension. Ultimately the hip will become stiff in a flexed, adducted and externally rotated position, and the patient will be unable to put on his own shoes and socks, cut his toe nails, etc.

Treatment in the early stages is usually conservative—namely, weight reduction, physiotherapy, analgesic drugs, advising the patient to use a stick and to have a slight raise on his shoe. If, however, in spite of this the condition is progressive, then operation is usually advisable. In the fairly early stages while the hip is still mobile, intertrochanteric osteotomy with internal fixation is still a very successful operation particularly in young patients (Fig. 19.22). Previously it was necessary to immobilize the patient in a plaster spica following an intertrochanteric osteotomy. This had the disadvantage that the hip might become stiff and there might also be permanent stiffness of the knee and therefore recovery was slow, but nowadays, providing the bone is of good texture and infection can be avoided, the results of internal fixation are very good and the patient does not need to stay in bed for any prolonged period; the risks of knee stiffness and increasing hip stiffness are minimal and, in fact, the range of hip movement is usually improved. If, however, the disease is advanced and the hip has already become stiff, a total replacement arthroplasty is indicated.

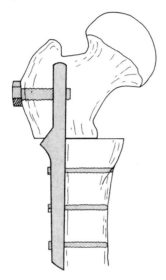

Fig. 19.22   Intertrochanteric osteotomy of the femur, with internal fixation.

The relevant nursing management of patients with osteoarthritis of the hip joint

The patient with osteoarthritis of the hip who enters hospital for treatment is most likely to have a surgical operation. The pre-operative preparation of the patient is similar to that of any other orthopaedic patient and this is discussed in Chapter 27. The patient is often someone who has suffered severe pain over a period of months or years and is relieved that something positive is about to be done to help her. A few days spent in the ward before operation will help her to orientate herself to the ward atmosphere and to meet other patients and staff; this period also enables her to rest from work and responsibility. A full clinical examination is required and her general health improved if this is possible.

Post-operative management

This is related to what has been done for the patient. The post-operative management of the patient who has undergone an osteotomy of the femur with internal fixation is different from that of the patient who has had an arthroplasty with total hip replacement.

Displacement osteotomy of the femur with
internal fixation (see Fig. 19.22)

In this operation the upper end of the femur is detached from the shaft and then re-attached in a new alignment. The fixation used is a specially designed device which holds the two cut surfaces firmly together. This has the advantage that the patient is made ambulant much sooner than if she has no internal fixation and had to be nursed in a hip spica.

With an uncomplicated post-operative phase the patient is allowed out of bed within a few days of operation and commences walking with help and the use of sticks a few days afterwards.

A post-operative regime for such a patient, subject to modification for each person, could be:

1 *Twenty-four hours after operation.* The patient sits with her knee flexed and her lower leg hanging over the edge of the bed. With the physiotherapist to supervise exercising the knees by moving the legs by both passive and active exercises.

2 *Three days after operation.* With two people assisting, one on each side, the patient stands. She is taught to balance using a walking stick in each hand to support her. Crutches are only needed for patients who are very unstable.

3 *Walking* is encouraged as soon as possible after this and at seven days many patients can walk around the ward. The patient may be able to reach the lavatory at this stage.

4 The patient is discharged from hospital about three weeks after operation.

After discharge from hospital

The patient is to be discouraged from staying in bed and incentive to further achievements in ambulation are given.

This is, of course, all subject to modification related to the general health and obesity of the patient. She must not be exhausted by strenuous efforts; the day-to-day activities of living are usually enough to improve the musculature. The range of activity of the hip is limited until union of the bone has occurred.

The patient does not return to manual employment or lifting weights for some months after operation.

Some oedema may occur around the ankles but this tends to disappear after two to three weeks; it must be reported to the doctor however.

Hip replacement arthroplasty

The explosive development in artificial joints—particularly the hip—has been due to improved knowledge of materials and the introduction of new materials. The ideal material should neither act on or be acted on by the body, should be strong and have a low wear rate and a low coefficient of friction. New materials are constantly being developed and possibly in the near future ceramics will be used as the ideal joint liners.

The post-operative management of this patient again depends upon which operation has been performed and the wishes of the surgeon. There are certain principles which apply to all operations on the hip, however, and these are:

1   The operation usually consists of a plastic replacement both of the lining of the acetabulum and a metal replacement of the upper end of the femur (Fig. 19.21b). The congruity of the two parts of the prosthesis depends not only on the strength of the repaired fibrous capsule but also on the musculature of the patient. When the patient is unconscious immediately after operation she gives no muscular support to her hip. It is therefore considered wise to support the affected leg against the unaffected leg until she recovers consciousness. In the operating theatre, therefore, a layer of wool is placed between the legs and two triangular bandages are used to fix the legs together; one in a figure-of-eight formation around the feet and ankles; the other is placed around the thighs above the level of the patellae in a double broad fold with the knot on top of the first turn. These bandages are kept in position until the patient has recovered consciousness and the leg is supported by suspension or pillows to prevent lateral rotation of the thigh.

2   The affected limb is supported when the patient has returned to bed by the use of:

(a) A Thomas' splint with a Pearson knee flexion piece supported by traction cords and counter-weights (see Chapter 28, p. 482).

(b) Hodgen splint with Pearson knee flexion piece (see Chapter 28, p. 481).

(c) Hamilton–Russell traction (see Chapter 28, p. 464).

(d) By using a pillow placed between the internal malleoli with another pillow on the lateral surface of each ankle.

(e) By using a triangular turning mattress which fits between the legs and is especially devised for this purpose.

The objective of these supports is to maintain the thighs in abduction and to discourage lateral rotation of the thigh before the musculature has recovered.

3 Extreme care is necessary in placing the patient on a bedpan. Enough nursing staff must be available to lift her and a handle on a supporting chain above the head of the patient will aid the patient to contribute to the lifting.

4 The wound is often drained by a vacuum drainage bottle through a fine polythene tube. This is described on p. 210, fig. 13.4.

5 The ring of a Thomas' splint may impinge upon the wound and dressing. The half ring of the Hodgen splint may be more convenient in use.

6 There is a danger that complications will occur if the patient is allowed to remain static in the bed. The physiotherapist will give the necessary passive and active exercises but additionally the patient must be encouraged to move about the bed as much as she is able. A bed cradle should take the weight of the bedclothing and pillows should not compress the tissues of the legs.

7 The complications which may occur if stasis is allowed include:

Pneumonia, bronchitis and other chest complications.

Phlebothrombosis and thrombophlebitis of the legs which may result in cerebral or pulmonary embolus and infarct.

Joint stiffness and decubitus ulcers.

Constipation and digestive problems.

The two main complications of hip replacements are:
(a) Infection
(b) Thrombophlebitis and pulmonary embolism.

Infection is minimized by using special air-conditioned theatres and special theatre masks, by special operative techniques and meticulous wound closure and drainage. Opinions differ about the routine use of antibiotics in clean wounds.

Thrombophlebitis is still an unsolved problem, the risk is greater in men.

There is some evidence that prophylactic heparin reduces the incidence of pulmonary embolism.

Final comment

The success of this operation is related to the attitude of the patient; one who is normally optimistic and willing to strive hard for recovery from her disability will gain more from the operation than others. The surgeon will take this into consideration when assessing the patient's suitability for operation.

Hip deformities

(a) *Real shortening*. One leg may be shorter than the other due to causes such as poliomyelitis, malunited fractures, premature epiphyseal fusion or congenital factors.

It is customary to measure the length of the leg from the anterior superior iliac spine to the medial malleolus; such a measurement is known as the 'real length' and any difference between the two legs is known as 'real shortening'.

(b) *Apparent shortening*. Either with real shortening or without, one leg may appear shorter than the other if the hip is fixed in a flexed and/or adducted position—for instance, following tuberculosis, infective arthritis, osteo-arthritis, poliomyelitis or a dislocation.

It is customary to measure apparent length from the umbilicus or the xiphisternum to the medial malleolus; any difference in the apparent length is known as 'apparent shortening'. If the apparent shortening is greater than the real shortening, then either the hip is held in an abnormal position (flexed and/or adducted closed position), or there is a fixed lumbar scoliosis or asymmetry of the pelvis.

When one examines a patient who appears to walk with one leg shorter than the other, the first thing is to discover whether this is due to real shortening of the leg or to apparent shortening, or both.

As a general rule the treatment of apparent shortening is to correct the hip deformity if this can be safely done. If there is in addition real shortening, or the deformed position of the hip cannot safely be corrected, then one can either compensate for the leg discrepancy by building up the shoe on the short side, or by performing an operation. There are three types of operation:

1   Lengthening the tibia of the short leg (see Chapter 26).
2   Shortening the femur of the longer leg (see Chapter 26).
3   Inhibiting growth of the longer leg by surgical intervention on the growth cartilages around the knee (see Chapter 26).
4   Lengthening the femur is more difficult and has more complications. It is usually only done by surgeons with special expertise.

20

Foot Deformities

Relevant applied anatomy and physiology

Animals which stand erect on their two hindlimbs and use their forelimbs as prehensile instruments by comparison with four-legged animals, have specially constructed feet. They have a forefoot; which serves to lever the body backwards against the forward tilt of the body; the hindfoot acts similarly when the body tilts posteriorly. The foot and toes are also capable of applying some lateral or medial leverage against sidewards sway. The foot must therefore be considered as a mobile flexible appendage which functions in such a way as to maintain the body upright under constantly changing circumstances, for example, when walking over rough irregular ground; it is not simply a stable platform upon which the body can rest. It is a mobile structure capable of altering the position of the centre of gravity so that the erect posture is maintained.

To perform the many intricate stabilizing movements the foot has a number of small bones, many synovial joints, muscles to move the joints and nerves which control the muscles. The nerves also convey impulses to the central nervous system which indicates the position of the foot and the pressure of the ground.

The bones of the foot

These consist of seven tarsal bones which form the posterior of the foot, five metatarsal bones, and fourteen phalanges.

The tarsal bones. These are strong and capable of withstanding the direct weight of the body; the highest of the tarsal bones, the talus, forms a joint with the distal end of the tibia and fibula, namely, the ankle. Three other joints in the tarsus are relevant to this chapter; these are the sub-talar joint, the talo-navicular joint and the calcaneo-cuboid joint. Arthrodesis, or the fusion, of any two of these joints converts the posterior foot into one bone as the three joints normally move synchronously.

TABLE 20.1

Group and name of muscle	Point of attachment on the foot	Functions	Nerve supply
ANTERIOR GROUP			
1 Extensor hallucis longus	Terminal phalanx of great toe on its superior surface.	1 Dorsiflexion of foot. 2 Elevation of great toe.	Anterior tibial nerve.
2 Extensor digitorum.	Four tendons, one each to a small toe.	1 Dorsiflexion of foot. 2 Elevation of toes. 3 Eversion of foot.	Anterior tibial nerve.
3 Tibialis anterior.	Inferior surface. Medial side of tarsal bones.	1 Dorsiflexion of foot. 2 Inversion of foot. 3 Elevation of 1st metatarsal. All three muscles are postural. They tend to pull the body forwards.	Anterior tibial nerve.
LATERAL GROUP			
1 Peroneus longus.	Down lateral surface of ankle and foot to be inserted on inferior surface	1 Eversion of foot. 2 Depresses the 1st metatarsal and plantar-flexes the foot.	Peroneal nerve; a branch of the lateral popliteal nerve.
POSTERIOR GROUPS			
Superficial			
1 Gastrocnemius. 2 Soleus. 3 Plantaris.	Tendo achillis and then on to calcaneum.	Plantar flexion. All three muscles are postural; they tend to pull the body posteriorly.	Posterior tibial nerve.
Deep			
1 Flexor hallucis longus.	Inferior surface of great toe.	1 Flexion of great toe. 2 Plantar flexion of foot.	Posterior tibial nerve.
2 Flexor digitorum.	Four tendons, one to inferior surface of each small toe.	1 Flexion of toes. Plantar flexion of foot.	Posterior tibial nerve.

3	Tibialis posterior. Inferior surface.	1 Inversion. 2 Plantar flexion. All three muscles are postural, they tend to pull the body towards its posterior surface.	Posterior tibial nerve.

The metatarsal bones. The five metatarsal bones project anteriorly from the tarsus; they each diverge slightly so that the forefoot is wider than the hind-foot; a line drawn along the centre of the length of a metatarsal bone is a 'metatarsal ray'. Although the first metatarsal ray which contributes to the great toe, is the stronger; it is the second metatarsal which is longer than the first which accepts most of the weight of the body, as the ball of the foot, in walking. The first (or medial) ray is relatively mobile; the fifth (or outer) ray is almost fixed.

The phalanges. The main function of the toes is to help to push the body off when walking or running. They also serve for the insertion of some important muscle tendons which help to stabilise the stance of the body. Normally they relieve pressure on the metatarsal heads and help in balance.

The arches of the foot. The bones of the foot are normally arranged in arches. Two arches are arranged longitudinally, from the heel to the heads of the metatarsals. The outer arch is low, the inner arch is higher. In addition, when the two feet are placed together they form a transverse arch in the tarso-metatarsal region. These arches which are supported by ligaments and muscles, help to give spring to the walk and act as shock absorbers.

Muscular control of the foot

As in the hand, if all the muscles which cause foot movements were placed directly on it the foot would be a bulky, clumsy affair. There are some small muscles in the foot but most of the foot control is carried out by muscles situated in the calf. These are classified as shown in Table 20.1.

These muscles act by pulling upon long tendons which cause movement at some distance from their site. These tendons pass downwards across the ankle joint and into the foot. Each tendon is surrounded by a sheath of synovial membrane which secretes synovial fluid inside the sheath. The tendons and sheaths are held against the ankle by fibrous bands known as retinacula. Injuries which sever the tendons around the ankle will thus impair the movements of the foot.

The nerves

The two main nerves controlling the function of the foot are the *anterior tibial nerve* and the *posterior tibial nerve* (Fig. 9.1, p. 113).

The anterior tibial nerve. This is a main branch of the lateral popliteal nerve. It supplies the muscles which dorsiflex the foot. Paralysis of these muscles, resulting from a lesion of the nerve, results in a deformity in which the foot hangs downwards; this is called a 'drop foot'.

The posterior tibial nerve. This nerve supplies the muscles which plantarflex the foot. Paralysis of these muscles, when a lesion of this nerve exists, results in a deformity in which the forefoot is pulled upwards; this is called a calcaneal deformity because the heel projects downwards.

The infant foot

The fetus within the uterus must be malleable and plastic to permit moulding during its passage through narrow openings at birth. After birth, growth in size of every structure (including bone) is rapid and continues until ossification is complete. To permit these processes, all the bones of the fetus and young infant are cartilaginous. Cartilage is soft and flexible, and is capable of rapid growth and alteration in shape. The foot is no exception and the skeleton of the foot of the newly born infant is entirely cartilage.

As long as the cartilaginous state exists the foot can be re-shaped. In the majority of congenitally deformed feet which are treated soon enough, i.e. as soon after birth as possible—and, provided correction is maintained, the bones of the foot will ultimately ossify into a reasonably functional shape. If the foot of the infant is left untreated for too long the deformed cartilage will ossify into deformed bone.

Deformities of the foot

It is convenient to divide deformities of the foot into *congenital* and *acquired*.

Congenital deformities

(a) *Congenital talipes equinovarus.* The most common congenital deformity is talipes equinovarus (Fig. 20.1). In this deformity the foot is adducted and

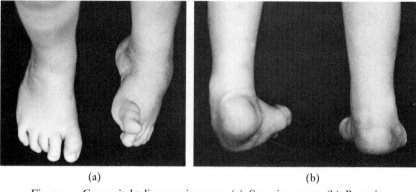

(a)   (b)

Fig. 20.1   Congenital talipes equinovarus. (a) Superior aspect. (b) Posterior aspect.

inverted; the heel is inverted, and the whole foot is held in equinus. This may be due to a variety of causes and may be associated with other conditions, e.g. arthrogryposis. It is commonly bilateral and is often inherited. In the earlier stages the best treatment is frequent gentle manipulation of the foot and holding it in the retained position. It is important that the adduction of the forefoot should be corrected first, then the inversion of the forefoot and heel; and only after this should the equinus be corrected. It is also essential that these manipulations should be very gentle, but should be repeated often, and that the splinting should not be so tight as to cause pressure sores on the baby's skin. In other words, the splint should be applied with the foot not quite as fully corrected as it was possible to obtain by manual manipulation. If treatment is performed regularly, e.g. twice a week, the majority of cases can be fully corrected; the foot should then be held in the corrected position until the child starts to walk. Provided the child's foot is corrected before he walks, relapse is unlikely. If, however, the foot is not fully corrected and the child is allowed to walk on the uncorrected foot, relapse is extremely likely. Under these circumstances it may be necessary to operate to divide the contracted ligaments and tendons on the medial side of the foot.

It often happens that the forefoot corrects easily but that the heel remains in equinus. Under these circumstances it is wise to elongate the tendo calcaneus. Forcible dorsiflexion of the foot with a tight tendo achillis leads to pressure on and deformity of the talus with later a stiff ankle.

The conservative regime outlined here is successful in the majority of patients. Bi-weekly attendance at hospital does however throw a great strain on the mother, particularly if she has other children and/or lives a long distance away. If regular attendance is impossible, it is better to correct the foot by dividing contracted ligaments and tendons and this is less traumatic than occasional forcible manipulations. If open operation is performed, it is important to avoid sepsis and haematoma formation both of which lead to fibrosis and relapses. It is also important to ensure that there is a true correction not just an apparent one. If the bones are not in normal alignment the altered axis of muscle action will cause a relapse.

If by the age of three the heel is inverted this should be corrected by a calcaneal osteotomy. Following this, a similar regime of repeated gentle manipulations and retaining the foot in the corrected position is necessary. If the deformity is more pronounced, it may be necessary also to excise a wedge of bone from the outer side of the calcaneo-cuboid joint during the operation.

In all forms of treatment the essential is to reduce the navicular to its corrected position in relation to the head of the talus, as the common feature of all forms of club foot is medial dislocation of the navicular—that is, a subluxation of the talo-navicular joint.

(b) *Congenital calcaneovalgus.* Children are often born with excessive dorsiflexion of their feet with the heels pointing downwards. This is usually a comparatively benign condition which responds to treatment by stretching and splinting. There is, however, a more severe form known as vertical talus. This is often associated with other lesions such as myelomeningocele, spasticity, etc. It is a much more difficult condition to treat. Basically it should be treated by repeated plantiflexion of the forefoot until the scaphoid once again articulates with the head of the astragalus. The foot should be held in this position for some weeks and then the tendo Achillis should be lengthened, allowing the foot to resume a neutral position.

Acquired deformities

(a) *Pes cavus.* In childhood, pes cavus (or excessive arching of the foot) is not uncommon. The basic anatomical feature is dropping of the forefoot and clawing of the toes. This deformity is usually caused by a neurological disorder, for example, poliomyelitis, peroneal atrophy, myelomeningocele, spinal dysplasia, Friedreich's ataxia, etc. As with other progressive neurological disorders, treatment is extremely difficult, but basically the surgeon aims at weakening the over-active muscles and strengthening the weak ones.

In the older child, pes cavus may arise in which the cause cannot be identified. The best treatment is osteotomy of the os calcis (Fig. 20.2).

(b) *Other acquired deformities.* A variety of foot deformities may arise following other neurological disorders, e.g. poliomyelitis or cerebral palsy. According to the muscles involved, the foot may be held in equinus (that is, extreme plantarflexion, Fig. 20.4); in calcaneus (that is, in extreme dorsiflexion, Fig. 20.5); inverted or everted.

Generally during the growing period an effort is made to balance an unequal muscle pull by tendon transfer, but once growth is complete, a severe foot deformity is best treated by arthrodesis of the three main joints of the foot—the subtalar, talo-navicular and calcaneal cuboid joints, with the foot placed in a plantigrade position.

Minor foot deformities

Hammer toes (Fig. 20.6) are extremely common and may be associated with pes cavus or occur in isolation. In adolescence and early adult life hammer

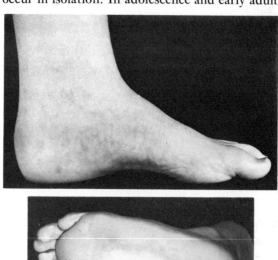

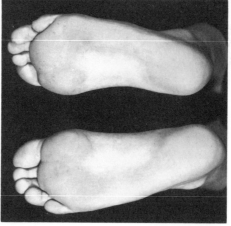

Fig. 20.2　(*Top*) Pes cavus. Left foot; medial aspect. (*Bottom*) Same patient photographed from below standing on a glass sheet. Note shorter length of left foot.

toes are best treated by arthrodesis of the interphalangeal joints, but in older patients with severe clawing of the toes and prominent metatarsal heads, the best treatment is excision of the metatarsal heads.

Overlapping of the fifth toe (Fig. 20.7) is also a common condition. If this gives rise to symptoms, e.g. pain and ulceration—it is best treated by Butler's operation in which an incision is made around the base of the toe; the skin, tendon and joint capsules are divided, but the digital nerves and vessels are left intact. The incision is then prolonged on to the sole of the foot and the toe is then placed in the corrected position where it is anchored by sutures.

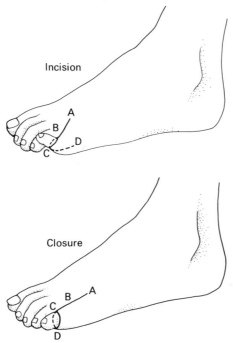

Fig. 20.3   Butler's operation for an overlapping little toe. The incision is made straight on the dorsal surface of the foot, round the base of the little toe and straight on plantar aspect. The toe is mobilized by dividing the extensor tendon and the joint capsule, and is then shifted into the plantar portion of the incision and the skin is sutured as in the diagram.

Hallux valgus. Hallux valgus deformity is very common and may be associated with hammer toes and flat feet (Fig. 20.8). It is nearly always associated with splaying of the metatarsal heads, and a painful exostosis over the medial aspect of the first metatarsal head. In young people the deformity is best treated by detaching the adductor hallucis longus muscle from the base of the proximal phalanx and attaching it to the metatarsal head.

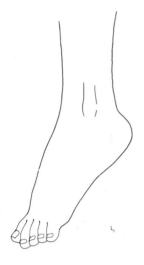

Fig. 20.4   Extreme plantarflexion.

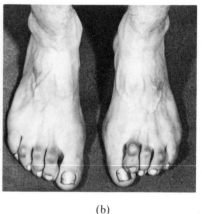

Fig. 20.5   Extreme dorsiflexion.

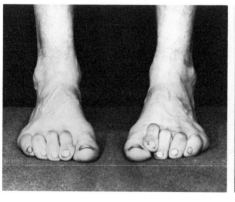

(a)   (b)

Fig. 20.6   (a) and (b) Patient with hammer toes.

In early adult life an osteotomy of the first metatarsal head (Mitchell's operation) is the best treatment. In middle-aged people the best treatment is a Keller's operation (excision of the base of the proximal phalanx and removal of the prominent exostosis). In very old patients with severe deformity and a prominent metatarsal head, Mayo's operation (excision of the metatarsal head) is very successful.

Metatarsalgia. Pain under the metatarsal heads may be due to prominent metatarsal heads, as for instance in claw feet with hammer toes. Most

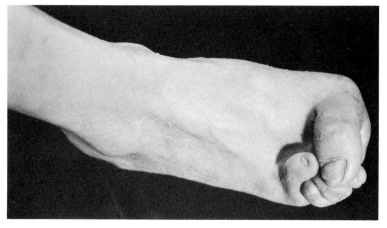

Fig. 20.7   Patient with overlapping toes.

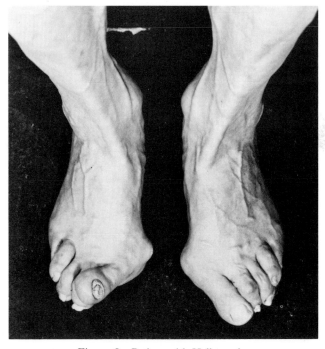

Fig. 20.8   Patient with Hallux valgus.

patients are improved by conservative treatment—that is, a well fitting and well placed metatarsal insole, but if, in spite of this, severe pain continues, excision of the metatarsal heads usually gives relief.

If a metatarsal insole is to be effective it is inevitably bulky. It is therefore important that the shoes be deep enough so that the toes are not constricted. In feet with severe claw toes specially made deep shoes may be necessary.

There is a special variety of metatarsalgia due to a neuroma developing on one of the digital nerves; in this condition the patient suffers from intermittent spasms of severe pain in the adjacent areas of the toes supplied by the affected digital nerve (usually the nerve supplying the cleft between the third and fourth toes). Fortunately, this condition is cured by exercising the affected nerve.

Other causes of pain in the feet are spurs on the os calcis, chronic foot strain, acute foot strain with muscle spasm (spasmodic valgus) and, of course, pain in the feet is very common in peripheral ischaemia, diabetes and rheumatoid arthritis.

Conditions affecting the toe nails

Subungual exostosis. This is a very painful condition but which fortunately can be cured by excising the nail.

Onycogryphosis. This is a curious deformity of the nail which becomes thickened and discoloured. It can be treated palliatively by filing down the nail, or radically by excising the whole of the nail and the nail bed.

Ingrowing toe nail. In this condition chronic inflammation appears down the side of the nail which becomes bent and pressed into the adjacent flesh. A mild degree can be treated by relieving pressure on the nail, or by excising the adjacent side of the nail and adjacent soft tissues. A severe degree of recurrent infection is best treated by total excision of the nail and nail bed.

Glomus tumours. As in the fingers, glomus tumours may give rise to severe pain and tenderness in the region of the toe and toe nails, but this can easily be cured by excision of the tumour.

The nursing management of infants with deformities of the feet

Club foot (Fig. 20.1)

This is a condition where close collaboration between the parents of the patient and the hospital staff can result in the cure of a condition which is seriously disabling for the patient's whole life if left untreated. The treatment of club feet (congenital talipes equinovarus) is rewarding, provided that it is efficient and consistent over several months. If the treatment lapses or is inadequate, the growing child and its parents will be faced with the patient's admission to hospital and surgical treatment, possibly when schooling has commenced and the interruption may be serious.

It is essential that the patient should be seen for manipulations and immobilization of the feet at least weekly and preferably twice weekly until the shape of the feet is as normal as it is possible to achieve. This may be accomplished in the following ways:

1 Attendance as an out-patient at a hospital.

2 Attendance at an orthopaedic peripheral clinic organized by After Care staff from the parent hospital.

3 Attendance at a clinic organized by the Medical Officer of Health of the area.

4 If regular out-patient attendance is impossible, the baby should be admitted to hospital.

This last method may be the only way when the family live at a great distance from a doctor or hospital, it is this last situation which presents the greatest number of untreated cases; club feet are common in remote 'undeveloped' parts of the world where little or no medical facilities exist.

It is often a hardship for the parents to attend hospital frequently and consistently but the disastrous results of inadequate treatment must be explained to them. The follow-up is the most important part of treatment.

Methods of manipulation and splintage. Treatment must commence as soon as possible after the birth of the infant; thus the orthopaedic surgeon and his staff will see the patient in the maternity unit. At this stage manipulation of each of the deformities separately and in turn into the over-corrected position is most likely to be successful, although the application of splintage to hold the position is difficult. *It is vitally important that the forefoot should be corrected before attempting to correct the heel.*

Splintage for congenital talipes equinovarus. The infant's foot is so small that the application of any immobilization, which is effective and yet does not constrict, requires considerable skill. As the child increases in size and treatment is established and is consistent, larger splints are required and are easier to apply.

1 *Zinc-oxide strapping.* This may be used in the first days of treatment. Pieces of waterproof zinc-oxide plaster 5 cm wide are prepared with lint sufficiently long to encircle the foot; this is fixed on to the adhesive surface

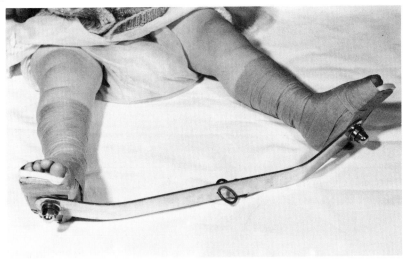

Fig. 20.9   A Bell-Grice splint applied to a patient.

leaving about 3 cm of adhesive uncovered at the beginning of the strip which is fixed on to the middle of the sole of the foot with the length of the strip pointing to the lateral side. The strip then encircles the foot and is carried up the lateral side of the leg to pull the foot into eversion. A further piece of zinc-oxide plaster 2·5 cm wide encircles the leg above the malleolus to hold the lateral strip in position.

The foot can be conveniently strapped to a metal 'tongue depressor' applied to the lateral aspect of the leg and foot, thus holding the forefront in the corrected position. Later the splint can be bent so as to hold the forefoot in the over-corrected position.

2   *Bell-Grice splint* (Fig. 20.9). These are supplied in a wide range of sizes small enough to fit the tiniest foot and large enough to continue in use to the conclusion of treatment. The crossbar is also supplied in various lengths to suit. Another advantage is that the footplate can be moulded to the shape required and only a thin layer of adhesive padding is required between the metal and the skin on the sole of the patient's foot.

Application of the soleplates. Two bands of 2·5 cm wide zinc-oxide water-proof strapping are used around the foot. The area of the zinc-oxide plaster to be in contact with the skin of the infant is covered with another piece of the adhesive with the two sticky surfaces in contact. These two bands are first stuck on to the base of the soleplate pointing laterally. They are then carried over the top of the soleplate and over the adhesive felt. The soleplate is now placed in position on the patient and the bands are carried firmly over:

(a) the base of the soleplate;

(b) the superior surface of the foot from the lateral to the medial side;

(c) the base of the soleplate from the medial to the lateral side.

One band is arranged at the level of the junction of the tarsal bones and the metatarsal bones; the other at the heads of the metatarsal bones. A third piece of zinc-oxide plaster passes up the back to hold the soleplate on to the patient's heel; it is carried up to mid-calf level.

Application of the crossbar. The crossbar of the splint is an important factor in treating this deformity. The degree of (a) abduction is controlled by the position in which the sole plates are bolted into position on the cross bar (which is altered weekly), and (b) eversion by the amount of bend in the cross bar. A hole and an 'S' hook enables the suspension of the splint to an overhead beam so that the infant can kick and exercise.

The splint may be applied when the baby is a few days old and treatment is continued for about six months. After discontinuation of this splintage, Bell-Grice boots attached to a cross bar may be worn by the patient as night splints for up to eighteen months of age.

3   *Dennis Browne splints.* These are unmalleable splints with rectangular sole plates with a lateral upright on each and a short cross bar. Each sole plate is applied with built up layers of adhesive felt applied to cause the degree of eversion required (Fig. 20.10). The lateral plate serves to hold the tibia and fibula in position so that the degree of eversion is maintained; this has the disadvantage that it may compress the peroneal muscles. Dennis Browne boots are used as night splints after discontinuation of the corrective splints.

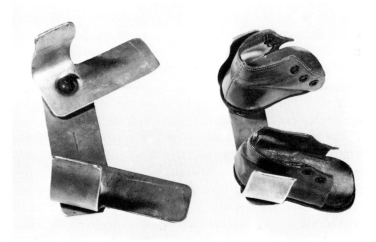

Fig. 20.10   Dennis Browne splints and boots.

The nursing care of infants with congenital talipes equinovarus and other deformities

The corrective splintage must be taken off and re-applied regularly. A minimum of attendance weekly for re-application is necessary and the mother must be instructed to return to the clinic if she has doubts about the efficiency of the splintage in the interval between visits. She must also be advised to avoid the soiling of the adhesive strapping by the infant's urine. The legs of the baby cannot be immersed when bathing.

At the orthopaedic clinic all splintage and waterproof adhesive is removed and the feet thoroughly washed. A suitable liquid for removing the zinc-oxide adhesive debris will be needed.

The feet will be examined by the orthopaedic surgeon or trained orthopaedic nurse or physiotherapist. This is also the opportunity for physiotherapy; the process of stretching during correction may affect the muscles of the leg, and it is important that the tone and strength of the muscles should be improved.

After physiotherapy the splints are re-applied or changed for a larger size after any further manipulation. A protective coating of either tincture benzoin compound or a silicone barrier cream may be used on the infant's skin under the adhesive. If possible the area of contact with the adhesive on the skin should be altered at each renewal of splintage. It is most important that splintage and over-correction is maintained constantly to the culmination of treatment; a lapse can retard progress.

When splintage is discarded, extensive physiotherapy is necessary. Walking, gait, balance and muscle re-education are necessary.

Plaster of Paris splintage for the treatment of congenital talipes equinovarus

1 *Serial plasters.* The feet are manipulated and plaster of Paris used to hold the over-corrected position. This is applied with the knees in flexion (the plaster bandages include the knee). The plaster splints are replaced at frequent intervals as the infant grows.

2 *Wedge (kite) plasters.* After the method of treatment with zinc-oxide plaster described on p. 349 has been discontinued, below-knee plasters are applied to retain the amount of correction already achieved. These are gradually wedged to increase the amount of correction of each of the deformities at subsequent visits to the clinic by the patient. Each deformity—inversion, adduction, and equinus—is wedged separately.

3 *Plaster of Paris shells*. If, despite all efforts, the Bell-Grice or Dennis Browne splintage described on pp. 351–352 cannot be retained because of breakdown of the skin under the adhesive, plaster of Paris shells may be used during the process of healing the skin (see Chapter 30, p. 519).

Surgical procedures

If the foot cannot be completely corrected by conservative means before the child starts to walk it is desirable to achieve this by operation. If the foot is very rigid operative division of ligaments is less traumatic than forcible manipulation which can do irreparable damage to a child's delicate bones and lead to permanent ankle stiffness due to a misshapen astrugulus. In the simpler cases where the forefoot has been corrected but an equinus deformity persists it may suffice merely to lengthen the tendo Achillis. In slightly more resistant cases it may be necessary to divide the plantar fascia: this may be combined with corrective osteotomy of an inverted calcaneus.

There are surgeons who now advocate and practise early surgical operations on the feet of the infant instead of using manipulative splintage. This is to overcome the 'tethering' effect of the soft tissues on the cartilaginous bones and thus permit them to grow in a normal shape.

If the forefoot cannot be corrected by gentle conservative measures it is less traumatic to divide the ligaments and tendons on the medial side of the foot than to resort to violent manipulations. Finally if the bones have already become misshapen it may be necessary also to excise a wedge segment of bone from the lateral aspect of the calcaneo-cuboid joint. It must be remembered that every operation leaves an internal scar. This fibrous tissue may contract (it almost inevitably does not grow normally) and the scar tissue is a frequent cause of relapse. Therefore, after any of these operations prolonged splinting is necessary.

Footwear in orthopaedic care

(a) General comments in the management of orthopaedic patients

The orthopaedic surgeon, nurse and physiotherapist must always be conscious of the footwear of the patient: in hospital the shoes worn by the patient may affect his rate of progress when he becomes ambulant after surgery; the aged patient may be unstable and liable to slip and fall with unsuitable shoes on the feet; the growing infant and child may retain the deformities caused by bad footwear for the rest of his life; alterations to shoes may form part of the treatment of the patient—for example, metatarsal bars on the sole of the shoes, or crooked and elongated heels.

(b) **The patient in hospital**

The nurse should ask the relatives of the patient to bring his footwear to hospital long before he is due to become ambulant after being bed-fast. Slippers, particularly if loose, are the *least* desirable form of footwear and no patient should be allowed to wear them constantly in the ward; the physiotherapist will reject them as unsuitable for re-education of the patient in walking and gait. Other obvious abnormalities to be rejected in footwear are high heeled or stiletto heeled shoes; sandals with no supporting uppers or heels; shoes of poor quality which do not support the foot. Footwear either too large or too small will not do; a check must be made to see that the bed-fast patient's shoes have not become too small in size because of growth of the feet.

(c) **Modifications to shoes**

The patient's shoes may require modification for therapeutic reasons or for the attachment of splintage. A strong leather shoe of good fit is essential for this; if the patient has none or has outgrown them, a new pair must be obtained. Examples of such modifications are listed below.

1 *Fitting a Rizzoli splint* (see Chapter 11, p. 181).

2 *Sockets into the heel of the shoe.* These are required for the fitting of a caliper or a below-knee iron or a weight-relieving caliper (see Chapter 11, p. 182). There may be:
(i)   circular;
(ii) circular with anterior stops;
(iii) circular with posterior stops;
(iv) circular with one anterior and one posterior stop;
(v)   rectangular.

3 *Shoe-raising to match the length of the opposite limb.* This may be required because of a deformity or to match the height of a Thomas' patten ended caliper.

4 *To produce inversion of the foot*
   (i)   *Crooked heel.* A piece of leather shaped like a wedge is inserted into the layers which form the heel of the shoe from the medial side.

(ii) *Crooked and elongated heel.* The heel in (a) is carried forwards towards the toe to increase the degree of inversion.

(iii) *Long Thomas' heel* (Fig. 20.11). The heel mentioned in (a) and (b) is carried still further forwards.

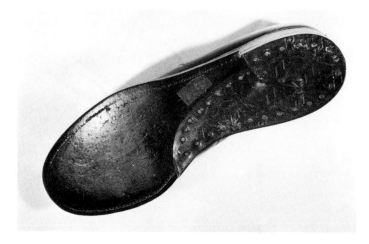

Fig. 20.11 A long Thomas' heel.

(iv) *Float-out heel* (see Fig. 20.12). The lateral surface of the heel of the shoe is extended outwards.

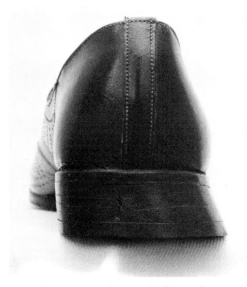

Fig. 20.12 A float-out heel on a shoe.

5   *To produce eversion of the foot.* The lateral side of the shoe may be raised by inserting extra layers of leather on the lateral edge of the shoe.

6   *Metatarsal bar* (Fig. 20.13). This is a bar of leather nailed across the sole of the shoe behind the heads of the metatarsal bones to relieve pressure on them.

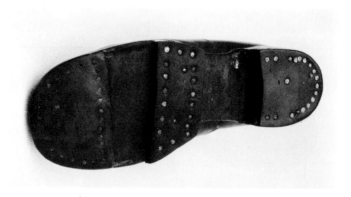

Fig. 20.13   Metatarsal bar on a shoe.

All these alterations require the attention of an expert shoemaker with experience in making surgical footwear. The orders given must be precise and leave no room for error; each alteration is expensive as it must meet the needs of the individual patient; repeated work is wasteful of time and money and retards the progression of the patient.

(d) Insoles
These are worn inside the shoes. Their advantage is that they can be transferred to different footwear as required. A cast is taken of the foot and the leather insole moulded from it.
    The order for the insole may request:
(i)   Moulded leather insole to the shape of the base of the foot.
(ii)   Insole with metatarsal dome, bar or button.
(iii) Insole with prominence under the calcaneo–cuboid joint.

(e) Children's footwear
The foot of the child grows constantly and rapidly. Replacement of footwear is necessary and costly, but the foot must not be forced into shoes which are too short or too narrow.

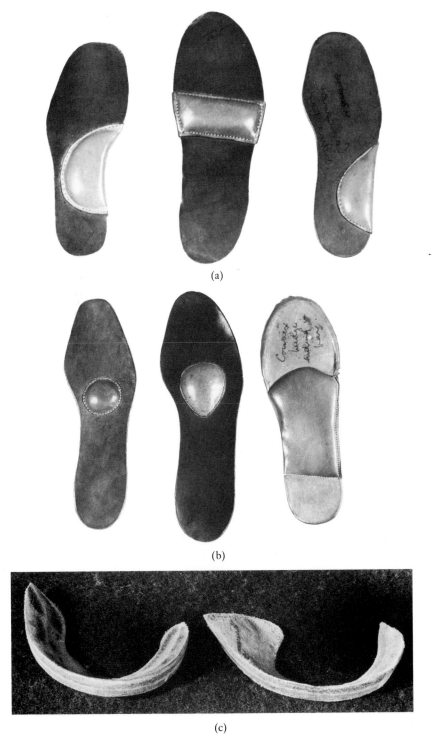

Fig. 20.14　(a) and (b) Various insoles. (c) Schwarz heels used for pes planus.

Most shoe manufacturers make a wide range of sizes in width and length in many style of shoe; they also train sales staff in the correct method of fitting children with footwear.

Orthopaedically it is always wise to regard money spent in buying the best children's footwear as money well invested.

21

Hand Deformities

The hand

A person's hands often reflect their personality, occupation and temperament and are a valuable indication of their state of health. Observation of a patient's hands is therefore always of importance—the colour, shape of the nails, state of the skin, presence or absence of sweating, tremor, presence or absence of swelling of joints, discoloration of the skin (e.g. from cigarette smoking) must all be observed in every patient. In addition, as our hands are one of the most useful parts of the body and the means by which most people earn their living, deformities of the hand are of great personal and economic importance.

Congenital deformities

There are a large number of congenital deformities of the hand. Some of these are inherited, as for instance, the typical lobster-claw hand, which, it is well known, runs in certain families. Others are due to adverse intrauterine influences, e.g. congenital amputation of the fingers, constriction bands, etc. In addition, congenital fusion of the fingers (syndactyly, Fig. 21.1) is not uncommon. This condition is easy to improve in so far as it is amenable to surgical correction. The simplest way of correcting this condition at the age of three or four years is to divide the fingers which are joined together and coat the subsequent raw surfaces with a free skin graft (Fig. 21.1).

In addition there are a number of other congenital anomalies of the hand—for instance, absence of the thumb, which may be associated with absence of the radius (Fig. 21.2). Congenital contracture of the little or of all the fingers and supernumerary digits. Supernumerary digits are best removed if they are unsightly or get in the patient's way. Occasionally a hypo-plastic thumb can be made more useful by inserting a bone graft, but usually small children adapt themselves very well to congenital anomalies of the hand and succeed

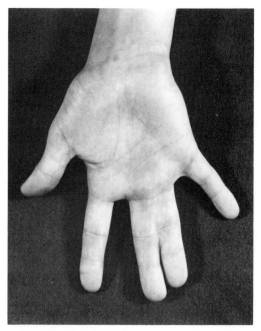

Fig. 21.1   Congenital fusion of the fingers – syndactyly.

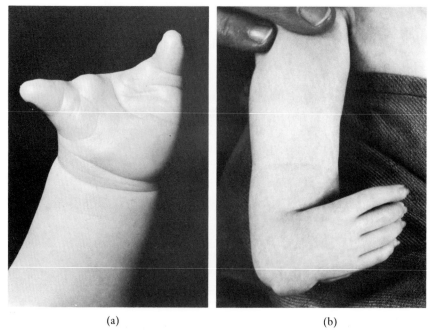

(a)   (b)

Fig. 21.2   (a) Congenital absence of digits. (b) Congenital absence of radius.

in acquiring excellent function, therefore surgical interference is of limited value.

Deformities of the hand may occur in association with a variety of nerve and tendon injuries which are considered in the appropriate section of this

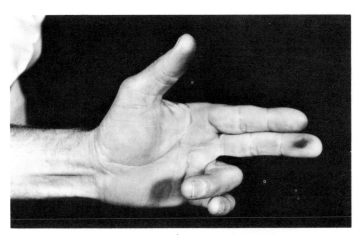

Fig. 21.3   Contracture of the palmar fascia (Dupuytren's contracture).

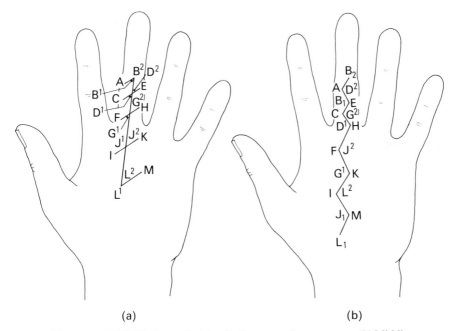

(a)   (b)

Fig. 21.4   (a) Middle finger, incision for Dupuytren's contracture. (b) Middle finger, closure of multiple 'Z' incision.

book. In addition, contracture of the palmar fascia (Dupuytren's contracture, Fig. 21.3) is an important common condition. If left untreated, this may lead to progressive deformities of the fingers, particularly of the ring finger, which becomes flexed at the proximal interphalangeal and metacarpophalangeal joints. This condition is often inherited and may be associated with similar contractures in the feet. Mild degrees of Dupuytren's contracture are not uncommon and if they are not progressive, do not necessarily require any treatment, although gentle passive stretching by the patient and the wearing of a night splint may be of use. If, however, the condition is severe and progressive, it is wise to perform an operation to excise the thickened fascia. This is best performed by a longitudinal multiple 'Z' incision (Fig. 21.4).

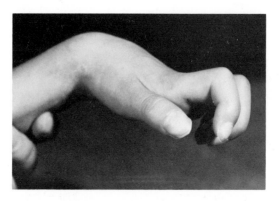

Fig. 21.5   Volkmann's ischaemia.

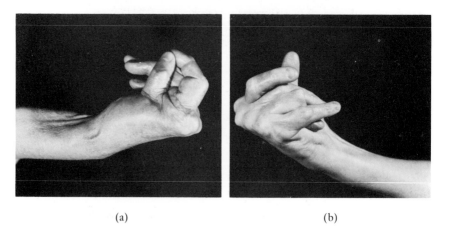

(a)   (b)

Fig. 21.6   (a–e) Series to show the hands of patients with rheumatoid arthritis.

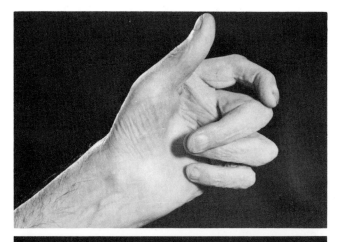

(c)

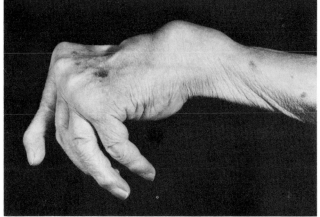

(d)

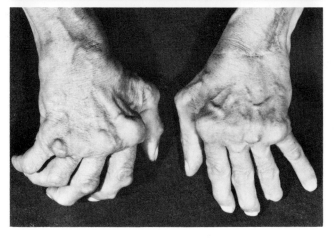

(e)

One of the problems after surgical correction of Dupuytren's contracture is poor skin healing. It is important that before operation the skin is made as soft and pliable as possible by the patient abstaining from heavy and dirty work and gently rubbing the skin with lanoline.

If the aponeurotic thickening is in the palm and this has been excised through a transverse incision there may be a large gap when the deformity is corrected. Some surgeons advocate leaving the wound open and allowing it to granulate and epithelialise. The results are surprisingly good!

Other surgeons advocate immediate skin grafting. In very severe, old-standing deformities where the finger joints are incurably stiff it may be necessary to anchor a finger whose skin can then be used as a pediclegraft to cover any defect in the palm.

Following injury or infection, a variety of hand deformities may occur, of which the two most common are:

1   *Volkmann's ischaemic contracture* of the long flexor muscles (Fig. 21.5). In this condition the flexor muscles are contracted, therefore the patient can only straighten his fingers when the wrist is flexed, and when he extends his wrist the fingers automatically close. Mild cases may be treated by gentle traction and splinting, but more severe cases are best treated by lengthening the tendons of the affected muscles.

Ischaemic contracture may also affect the intrinsic muscles when the opposite deformity arises—namely, hyperextension of the interphalangeal joints, and flexion of the metacarpophalangeal joints. This condition, if severe, is best treated by division of the tendons of the intrinsic muscles where they are inserted into the extensor tendons of the fingers.

2   *Rheumatoid arthritis* (Figs. 21.6a–e) commonly affects the joints of the hands and fingers, particularly the metacarpophalangeal and proximal interphalangeal joints; not only is there pain and limitation of movement, but ulnar deviation of the metacarpophalangeal joints is very common. This condition is best treated by excision of the thickened synovium and holding the metacarpophalangeal joints in a neutral position. If there is extensive destruction of the interphalangeal joints these may be treated by replacement arthroplasty (Fig. 21.7). Spontaneous rupture of finger tendons is not uncommon in rheumatoid arthritis. They should be repaired and the underlying cause—spike of bone, granulation tissue, etc.—removed.

Deformities of the fingers may also arise as a sequel to injury when the metacarpals or phalanges unite in a bad position, or due to disease of the bone such as chronic tuberculous infection or cartilaginous tumours

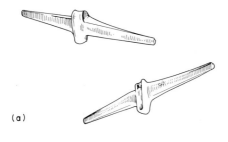

(a)

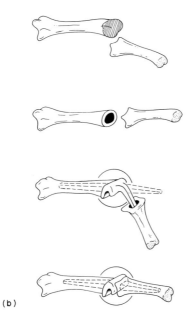

(b)

Fig. 21.7   Joint replacement using a one-piece plastic prosthesis. (a) Finger joint prosthesis. (b) Series of steps showing resection of metacarpal head and insertion of stemmed implant.

(chondromata). These give rise to swelling of the bone and occasionally to spontaneous fractures.

Tendovaginitis
Another common condition is thickening of the tendon sheath giving rise to 'clicking', locking, limitation of movement, pain and a localized swelling. The common sites are the extensor tendons of the thumb on the lateral side of the lower end of the radius, and the flexor tendon of the fingers opposite

the metacarpophalangeal joint. In babies the tendon sheath of the thumb flexor tendon is often affected. In addition, thickening of the tendon sheaths of the flexor tendons due either to tuberculosis or rheumatoid arthritis is fairly common and should be treated by excision of the thickened tendon sheath.

Another common swelling around the wrist is a ganglion, which is a gelatinous degeneration of a tendon sheath or joint. On rare occasions these may press on nerves, causing paralysis and muscle wasting and deformity, but usually the patient comes complaining either of pain or the fact that they are unsightly. If the symptoms warrant it, they may be treated by excision of the ganglion.

Lastly, certain painful tumours known as glomus tumours of the fingers may occur around the finger nails. These are extremely tender and painful and must be treated by surgical removal.

Burns involving the skin of the hand may lead to severe fibrosis and contracture and require treatment by extensive skin grafting. Prevention of deformity by splinting in the early stages is essential.

22

Affections of the Knee

Relevant applied anatomy and physiology

The knee is a hinge joint with a large area of synovial membrane. This is the optimum type of articulation for its particular situation in the body. It would be most inconvenient to have, for example, a ball and socket joint there! The hip, with the knee and ankle together considered as a unit, are the ideal structures for the functions which the leg performs—standing, sitting, walking, running, etc; just as the unit formed by the shoulder, elbow and wrist are the most suitable for the arm.

Muscular control of the knee

Because flexion and extension are the principal movements (a small amount of rotation of the tibia also occurs) only two main groups of muscles are required to cause them—the flexor group (hamstrings and gastrocnemius) to bend the knee and the extensor group (the quadriceps femoris) to cause it to straighten. A major function of both the groups, however, is to hold the knee still in any desired posture, so that the knee is a stable, reliable supporting structure.

An important duty of an orthopaedic nurse, in collaboration with the physiotherapist, is to encourage the patient to maintain the strength and efficiency of the muscles controlling the knee; by exercising them regularly for the whole time the patient is in bed. When the time comes to get up and stand, his legs should be capable of supporting his body weight in a short time; if these muscles are allowed to atrophy, long tedious periods of exercise lie before the convalescent patient.

The nerves of the knee

The muscles of the knee and the joint itself, are supplied by the femoral nerve on the front of the thigh (supplying the quadriceps) and the sciatic nerve with its main divisions on the posterior surface (supplying the hamstrings and gastrocnemius). Division of either or both of these nerves will therefore seriously impair the action of the knee (see also Chapter 11). The knee, like any other joint, may also be deprived of its sensory nerve supply as a result of disease; it is then vulnerable to repeated trauma because no pain is felt; the flail, swollen joint which results is known as a neuropathic joint, but is often called a 'Charcot joint' after Charcot, the great French neurologist.

The bursae of the knee

The knee is supplied extensively with protective bursae; these are pouches of synovial membrane, containing synovial fluid situated between muscle tendons and capsule, and on the anterior surface of the patella. One of these extends up for about one third of the length of the thigh behind the quadriceps; another is on the anterior surface of the tibia. As the result of infection, or surgery, or trauma, these bursae can become distended with the products of the lesion—blood, pus, or increased synovial secretion. It is necessary, when an effusion is expected, to maintain firm compression on the bursae. This is the reason for the application of the Jones pressure bandage (see p. 379) which must extend from mid-calf to mid-thigh, well below and well above the bursae to prevent their distension.

The menisci

These are two incomplete rings of cartilage placed on the plateau of the tibia in direct relationship to the condyles of the femur (Fig. 22.1). They are aptly named as each forms a perimeter, similar to the shape of the surface of water

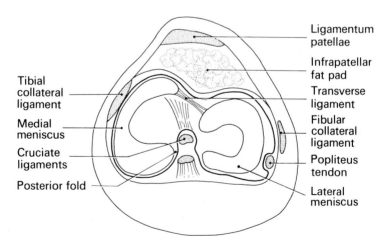

Fig. 22.1   The menisci.

in a glass, in which the condyle is cupped. Their exact function is uncertain but many anatomists believe that they guide and control the tibia as it slides around the femoral condyles. They may also control the movement of synovial fluid.

The cruciate ligaments
These are two strong ligaments (Fig. 22.1) which serve to hold the femur in the correct relation to the plateau of the tibia; they thus assist the function of the menisci. 'Dashboard injuries' may cause a rupture of the cruciate ligaments with anterior or posterior subluxation of the joint.

The extracapsular ligaments
The capsule of the knee is strengthened on all surfaces by ligaments. These are strong bands which pass from femur to tibia. As a result of trauma the ligaments may be strained or ruptured. In particular there are strong ligaments on the lateral and medial aspects. The stability of the knee depends to a large extent on the ligaments.

Congenital abnormalities of the knee

Congenital genu recurvatum
Congenital abnormalities of the knee joint occur in three main forms. A baby may be born with congenital hyperextension of the knee, sometimes referred to as congenital genu recurvatum; this is due to congenital shortening of the quadriceps muscle (Fig. 22.2). It may be part of a generalized muscle fibrosis as in arthrogryposis and may be associated with other lesions such as dislocation of the hip. It may also occur as an isolated phenomenon. The condition may be associated with disorders of the spinal cord, and in particular with myelomeningocele (Chapter 18). The treatment is to lengthen the rectus femoris tendon and thus restore flexion movement of the knee joint. If this is done in early infancy the prognosis is good, though there may not be full restoration of knee flexion.

Congenital dislocation of the patella
Another congenital abnormality of the knee is that of congenital dislocation of the patella, when the patella is permanently dislocated to the lateral side. In infancy there is relatively little functional disability from this condition, though of course, the appearance of the knee is ugly and this naturally distresses the parents. It is possible to reduce the dislocation of the patella by

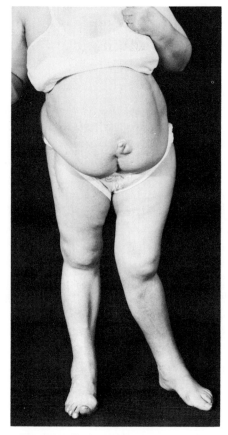

Fig. 22.2   Patient with genu recurvation.

dividing the contracted capsule on the outer side of the joint and transplanting the ligamentum patellae to a more medial site. Whether this leads to a better functioning knee is doubtful, however, but the cosmetic improvement probably makes it a worthwhile operation.

Congenital genu valgum, genu varum and flexion contracture

Occasionally children are born with widespread deformities of the leg associated with either gross knock-knees (Fig. 22.3), bow-legs (Fig. 22.4), or flexion contracture of the knee. These conditions are not uncommon in association with absence of either the tibia or fibula. Treatment of both these conditions is essentially unsatisfactory, but it is usual if the tibia is absent to place the fibula in contact with the lower end of the femur so as to try to

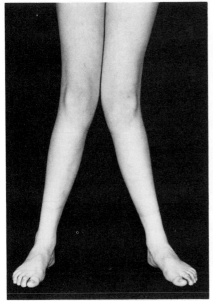
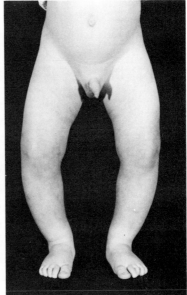

Fig. 22.3   Patient with knock-knees.   Fig. 22.4   Patient with bow-legs.

restore some sort of stability to the leg. The patient, however, will usually need to wear a supporting caliper.

Lesions in childhood

Fibrosis of the quadriceps muscle. A recently recognized condition of the knee which occurs in early childhood is fibrosis of the quadriceps muscle leading to progressive limitation of knee flexion. Again, this may be part of a generalized condition such as arthrogryposis, but it appears most commonly to follow repeated intramuscular injections into the thigh—for example, if the child has had a severe infection in early infancy.

The treatment is to divide the muscles which are the site of the fibrosis; this restores full flexion of the knee but there may be some permanent limitation of the strength of knee extension.

Lesions in adolescence

Osteochondritis of the tibia. In adolescents—boys especially—pain and swelling in the region of the insertion of the ligamentum patellae are likely to develop; this is known as Osgood-Schlatter's disease, or osteochondritis. It is essentially a benign condition which will settle down with a short period of rest and abstaining from strenuous athletics; drastic treatment is seldom—if ever—indicated. The patient may, however, be left with slight permanent prominence of this region, but no functional disability.

Osteochondritis dissecans. During adolescence another fairly common condition is osteochondritis dissecans. This is characterized by small areas of bone and cartilage separating from the main articular surface of the femur and ultimately forming loose bodies in the joint (Fig. 22.5). In the early stages the symptoms are relatively mild, there are occasional attacks of pain with some synovial effusion and occasional 'giving way', but once there is an established loose body the patient complains of periodic locking of the knee, rather similar to cartilage trouble, and the patient may also feel a loose body coming to the surface in various situations. The diagnosis is clinched by the surgeon feeling the loose body and by radiological examination, and the treatment is to remove the loose body. The treatment of osteochondritis dissecans—that is

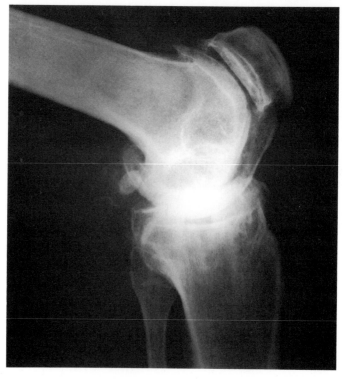

Fig. 22.5   Osteophyte of the knee with loose bodies.

before a loose body has separated—is somewhat controversial. Ther those who believe that it is best to remove the affected area, and others believe that it is best to try to re-attach the area; this is done by drill through the area into the underlying bone and hoping that a new blood supply will form. Some surgeons also fix the affected area in place either with small metal pins or small bone grafts.

Lesions of the menisci (cartilages)

These are undoubtedly the most common lesions occurring during the most athletic period of life between the ages of seventeen years and thirty years. In the United Kingdom it is most common for the medial meniscus to be affected. The classical symptoms are, that following a twisting injury, the patient is unable to straighten his knee and an effusion develops. The cartilage has to be reduced—usually under an anaesthetic—but further attacks occur with the knee locking in some twenty degrees of flexion—that is, the patient is unable to extend the knee fully but can usually flex the knee. This is accompanied by pain in the region of the medial meniscus. In less typical cases the patient may merely complain of intermittent giving way of the knee, or merely of intermittent synovial effusion. The diagnosis is made from the history and by excluding other causes such as loose bodies and osteochondritis. Provided the diagnosis is correct, treatment by removing the torn meniscus is very successful in relieving the symptoms, though it is now recognized that following removal of a meniscus the knee is likely to develop degenerative changes some fifteen or twenty years later.

Lesions of the external meniscus are less common; they may present in the above classical form—that is, attacks of locking, or they may present as a cyst which is painful, especially at night, and is visible and palpable on the outer side of the knee (Fig. 22.6).

There is another syndrome associated with a congenital abnormality in the shape of the lateral meniscus—the so-called discoid cartilage—which gives rise to periodic clunks and instability of the knee. Such menisci are very liable to become torn and the classical symptoms of locking as detailed above will then become manifest.

Chondromalacia patellae

Another syndrome which occurs at all ages but starts in adolescence is chondromalacia of the patella. In this condition degenerative changes occur in the articular cartilage of the patella, leading to pain, recurrent effusions and attacks of locking and giving way which may closely mimic a cartilage lesion. This is a very common condition and, in older patients some degree

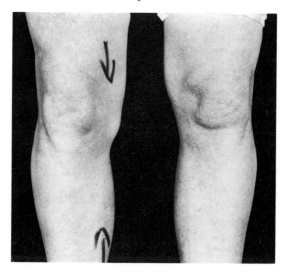

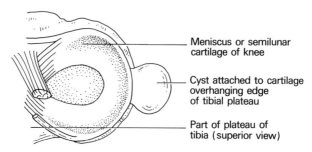

Meniscus or semilunar
cartilage of knee

Cyst attached to cartilage
overhanging edge
of tibial plateau

Part of plateau of
tibia (superior view)

Fig. 22.6 A cyst on the medial cartilage of the knee.

of degeneration of the patellar articular cartilage is almost universal. If the symptoms are severe, the condition can be treated either by excising the whole patella, or by excising the affected portion of articular cartilage if the disease is relatively localized. Surgeons differ as to whether it is best to perform a localized excision of the articular surface or a total excision of the whole patella. An alternative procedure is anterior transposition of the fibial tubercle which lessens the pressure between the patella and the femur and may relieve symptoms and prevent the condition getting worse.

Recurrent dislocation of the patella

Recurrent dislocation of the patella is also not uncommon and is mainly a disease of adolescence. In this condition the patella dislocates laterally from time to time, leading to pain, collapse of the knee, inability to move the knee, and obvious deformity in a sense that the patella can be seen and felt in an abnormal position on the outer side of the joint. In time, degenerative changes occur on the articular surface of the patella. In young children—that is, before growth is complete—the condition is best treated as for congenital dislocation of the patella, but in older patients—that is, after growth is complete—the most successful treatment is to transplant the insertion of the ligamentum patellae to a more medial position. It is, however, important that this operation should be done before the changes in the articular cartilage are too marked. If there is already extensive degeneration of the articular cartilage, excision of the patella may be required at a later date.

Torn ligaments

Tearing of ligaments of the knee is very common, especially in boys or men who play football. Severe tears of the medial or lateral collateral ligaments nearly always require immediate repair when the results are good. Late repairs are less satisfactory. Angulation of more than 40 degrees (if necessary under anaesthesia) is usually an indication for repair. Tears of the cruciate ligaments are not usually amenable to surgical repair and, if severe, give rise to chronic instability of the knee. The classical sign of cruciate instability is antero-posterior gliding of the tibia on the femur. Treatment in the first place is to build up the quadriceps and give the patient some external support of the knee. In spite of this, severe symptoms may persist and the condition ultimately leads to gross degenerative changes in the knee joint. In this case the alternatives are either for the patient to wear a walking caliper or to have an arthrodesis of the knee performed. Before the surgeon considers arthrodesis of the knee the patient should always wear a plaster cylinder for some four to six weeks so that he will be aware of the disadvantages of having a permanently stiff knee. Provided he is prepared to accept these and understands the position, arthrodesis of the knee is a good pain-relieving procedure.

Neuropathic disorders

In certain neurological conditions—especially tabes dorsalis—the knee becomes swollen and unstable due to laxity of the ligaments and capsule. Abnormal movements—e.g. lateral laxity and hyperextension occur. Ultimately the knee becomes disorganized. The treatment is to wear a caliper.

Synovial chondromatosis

This is a rare, ill-understood condition in which multiple small cartilaginous bodies form in the synovial membrane. Typically the patient presents with pain, recurring effusions in the knee joint, and chronic swelling of the synovial membrane. In advanced cases the cartilaginous bodies may be visible on radiological examination but in early cases the diagnosis is often only made at operation. The treatment is excision of as much of the synovium as possible.

Another, but relatively rare, condition is a tumour known as synovioma. In the early stages it mimics villous synovitis but there is a strong tendency to malignant changes later so it should be excised.

Villous synovitis

A rather similar condition is villous synovitis which typically affects middle-aged women. The synovial membrane becomes thickened, red and inflamed with small areas of erosion. The patient complains of pain, recurring effusions and swelling of the knees. The condition may respond to conservative measures, e.g. physiotherapy and quadriceps exercises, but if it persists a sub-total synovectomy usually gives relief.

Rheumatoid arthritis

Rheumatoid arthritis presents in the knees with a very similar syndrome, but the various serological tests (e.g. the Latex and Rose-Waaler tests) are usually positive and there is evidence of polyarthritis elsewhere in the body. For early cases of rheumatoid arthritis of the knee sub-total synovectomy is a good operation. If left untreated, the synovial membrane ultimately grows over the articular surface—as so-called 'pannus'—and leads to erosion of the articular surface, destruction of the articular cartilage, and finally disintegration of the joint. If a synovectomy is to be successful in rheumatoid arthritis, it is essential that it should be done before the condition is too advanced. Occasionally in rheumatoid arthritis confined to the knees, an arthrodesis is indicated. This has the disadvantage, especially if it is bilateral, that it may be difficult for the patient to sit with comfort, and if other joints are affected later on, this may be disastrous for the patient. Therefore, in rheumatoid arthritis arthrodesis of the knee should only be undertaken on very rare occasions.

The results of knee replacement by prosthesis are usually good in rheumatoid arthritis. This is usually the treatment of choice when all else fails.

Degenerative arthrosis

Degenerative arthrosis of the knees, or so-called osteoarthritis, is very common, especially in elderly people. The symptoms are usually intermittent, may go on for years without leading to very severe disability and in the main, treatment should be conservative by physiotherapy, quadriceps exercises, and suitable analgesic drugs. If, in spite of these, the pain is disabling, then a tibial osteotomy performed just below the articular surface of the tibia is usually very successful in relieving symptoms. The reason for this is unknown but it probably alters the blood supply to the joint. If, in association with the osteoarthritis, there is either genu valgum or genu varum, correction of the deformity can be appropriately undertaken at the time of the tibial osteotomy (Fig. 22.7).

Knee replacement is less often indicated in degenerative arthrosis than in rheumatoid arthritis.

Tuberculosis of the knee
This may affect the knee, as other joints. The patient will present with pain, swelling of the joint and some constitutional disturbances. In the early stages it may be hard to differentiate tuberculosis from rheumatoid arthritis and for this reason a synovial biopsy may be essential to establish the diagnosis.

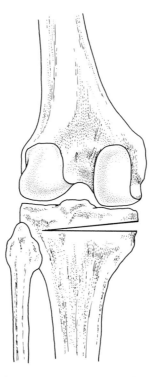

Fig. 22.7   Tibial osteotomy for osteoarthritis of the knees.

Treatment is essentially by the administration of antibiotics and chemo-therapy, but in addition, if the synovial membrane is thickened, a sub-total synovectomy is usually helpful. In old standing cases or where there has been extensive destruction of the knee joint, arthrodesis is sometimes required. This was commonly needed before the days of streptomycin but is rarely required nowadays.

Haemophilia

Haemophilia, i.e. bleeding into the knee due to a failure of blood clotting—is not uncommon. It results in chronic arthritis of the knee with pain, swelling, typical radiological changes and ultimately limitation of movement. Basically the treatment is to treat the acute haemorrhagic episode by the administra-tion of anti-haemophilia serum, and also aspiration of the blood from the knee joint. In severe cases the patient may need to require a supporting caliper. Occasionally the arthritis may be so severe as to lead to severe deformities which require correction.

Flexion deformities of the knee

Flexion deformities of the knee are seen in a variety of conditions, either in certain disorders of the central nervous system—for instance, spastic paresis, or secondary to diseases of the knee joint, either chronic or acute arthritis. Mild cases can be treated by active exercises, assisted movements and splinting. More severe cases require division of the hamstring muscles followed by slow correction of the deformity by passive stretching and assisted exercises. Usually the divided hamstring muscles are re-attached to the femur. In very severe deformities a supracondylar osteotomy may be required. In all cases slow correction is essential to avoid damage to the circulation.

Arthroscopy

During recent years a small bore arthroscope has been developed which enables the surgeon to inspect the inside of the joint through a small stab incision. Where the diagnosis is in doubt this often enables an accurate diagnosis to be made and the right treatment, operative or non-operative, to be prescribed.

Operations on the knee

(a) *Bloodless field of operation* (see also Chapter 27, p. 440). The surgeon prefers to operate on the hand, wrist, elbow or the foot, ankle and knee without bleeding obstructing the field of vision. Blood reduces the speed of the operation and cannot be completely removed from a joint; it will clot within the capsule and tend to cause adhesions between the structures within the joint.

On the operating table it is therefore usual to adopt this procedure.

(i)   elevate the leg above the level of the trunk;

(ii)   apply a rubber bandage from the toes to the mid-thigh on the patient;

(iii)   apply a pneumatic tourniquet above the level of the bandage on the thigh;

(iv)   remove the rubber bandage before the operation, leaving the inflated tourniquet in position.

Thus the blood will not flow into the joint capsule before the release of the tourniquet, by which time a Jones compression bandage will be in position to prevent the effusion of blood (haemarthrosis).

(b) *The position of the knee at operation.* Many operations on the knee do not require any modification of the position of the patient lying supine on the operating table. For some operations the surgeon prefers to operate with the patient's knee in flexion, the degree of flexion related to the site of operation. For example, to reach the attachments of the cruciate ligaments, either on the plateau of tibia or in the intercondylar notch on the distal end of femur, complete flexion of the knee into a hairpin position is required.

To achieve and hold these positions the leg must be bent at the knee over the end of the operating table. Care must be taken to avoid pressure on structures such as nerves or arteries which may be damaged by crushing. The following areas must be guarded by the use of foam-rubber or gamgee pads:

(i)   The popliteal space behind the knee.

(ii)   The lateral surface of the leg near the neck of fibula.

(iii)   The ankle.

(c) *The Jones compression bandage.* To prevent effusion into the knee after surgery, the Jones compression bandage is applied before removal of the pneumatic tourniquet around the thigh. The method is as follows:

(i)   A sterile dressing is applied to the wound and held in place by a suitable adhesive. There are many new developments in the field of surgical dressings and adhesives so that it is hard to be specific about the wound dressing. A plastic spray-on dressing or micro-porous tape may be used according to the surgeon's wishes.

(ii)   A thick layer of sterile surgical wool is applied from mid-calf to mid-thigh. This is fixed by 10 cm wide calico bandage.

(iii)   A thick layer of splint wool is applied over the first bandage and this is firmly bandaged in position.

(iv)   A further layer of splint wool and calico bandage is applied. The original bandage described by Sir Robert Jones recommended six alternating layers of material—surgical wool, calico bandage, splint wool, calico bandage, more splint wool and a final calico bandage. Each bandage is firmly applied and is secured by a large safety pin.

This will be modified according to the surgeon's wishes; examples of these modifications are:

(i)   To incorporate a large pad of wool behind the knee to create 5 degrees of flexion; or

(ii)   To incorporate the pad of wool and an aluminium gutter splint which should be as long in length as the finished supporting bandage; the final bandage holds this in place.

The many layers are applied so that the pressure on the knee joint can be maintained even though the top layers of bandage and wool are removed for checking and reapplication. When this is done the inner layer of wool and bandage is left untouched; it must not be removed before some healing of the tissues has occurred and bleeding into the joint is not likely to happen. Most surgeons require that it remains in place for ten days but this length of time is now modified by some.

The gutter splint is incorporated into the bandage when the surgeon wishes the patient to walk with the compression bandage in position, soon (perhaps twenty-four hours) after the operation; flexion and extension of the knee are then not possible as the patient walks.

Another concept is that the patient must not apply weight to the leg until the compression bandage has been removed and physiotherapy has regained full quality of musculature. He is allowed out of bed into a wheelchair or on to crutches.

(d) *Quadriceps drill.* The word DRILL is deliberately used. The quadriceps and hamstrings are the powerful muscles which move and stabilize the knee. If these are permitted to become weak and inefficient, the movements of both the hip and the knee are affected. The patient will be unable to stand after rising from his bed and may be left with an ugly limp which will take some months to vanish. If he is an active sportsman he will be limited in his abilities. As patients with lesions of the knee are often youthful, it is unkind to allow them to lapse into a state where the muscles are wasted when a fair amount of 'bullying' will keep them exercising their legs when lying in bed or when sitting in a chair or wheelchair.

All ages of patient are therefore encouraged to exercise their muscles without direct supervision, to a specific routine. This is to tense both quadriceps and hamstrings groups of muscles, and then relax them, repeatedly for the first five minutes of every hour they are awake. The patient can be taught to 'pull up' the patella, particularly if it is visible.

Additional to this the physiotherapy staff may encourage 'group activities' among a number of patients with knee lesions in the same orthopaedic unit. This includes removal of the top bedclothes and lifting and lowering each leg (whether affected or not) in turn.

Physiotherapy for the knee

For the recumbent patient the exercises are mainly those described above. Once the patient is out of bed the exercises may become more active and may take the following forms:

(a) Seated flexion and extension exercises, using pulleys and cords with varying weights attached. The patient has the cord attached to the foot and ankle and applies effort against the weight by either flexion or extension as required. As the musculature improves, the weight is increased.

(b) Stationary bicycle: the patient cycles a distance as recorded on the meter of the stationary bicycle. The effort required of the patient may be increased or decreased by varying the friction to be overcome as the wheels turn.

(c) Walking, running, cycling, dancing are obviously excellent for exercising the knee.

(d) Rehabilitation in industry: firms which have a rehabilitation programme for their employees may employ the worker on a machine or device which is operated by the use of the legs; a treadle loom or sewing machine is an obvious example.

Splintage for the knee

1   *Plaster of Paris*
    (a) *Plaster leg cylinder.* See Chapter 9, p. 141.
    (b) *Plaster back splint.* See Chapter 9, p. 141.
2   *Plastazote back splint.*
3   *Aluminium gutter splint.*
4   *Thomas' bed-knee splint.* See Chapter 9, p. 137 and Chapter 28.
5   *Thomas' walking caliper.* See Chapter 9, p. 139.
6   *Weight-relieving caliper.* See p. 324.

7   *Other calipers.* See Chapter 31.

8   *Knee cage* (Fig. 22.8). This is a hinged device which limits the movements of an unstable knee by supporting it in the actions of flexion and extension only. Thus lateral or medical strain on the knee is relieved. It is, however, cumbersome and easily slips out of position. Relatively few patients like it.

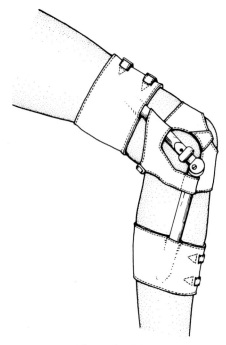

Fig. 22.8   A knee cage.

23

Affections of the Shoulder

Relevant applied anatomy and physiology

The freely movable synovial joints of the body are designed so that they best serve the function of the part in which they are situated. Thus hinge joints occur where a hinge is needed; pivot joints are found where a pivot action is required; gliding joints where a limited amount of movement on a flat plane is needed. A ball and socket joint such as the shoulder is an excellent example of the correct siting of a joint; the ball and socket design which offers the widest possible range of movements in any joint, allows placement of an arm in many different positions. Thus we may carry the arms above the head to reach a high shelf, or forwards to push a car, or downwards to lift an object from the floor; the arms can also reach out to the side or describe a circle, as in throwing a ball.

To permit this wide range of movements modifications exist in the design of the joint which make it different from other joints:

1 A large bony ball (the head of the humerus) fits into a relatively shallow socket (the glenoid cavity of the scapula).

2 The glenoid cavity is deepened by the presence of a cartilaginous lip; this creates a larger surface for contact with the head of the humerus.

3 The capsule of the joint is large and loose. It is large enough to allow a tuck of fibrous capsule to hang down when the arm is by the side. Without supporting structures the capsule does not give stability to the joint.

4 The fibrous capsule is supported by:

    (i) A layer of extracapsular ligaments, and external to this

    (ii) A layer of muscles situated between the humerus and scapula, called the rotator cuff.

5 The function and stability of the shoulder depends upon the efficiency of the rotator cuff muscles. No matter what posture is adopted, placing the arm in any of many different positions, the muscles contract to maintain the head of the humerus in close contact with the glenoid cavity of the scapula. Paralysis of these muscles causes instability of the joint with frequent recurrent dislocations of the joint.

The main nerve supplying the capsule of the shoulder and the important deltoid muscle, is a nerve which winds around the surgical neck of humerus after it leaves the brachial plexus. This nerve (the axillary, or circumflex nerve) may be crushed in a fracture of the surgical neck of the humerus.

The wide range of movements available at the pectoral girdle and at the shoulder is not solely because of the ball and socket joint. Two other joints contribute to arm movement:

    (i)   The sternoclavicular joint and,

    (ii) The acromioclavicular joint.

Loss of function of these joints can cause restriction of, primarily, scapular movement and, secondarily, arm movement.

Affections of the shoulder

Congenital lesions

Sprengel's shoulder. The commonest congenital lesion of the shoulder is the so-called Sprengel's shoulder which is characterized by the scapula on that side being smaller, of an abnormal shape, elevated, and bound down to the chest wall (see Fig. 18.12). This syndrome is often associated with congenital lesion of the cervical spine such as congenital fusion of the cervical vertebrae. In addition there may be a bar of ectopic bone stretching from the spine to the scapula, often known as the omo-vertebral bone. Even if there is no bar of bone there are often strands of fibrous tissue.

In the earlier stages the treatment should be by passive movements to mobilize the scapula as far as possible, but if the deformity is severe and the limitation of movement is marked it is best treated by excision of the upper part of the scapula, including any bony or fibrous bands passing from the scapula to the spine. Following this the scapula slowly drops to a more normal position, the cosmetic appearance is much improved and there is often, but not always, some improvement in the range of shoulder movement.

Erb's palsy. Another congenital lesion, in the sense that it may be present at birth, is Erb's palsy. This is paralysis of certain muscles of the arm due to damage of the brachial plexus at birth and is therefore more common when labour has been difficult or prolonged. In a characteristic case there is paralysis of the abductors and external rotators of the shoulder, of the flexors of the elbow and of the extensors of the wrist and fingers; the whole arm being held in the characteristic 'waiter's tip position' (Fig. 23.1).

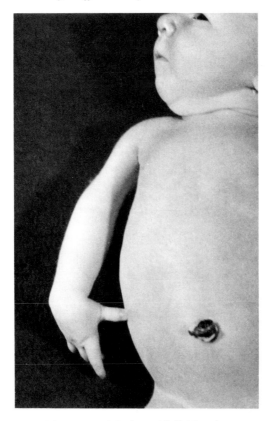

Fig. 23.1   (a) Patient with Erb's palsy.

The treatment in the early stages is by means of passive stretching and assisted movements to avoid contracture of the joints and muscles and the arm being fixed in a permanent position of deformity.

The prognosis for a certain amount of recovery of the muscles is good, but full recovery of the external rotator muscles is unusual. If this remains paralysed the patient cannot lift the arm in a normal way or rotate the arm externally, which makes the patient appear awkward in certain movements— e.g. shaking hands, eating, etc.

The best treatment is to divide some of the internal rotator muscles of the shoulder, e.g. the pectoralis major and latissimus dorsi and transplant these to the back of the humerus to act as external rotators.

Simple division of these muscles without transplantation is not very successful and the disability usually returns. Similarly, external rotation

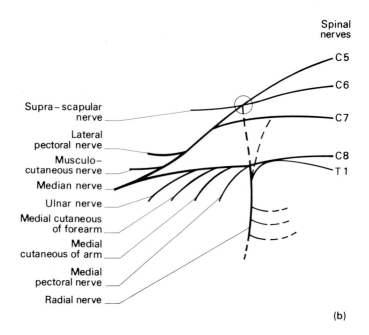

Fig. 23.1 (b) A diagram of the brachial plexus.

osteotomy of the humerus, which is often advised, is disappointing in the long run, as the deformity recurs.

Paralysis of the shoulder
Paralysis of the shoulder may occur, as described above for instance, due to birth palsy, or it may occur following a brachial plexus injury, or following an infection of the anterior nerve roots such as poliomyelitis. If the disability is severe, arthrodesis of the shoulder is sometimes advised, but stiffness of the shoulder has certain disadvantages and should never be advised in the young child; it is only of advantage to the patient with good control of the scapula, elbow and hand. As many patients with paralysis of the shoulder develop excellent trick movements and learn to manage well even though the shoulder is flail, the operation of arthrodesis of the shoulder is only to be undertaken on the rare occasions when it is quite clear that it is

going to be a real functional advantage to the patient and the disadvantages do not outway the advantages. Transplantation of muscles, e.g. the trapezius from the scapula to the humerus is also sometimes performed.

Recurrent dislocation of the shoulder

This fairly frequently follows dislocation of the shoulder in young people. In older people, the risk of recurrent dislocation is small, but as the risk of recurrent dislocation in young people is high, it is usually advisable that, following a reduction of a dislocation in young people, the shoulder should be held in the fully internally rotated and adducted position for at least four weeks. However, if recurrent dislocation does occur, this is usually due to a tearing of the capsule or a separation of the glenoid labrum from the rim of the glenoid articular surface.

In older people the risk of recurrent dislocation is small and it is usually wise to commence early movement after reduction of the dislocation.

The treatment of recurrent dislocation is to repair the tear in the capsule or re-attach the glenoid labrum to bone. This can be done either by directly suturing the capsule to the bone or by reefing the capsule and shortening the subscapularis muscle. Following operation the arm is kept in full internal rotation for four weeks. The results are usually satisfactory though there may be some slight limitation of external rotation.

Suppurative arthritis

Infections of the shoulder joint are relatively rare but occasionally an acute infection does occur and this is treated as outlined in Chapter 13.

Tuberculosis of the shoulder

In the past, chronic infection in the form of tuberculosis of the shoulder has occasionally occurred. It was often associated with tuberculosis of the lungs and was characterized by a very slow insidious onset with pain, wasting and progressive limitation of shoulder movement. Nowadays it would usually be treated by antibiotics, chemotherapy and, if necessary, partial excision of the synovial membrane, but in the past it often went on to marked destruction of the shoulder and fibrous ankylosis; bony arthrodesis of the shoulder joint was often necessary.

Disorders of the shoulder joint capsule

The shoulder joint has a voluminous capsule which is vulnerable to a variety of disorders, the exact causes of which are ill understood. The most dramatic of these is the so-called supraspinatus tendonitis where the patient has acute pain under the acromion process, characterized by difficulty in abducting the shoulder and, if the patient tries to lower the arm to his side from the vertical position, there is an acute attack of pain in the middle range of movement and he has to drop his arm to the side. This supraspinatus tendinitis may be associated with evidence of calcification or with the formation of an enlarged bursa and, on rare occasions, with rupture of the tendon. The treatment in the first place should be conservative but if the pain persists then operation to remove any calcified material or an enlarged bursa is usually successful. If there is a complete rupture of the tendon it is wise to try to repair this in the younger age group, but the results are only moderately good as there is usually fairly wide degeneration of the tendon and the joint capsule.

The arm must be held in abduction for at least eight weeks after operative repair. It is probably wise to restrict operation to the relatively young and active.

Frozen shoulder

There is another condition known as frozen shoulder or adhesive capsulitis, in which extensive fibrosis occurs in the shoulder joint capsule with progressive loss of movement and pain. This is usually a self-limiting condition though it may take some six to nine months for the condition to subside. During the acute phase the patient should be treated with rest, heat and analgesic drugs and, during the recovery phase, he should be treated by active exercises and gentle assisted movements. Small doses of steroids for a limited period are very helpful but in a self-limiting condition, 'steroid addiction' must be avoided. Occasionally there is permanent limitation of movement, and under these circumstances a gentle manipulation of the shoulder may be helpful, though this should never be done in the early or acute phases as at that time it may lead to some exacerbation of the symptoms. Manipulation of the shoulder should always be performed very gently as otherwise there is a risk of producing a fracture of the humerus. Following manipulation the patient will require adequate analgesic drugs, heat and encouragement in the active exercises. For this reason it is usually wise to admit the patient to hospital for a day or two.

Nursing management of patients with affections of the shoulder

Rest and support for the shoulder

The optimum position of rest for the shoulder is usually with the arm supported in abduction. This is achieved by:

(a) The application of a plaster of Paris shoulder spica which may be complete or lidded (see Chapter 8, p. 105), or

(b) The use of the Littler-Jones abduction splint (see Chapter 8, p. 101). Full abduction of the arm is not always necessary or desirable and the surgeon may wish to modify it. It is more convenient to the patient if the hand can be carried to the mouth and face and when this is possible, part flexion of the arm as well as abduction may be arranged.

The position of abduction is, in either case, inconvenient for the patient: to put on a shirt or coat is a major physical feat when attempted without assistance. Comfort in bed is also hard to achieve without special supports and pillows. It is therefore part of the nurse's duty to enquire into the home circumstances of the patient who is to be sent home in an abduction appliance. There must be someone capable of giving reasonable assistance to the patient in his daily living activities. In fact, holding the arm in abduction is so inconvenient that it is usually restricted to indications where it is essential:

1   After repair of a torn supraspinatus muscle,

2   After arthrodesis of the shoulder,

3   In certain fractures which cannot be reduced with the arm hanging down and are not amenable to operative fixation.

Supporting the arm to the side and chest

A more comfortable method of immobilizing the shoulder, when possible, is by bandaging the arm to the trunk of the patient underneath his clothing. The method is as follows:

1   The skin on the side and front of the thorax and medial side of the whole of the arm and the axilla is washed, dried and powdered.

2   A thin layer of splint wool is arranged between the two skin surfaces.

3   The arm is placed across the thorax with the hand flat on the anterior surface near the opposite shoulder. It is supported there by an assistant.

4   Using 10 cm wide conforming bandages, the supporting bandage is commenced at the vertebral column, passed around the waist of the patient going towards the unaffected side first; this is anchoring turn.

5   The next turn of the bandage passes across the back of the hand of the patient as it rests on the front of thorax, and then to the affected shoulder.

6   It then passes over the affected shoulder, down to the posterior surface of the flexed elbow and up again on the anterior surface of the arm to the affected shoulder.

7   From the affected shoulder the bandage is carried across the posterior surface of the thorax to the waist on the unaffected side.

8   To complete one set of turns the bandage is taken around the point of the flexed elbow on the affected side and back to the starting point.

9   After carrying the bandage over the anterior surface of the thorax the whole set of turns are repeated. At least two bandages are required.

10   Regular daily removal of the bandages with an assistant supporting the arm in the correct position must be arranged. The skin is again washed, dried and powdered with talc. New splint wool is placed between the skin surfaces and clean bandages used to re-apply the support.

24

Low Back Pain and Sciatica

Relevant applied anatomy and physiology

The human vertebral column is adapted to support the body in the upright position. It has many functions but three are relevant to this chapter: (1) movement, (2) stability and (3) protection of the central nervous system. The spinal column is constructed so that it can protect the spinal cord, support the head, trunk and arms, and allow movement. As a corollary, if the vertebral column is affected by any pathological disorder, the resulting lesion is most likely to impair these functions.

The column is constructed of twenty-six bones placed vertically above each other (vertebrae) with an elastic shock absorber (intervertebral disc) between each pair of bones. Adjacent and posterior to each disc is the opening through which the peripheral nerves pass on their path from the spinal cord to their peripheral end organs (Chapter 11). The boundaries of this opening, the intervertebral foramen, include two structures which are essential for movement of one of the vertebrae upon the other; these structures are the intervertebral disc on the anterior surface and the interlaminar synovial joint on the posterior surface of the opening through which the spinal nerve leaves the neural canal.

The size of the opening may be reduced by the following factors:

1 A reduction in the distance between each pair of bones, or
2 An increase in the size of the intervertebral disc which then protrudes posteriorly into the intervertebral foramen, or
3 An increase in the size of the capsule of the interlaminar synovial joint which then protrudes anteriorly into the intervertebral foramen.

As a result of this decrease in the size of the orifice, the nerve passing through it is irritated and constricted; this is known as *nerve root pressure*.

This is not the only form of compression and irritation of a nerve root; any protuberance which impinges on the nerve (e.g. a tumour) has the same effect.

The structure and function of an intervertebral disc

The intervertebral discs are essential structures for the relatively wide range of movement of the normal vertebral column. These pads, which correspond in shape and size to the adjacent vertebral bodies, are malleable; they permit a small amount of movement of one vertebra upon the other in any direction. This range of movement is possible because the intervertebral disc has a special form of construction. The disc is basically a box containing a fluid core. The roof and floor of each box is formed by the cartilaginous end plates of the adjacent vertebral bodies; its walls are formed by an outer tough casing of interlacing supporting fibres (the annulus fibrosus). Inside the box is an inner gelatinous centre, the nucleus pulposus. In some people the cartilaginous end plate of the vertebra is weak and the nucleus pulposus protrudes into the bone of the adjacent vertebral body forming structures known as Schmorl's nodes.

The intervertebral ligaments

Each vertebra is attached to its neighbouring vertebrae by a number of ligaments. These contribute greatly to the stability and strength of the vertebral column. The most important are:

1 The anterior longitudinal ligament which runs down the whole length of the spine on the anterior aspect.
2 The posterior longitudinal ligament.
3 The ligamentus flavum between the adjacent laminae and
4 The interspinous ligaments between adjacent spinous processes.

Low back pain and sciatica

Literally, sciatica means 'irritation of the sciatic nerve', but it is commonly applied as a generic term for any pain which is felt to radiate down the leg. The possible causes of such pain can best be considered anatomically, starting with the most proximal lesions and ending with the more distal ones.

Disorders of the spinal cord such as intramedullary tumours, may cause pain in the leg. Similarly, any cause of cauda equina irritation may cause pain down the leg. Of these, pressure from a prolapsed intervertebral disc (Fig. 24.1) is the most common, but intra and extra dural tumours, dermoid cysts, adhesions, congenital abnormalities and ischaemic lesions of the cauda equina can all cause pain referred down the leg. Among the more distal causes of pressure on the sciatic nerve, one includes sacroiliac disease, tumours of the sciatic nerve and tumours adjacent to the nerve which press on it—for example, so-called ganglia arising from the superior

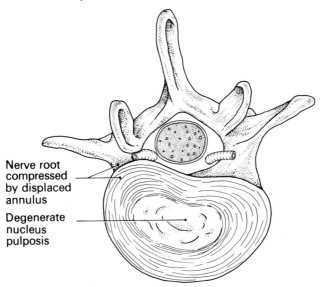

Nerve root
compressed
by displaced
annulus

Degenerate
nucleus
pulposis

Fig. 24.1 A prolapsed intervertebral disc causing nerve root pressure.

tibio-fibular joint may press on the nerve and cause pain in its area of distribution (Fig. 24.2).

Disorders of the lower lumbar joints, sacroiliac joints and hip joints may also give rise to pain which mimics sciatica, and the pain of ischaemic disease, for example due to occlusion of the aorta, also may cause pain in the leg (Fig. 24.2). Narrowing of the spinal canal or spinal stenosis may cause ischaemia of the cauda equina in older patients. This is another cause of pain in the legs.

The most useful approach to the problem of sciatica is to describe the typical features of a classical sciatica due to a prolapsed intervertebral disc (Fig. 24.1). The main symptom will consist of pain radiating down the leg as far as the ankle and sometimes into the toes. The signs include a tilt of the spine to the affected side (Fig. 24.3); stiffness of the spine; limitation of straight leg raising and also certain neurological signs, of which the most common are absence of the ankle jerk and weakness of the calf muscle (caused by a lesion of the first sacral nerve root), weakness of the extensor of the great toe and impairment of sensation on the antero-lateral aspect of the shin (caused by a fifth lumbar lesion). Naturally both the extent and exact type of physical signs will vary according to which nerve root is affected. Large central disc prolapses may interfere with bladder control.

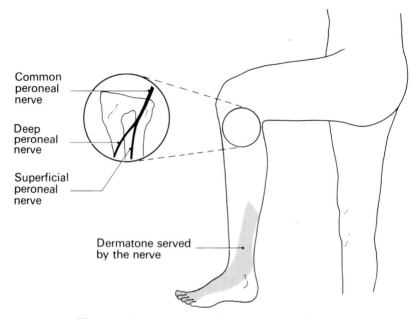

Common
peroneal
nerve

Deep
peroneal
nerve

Superficial
peroneal
nerve

Dermatone served
by the nerve

Fig. 24.2   Root pressure on the common peroneal nerve.

It will be seen that the most important step in examining a patient with sciatica is to exclude the serious causes such as tumours and arterial disease. If these can be excluded, the majority of causes of sciatica can be assumed to be due to pressure from a deranged intervertebral disc.

Most intervertebral disc lesions will settle down with a period of rest in bed with traction (Chapter 28) and the administration of suitable analgesics and sedatives. However, if the pain does not settle down within three weeks, or if there are frequent recurrent attacks, or if there is serious muscle weakness or interference with micturition, then operation for removal of the affected disc is indicated. Providing the diagnosis is correct and the whole of the abnormal disc is removed, these operations are nearly always completely successful. Accurate pre-operative diagnosis by radiculography and discography enables the surgeon to limit his operation to an interlaminal approach to one disc, thus reducing the incidence and extent of post-operative adhesions.

In young patients who do heavy work discectomy may be combined with fusion.

Back pain
There are naturally a great variety of pathological conditions which can give

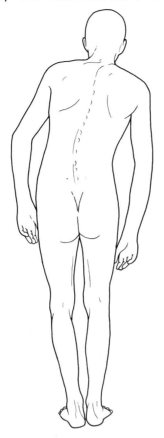

Fig. 24.3   Patient showing signs of sciatica.

rise to pain in the back. All the forementioned causes of sciatica can be associated with pain in the back. In addition, diseases of the vertebrae, intervertebral discs and ligaments may all present as back pain. Among these must be included Schmorl's nodes, osteochondritis (juvenile kyphosis or Scheurmann's disease), ankylosing spondylitis, tuberculosis, typhoid fever, staphylococcal infections, abortus fever and other infections of the intervertebral discs. Osteoporosis, hyperparathyroidism, primary tumours, both benign and malignant, secondary tumours of the vertebrae and discs, spinal tumours, disc degeneration, injury and damage to the ligaments and posterior articulations must all be considered in the differential diagnoses. In addition, abdominal extra-spinal conditions—for example, abdominal aneurysms, pancreatic neoplasms, penetrating ulcers of the stomach and duodenum and renal conditions—all may present as pain in the back.

Most of these conditions can be diagnosed or excluded by taking the history and carrying out a careful clinical and radiological examination of the spine.

If the diagnosis is still in doubt, radiological examination to estimate the uptake of Strontium 87 can be of great value in revealing early lesions—e.g. neoplasms or infections of bone. Osteoporosis is also a common cause of back pain either in its idiopathic form or secondary to hyperparathyroidism (Chapter 4) but when all these conditions have been excluded, there remains a number of patients who complain of back pain in whom the exact pathological cause is a matter of conjecture. These appear to present as three main syndromes:

1 *Recurrent lumbago.* This may be precipitated by unusual activity or strain, or by cold wind, damp, a change in the weather, or by emotional strain. The exact pathology is unknown but it is probably due to biochemical changes in the nucleus pulposus of the intervertebral disc. It is usual for the acute attack to subside with a period of bed rest, warmth and suitable analgesics. If an attack does not subside within three or four weeks it is important to exclude any of the more serious conditions listed above.

2 *Chronic backache.* Aggravated by standing, sitting and activity and relieved by rest, this condition is most common in women. It is usually the result of poor muscle tone and weak ligaments, and is usually relieved by measures to improve muscle tone such as abdominal and spinal exercises, and the wearing of a suitable supporting corset.

3 *Degenerative changes.* This third syndrome occurs in the older patient with degenerative changes in the intervertebral discs and posterior articulations. The main feature here is pain at night and relative absence of pain during the day. Some patients obtain relief by the application of heat and exercises, others are helped by wearing a supporting belt; most relief is obtained by the administration of suitable analgesic drugs, e.g. Butazolidine with stronger sedatives at night.

On rare occasions any of these three syndromes may be sufficiently severe to warrant surgical intervention—e.g. spinal fusion, but as a general rule they are best treated by the above mentioned palliative measures. In many patients the pain is episodic and, provided they are assisted by palliative treatment during an acute phase, they will usually have considerable periods without symptoms and will not require any medical attention.

In all patients with back problems attention to posture when standing, sitting or lying is important. A firm mattress at night is essential and long car rides should be avoided.

The nursing management of patients with acute low back pain and sciatica

Often these patients are seriously demoralized by their back lesion, particularly if there is a recurrence of the condition for which they have had a previous long course of treatment. There is a need for reassurance and a positive approach to their management; they must not be allowed to feel that nothing is being done or can be done. A clear explanation of what is wrong, and how they can co-operate in the diagnostic tests is invaluable. The stages of their treatment, the alternatives which must be tried, and their part in assisting and achieving recovery must also be explained. This is a condition in which the patient's work, hobbies and domestic conditions play a very important part in deciding the right treatment.

Complete bed rest
The first approach to the treatment of many lesions of the back is complete bed rest. This is now discussed.

(a) *The bed.* The least desirable bed for the management of any patient with a spinal lesion, is that with a soft flexible structure which will sag. A firm, even, hard mattress is the best. An orthopaedic bed has a solid unsprung base under a slim mattress. This is different from the patient's usual bed and it will take some time for him to accept. Patients with back lesions should be encouraged to modify their own bed similarly at home, by arranging a sheet of hardboard over the springs of the bed and under the mattress.

A firm bed maintains the spine in good posture during sleep, particularly if only a single pillow is supplied and when the patient is in the supine position.

(b) *Management of complete rest* (see also Chapter 27, p. 413). 'Complete bed rest' means exactly that—rest in bed without physical activity. When it has been ordered by the orthopaedic surgeon there is a reason and a need for it. The patient with a spinal lesion is often a patient who is tired and exhausted; the exhaustion may be physical—perhaps as the result of hard unrelieved effort lasting over a long period of time; a housewife with a family of young children, managing without aid and in poor financial circumstances may present such a state. It is often hard for the surgeon to know if the back pain is the cause or the effect of the patient's physical state; the only way to find out is to attempt to relieve the physical and mental weariness by insisting that the patient is taken out of her environment and that her responsibilities are given to others for a reasonable length of time.

(c) *Mental rest.* The patient on the complete rest regime must also be mentally at rest. The act of ordering a patient to bed in hospital does not ensure rest if the daily worries of the patient are not taken over by another person or agency acceptable to the patient. An obvious need for the young housewife is that a relative, trusted by the patient, takes over the running of her household during her stay in hospital. If the patient will have financial distress as a result of staying in bed, positive action must be taken by the social worker to prevent this distress. Physical rest cannot occur if the patient is worried and agitated; in extreme states it may be necessary for the surgeon to order the relevant barbiturate tranquillizer drugs to cause relaxation as well as analgesics. Mental rest is impossible if the patient is bored; suitable diversions are also necessary.

(d) *Physical rest.* Under the care of nursing staff the patient remains in the horizontal position for the whole period ordered by the surgeon. Sitting up in bed, or chair, standing, reaching into the bedside locker, or ambulation to bathroom and toilet are prohibited. Meals must be consumed lying flat and the patient must learn to transfer food from plate and cup to mouth in this position; most people learn to achieve this skill in a relatively short time.

As a direct result of the complete mental and physical rest, patients often feel relief from their symptoms, possibly due to the relaxation of muscles previously in spasm. Suitable diversional activities are a necessary part of treatment.

Leg or pelvic traction

If the patient with a back lesion does not respond to complete bed rest within a reasonable period of time the surgeon may order Pugh's traction, or weight and pulley traction, or pelvic traction (Chapter 28, p. 486). Frequently in order to save time and money, traction is ordered at once without trying simple bed rest if the patient has to be admitted to hospital.

Physiotherapy

After bed rest or traction, physiotherapy is necessary for the treatment of low back pain. This takes the form of applications of heat and massage to relax the muscles of the back. As the condition shows signs of responding to treatment the surgeon may order an increase in the tempo of physiotherapy to improve the musculature of the vertebral column. All of this is only on the direct instructions of the surgeon however; harm can be caused if the wrong form of activity is given at an unsuitable stage of treatment.

Intermittent traction

Many patients are considerably relieved by intermittent traction in the physiotherapy department which may have a dramatic effect during an acute attack. On a special traction table the patient is given increasingly strong pulls for 15–20 seconds with relaxation in between. In the early stages the treatment must be carefully monitored as sometimes it aggravates the pain.

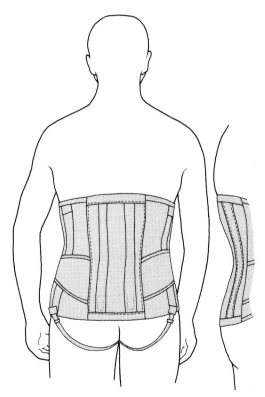

Fig. 24.4   A Goldthwait belt.

Injections

Sometimes injection of a local anaesthetic and hydrocortisone into a tender musculotendinous nodule gives relief.

The injection of a similar solution into the extradural space also gives relief to some patients.

Spinal supports

Belts vary from a light abdominal corset to heavy leather ones with a rigid steel plate in the back. Some patients with low back pain and/or sciatica may require a firm support, the purpose of which is to limit the range of movement of the spine and reduce muscular effort.

These consist of:

(a) Supporting belts or corsets. The Goldthwait belt is an example (Figs. 24.4 and 29.4); many variations of this design have been produced and manufacturers offer their own patents and designs (Chapter 29, p. 505).

(b) Posterior plaster slab with a tubular supporting bandage (Chapter 30, p. 525).

(c) Plaster jacket (Chapter 30, p. 529).

Surgical treatment

Various operative procedures have been devised for this condition. The relevant post-operative management is as defined by the surgeon. The principles of the surgical management of orthopaedic patients are described in Chapter 27.

In general, operations are performed (a) to remove any structure which is pressing on a nerve root, e.g. an intervertebral disc, (b) to fuse together (arthrodese) vertebrae whose connecting joints are irretrievably damaged.

25

Brachial Neuritis

A patient may experience pain in a given part of his body either because there is a local lesion such as inflammation or a tumour in this region, or because the sensory nerves which supply the region are being irritated at a more proximal level, e.g. by a lesion of the spine, or because a visceral stricture which is innervated by the same nerve root is also the site of a lesion; but because the brain's recognition of localization of visceral pain is poor, the patient's brain refers the pain to another region for which conscious localization is better. The classic example is irritation of the diaphragm which is often felt as pain at the tip of the shoulder—as the diaphragm (which is innervated by the phrenic nerve) has the same root value as the skin of the shoulder. In considering the clinical syndrome of brachial neuritis (pain in the arm) we may have to consider all three causes of pain.

For instance, shoulder pain may be due to a local lesion, supraspinatus calcification, to a lesion in the neck irritating the nerves supplying the shoulder, e.g. cervical spondylosis, or as already incidenced, it may be due to a diaphragmatic irritation. Brachial neuritis is not therefore a diagnosis, but is a useful descriptive term for a variety of clinical and pathological syndromes which have certain features in common. The various causes of brachial neuritis are arranged according to their anatomical situation, beginning with the most proximal lesions and ending with the most distal ones.

Disorders of the spinal cord

A variety of disorders of the spinal cord may give rise to pain referred down the arm, e.g. intramedullary tumours. Such disorders can usually be diagnosed by the associated neurological signs, e.g. the nerves of the leg will be affected also. In the same way various lesions of the spinal column may give rise to pain in the arm; of these the most common are cervical spondylosis or degenerative arthritis, which will give rise to pain in the arm as well as pain in the neck, and more rarely, involvement of the pyramidal tracts with spastic

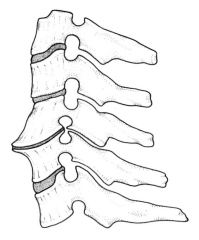

Fig. 25.1 Cervical spondylosis. Note the anterior and posterior osteophytes, narrowed disc and diminution in the size of the nerve foramina.

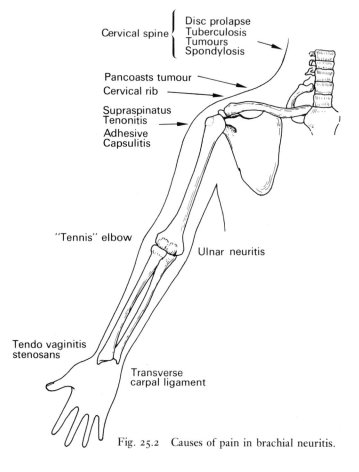

Cervical spine {
Disc prolapse
Tuberculosis
Tumours
Spondylosis

Pancoasts tumour

Cervical rib

Supraspinatus
Tenonitis

Adhesive
Capsulitis

"Tennis" elbow

Ulnar neuritis

Tendo vaginitis
stenosans

Transverse
carpal ligament

Fig. 25.2 Causes of pain in brachial neuritis.

paresis of the legs. Various tumours of the vertebral column, both primary and secondary, may also present as pain radiating down the arm.

Disorders of the nerve roots

A variety of conditions, particularly virus diseases, may affect the nerve roots of the cervical plexus and cause pain in the arm. Most of these are associated with some degree of lower motor neurone paralysis. Poliomyelitis, Herpes Zoster, and the so-called neuralgic amyotrophy are three examples of virus diseases characterized by severe pain in the arm, and the first and third of these almost inevitably lead to paralysis of certain muscles. The prognosis for spontaneous recovery in the last named is good, however, and in the course of a year to eighteen months full recovery usually occurs.

Disorders of the brachial plexus

In addition to injuries to the brachial plexus which are dealt with elsewhere, tumours of the brachial plexus may cause pain in the arm. These may either be true nerve sheath tumours, or the so-called Pancoast's tumour, which is a

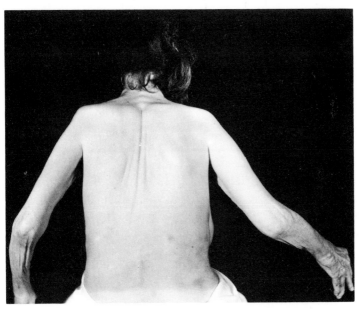

Fig. 25.3 Patient with paralysis of the shoulders and arms.

cancer of the apex of the lung which gives rise to intractable pain down the arm and may be difficult to diagnose in the early stages as neurological changes are usually comparatively late.

Cervical ribs (extra bony projections on the seventh cervical vertebra) are occasionally the cause of pain in the arm but more frequently cause pressure on the sub-clavian artery, giving rise to symptoms of ischaemia in the arm. It should be realised that cervical ribs are commonly present and are often symptomless; their mere presence does not indicate they are necessarily the cause of the patient's pain. The operation of removal of a cervical rib should not be undertaken lightly, it is easy to stretch or otherwise damage the brachial plexus and cause paralysis.

Shoulder lesions

There are a variety of lesions of the shoulder which are dealt with more fully in Chapter 23 but of these both supraspinatus tendonitis, supraspinatus calcification and the so-called frozen shoulder syndrome are all common causes of pain in the arm. Diseases of the bones of the shoulder also cause pain in the arm. In the past, tuberculosis of the shoulder joint was relatively common.

Tennis elbow

The commonest elbow lesion to cause troublesome pain is a condition known as tennis elbow. The exact pathology and aetiology of this condition is obscure, but it is almost certainly due to degenerative changes in the tendon of origin of the extensor carpi radialis muscle. Although this is a disabling condition, spontaneous cure nearly always occurs, though it may take several months. The process of cure may be accelerated by the injection of hydro-cortisone into the affected area, or by resting the elbow in plaster of Paris for some six weeks.

Ulnar neuritis

Another cause of pain in the arm—this time mainly on the ulnar side of the arm to the little finger—is ulnar neuritis. This commonly occurs due to irrita-tion of the ulnar nerve where it lies in the epicondylar groove at the back of the lower end of the humerus. This may be associated with deformities of the elbow or osteoarthritis of the elbow. Treatment is to decompress the nerve by surgical division of the overlying band.

Median nerve compression

Severe pain in the fingers and especially the thumb, index and middle fingers indicates compression of the median nerve where it passes under the carpal ligament, giving rise to the so-called carpal tunnel syndrome. This is characterized by severe pain at night which is only relieved by the patient getting up and waving her hands about. It is more common in women and may be associated with objective signs of median nerve dysfunction such as weakness of the thenar muscles and disturbance of sensation in the thumb and index finger. It is almost invariably cured by radical division of the volar carpal ligament.

A ganglion may press on the nerves in the arm, giving rise to pain, and is especially common in the palm of the hand pressing on the ulnar nerve with resultant pain and weakness of the small muscles of the hand.

Another cause of pain in the arm is tendovaginitis stenosans, particularly of the extensor tendons as they pass down the radial side of the lower end of the radius.

In addition, a variety of lesions of the peripheral nerves of the arm, of which in the whole world the most common is leprosy, may give rise to severe and intractable pain.

26

Leg Inequality

Real shortening

One leg may be shorter than the other due to causes such as poliomyelitis, malunited fractures, premature epiphyseal fusion, or congenital factors. Increase in leg length may be caused by either chronic infection or an arterio-venous aneurysm.

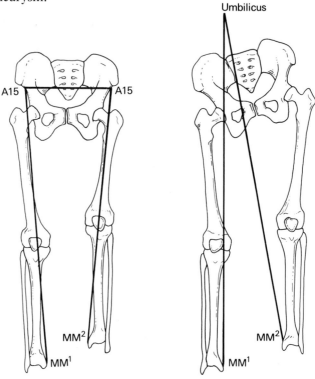

Fig. 26.1 (Left) Real shortening due to a short femur. The distance from anterior iliac spine to medial malleolus is less on the short side. (Right) Apparent shortening. If one hip is *add*ucted and the patient stands with legs parallel, i.e. the other hip *abd*ucted and although the bones are of equal length the umbilicus to medial malleolus distance is less on the *add*ucted side compared with the *abd*ucted.

406

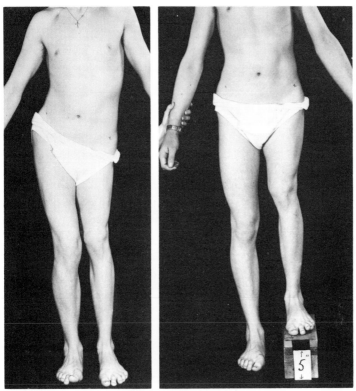

(a)   (b)

Fig. 26.2   (a) Patient with shortened left leg: note tilting of the pelvis. (b) Patient with shortened left leg. Tilt of pelvis corrected by raising the left foot 5 inches.

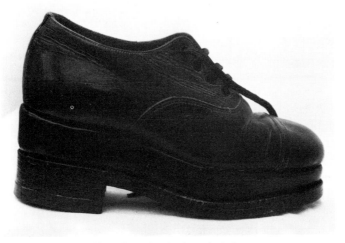

Fig. 26.3   A raised surgical shoe.

It is customary to measure the length of the leg from the anterior superior iliac spine to the medial malleolus; such a measurement is known as the 'real length' and any difference between the two legs is known as 'real shortening' (Fig. 26.1).

Apparent shortening

Either with real shortening or without, one leg may appear shorter than the other if the hip is fixed in a flexed and/or adducted position—for instance, following tuberculosis, infective arthritis, osteoarthritis, poliomyelitis or a dislocation.

It is customary to measure apparent length from the umbilicus or the xiphisternum to the medial malleolus; any difference in the apparent length is known as 'apparent shortening' (see Fig. 26.2a). If the apparent shortening is greater than the real shortening, then either the hip is held in an abnormal (flexed and/or adducted-flexed position) or there is a fixed lumbar scoliosis or asymmetry of the pelvis.

When a patient is seen who appears to walk with one leg shorter than the other, the first thing the surgeon wants to know is whether this is due to real shortening of the leg, or to apparent shortening, or to both.

As a general rule, the treatment of apparent shortening is to correct the hip deformity if this can be safely done. If there is in addition real shortening, or the deformed position of the hip cannot safely be corrected, then the surgeon can either compensate for the leg discrepancy either by building up the shoe on the short side, or by performing an operation. There are three types of operation:
1   Lengthening the short leg.
2   Shortening the long leg.
3   Inhibiting growth of the long leg.

The last method (epiphysiodesis) has not in general proved reliable and is seldom used nowadays as it may give rise to severe deformities. The second method—namely, shortening the femur of the longer leg, is a relatively safe method but has the disadvantage of diminishing the patient's total height.

The simplest technique is to divide the femur, allow the ends to overlap by the required amount and then fix them together by screws. This procedure seldom leads to complications and union is rapid and certain (Fig. 6.2).

If it is decided to lengthen the shorter leg, it is essential that this should be done slowly in order to avoid risk of damage to blood vessels and nerves. It is also important to avoid the development of severe deformities of the ankle during the process of lengthening, therefore, the operation is often done in two stages. At the first stage the tibia and fibula are joined together two inches above the ankle; at the same time a portion of the fibula is excised. This preserves the normal anatomy of the ankle. The principle is to insert four pins in the tibia and then divide it between the second and third pins, a special apparatus gradually increases the distance between the second and third pins over a period of time. Normally it is possible to obtain two inches of length without the risk of complications, but any further lengthening tends to introduce hazards and must be approached with care (see Fig. 26.6).

Lengthening of the femur is a more difficult procedure and is not recommended for routine use. It often leads to limitations of knee movement. In general it is far easier to lengthen a short leg due to poliomyelitis than one with normal muscles, e.g. after a malunited fracture or a congenital shortening. The latter are notoriously difficult.

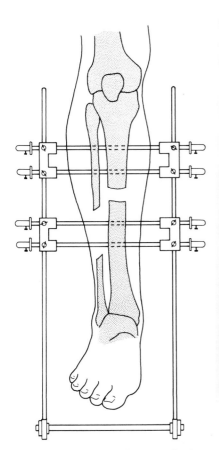

Fig. 26.4   Principles of leg-lengthening.

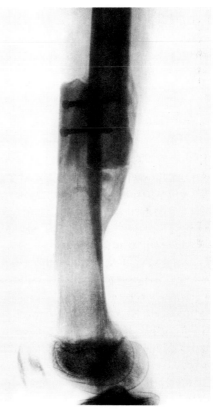

Fig. 26.5   Technique with femoral shortening with screws showing callus formation.

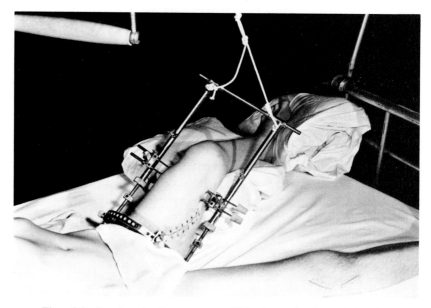

Fig. 26.6   Leg-lengthening apparatus. This shows the femur being lengthened which is more difficult than the tibia and fibula.

Finally, it should be remembered that many patients are quite able and
willing to accept up to one and a half inches of shortening without any
severe functional or cosmetic disability, and that leg equalization is usually
more of a cosmetic advantage than a functional advantage and does not
necessarily lead to any improvement in the patient's ability to walk.

Leg lengthening

Traditionally in this country leg lengthening apparati have consisted of
two lateral bars which are fastened to the bone by four transfixion pins and
the bone is then divided between the two middle pins and distraction is
commenced. Recently a new concept in leg lengthening has been developed
in the USSR. Basically this aims at lengthening the bone at the site of the
upper tibial growth cartilage without any operation on the bone in this
region. Two pins at an angle are inserted into the epiphysis and two into
the metaphysis of the upper end of the tibia. These are fixed to encircling
rings, and the two rings are then distracted. An obvious advantage of this
apparatus is that it is much more suitable because it is basically a three
dimensional, not merely a two dimensional, apparatus and as a result of the
stability which this provides there is far less pain (Fig. 26.7).

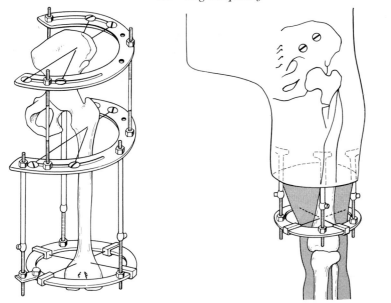

Fig. 26.7   Lengthening the leg at the site of
the upper femoral growth cartilage.

Fig. 26.8   Plaster of Paris single hipspica
leg-lengthening device.

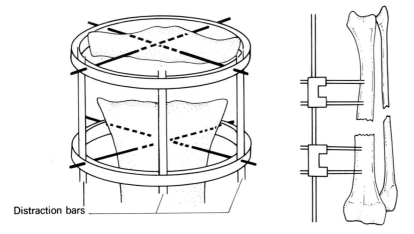

Distraction bars

Fig. 26.9   Distraction at site of growth cartilage.   Fig. 26.10   Judet leg lengthening.

The nursing management of the patient on
distraction apparatus

Distraction apparatus is used to increase the length of a leg. The equipment
must not be heavy as weighty equipment tends to restrict the movement of the
patient in his bed; this will lead to stiffness of the joints adjacent to the site of

lengthening through absence of use. Lightweight equipment which is suspended by counterbalancing weights, permits a wide range of movements to the patient and makes nursing management simpler.

As the patient has four pins passing through the leg, entering the skin on the medial surface and leaving on the lateral surface, these wounds may be points for the entry of infection. Therefore:

1 The patient must be free of infection when the operation is performed. Temperature recordings should be a four-hourly procedure during the forty-eight hours before operation. Any fluctuation should be reported to the surgeon.

2 The whole surface of the skin must be free of pustules and boils.

3 The skin preparation of the affected limb must be scrupulous. All skin folds, between the toes, in the groins, the perineum, and gluteal cleft must be carefully cleaned before and after operation.

4 Good personal hygiene of the patient and frequent replacement of bed linen will reduce the risk of infection.

5 The surgeon may order antibiotics as prophylaxis.

6 The wounds must be covered with a suitable dressing material. Aerosol spray-on dressings are excellent, provided they seal the wound on all surfaces.

During the lengthening period a careful watch must also be kept for the possible onset of damage to blood vessels or nerves by overstretching. While a certain amount of pain is inevitable, continued severe pain necessitating repeated strong analgesics suggests that damage is occurring. Ischaemia, pallor or blueness of the foot, loss of sensation or paralysis are indications that lengthening must be stopped and tension reduced.

Physiotherapy. Physiotherapy is necessary at all stages of the care of the patient. Whilst in bed the adjacent joints and muscles are exercised. Once the patient returns to bearing weight on the affected limb, retraining in walking with the variation in limb length, is necessary.

Nutrition. As callus formation is important, the patient must be given a high protein diet with a high mineral and vitamin content. Vitamins A and D are particularly important. Most patients have no dietary problems (they are usually young). There are some who will require special supplements however.

Section D

Practical Management of the Orthopaedic Patient

27

Comprehensive Patient Care

The general pattern of orthopaedic care

The orthopaedic surgeon is the chairman of the orthopaedic team. He co-ordinates all the facets of welfare and rehabilitation for the patient in a community.

As with all medical services, efficient communication between all concerned with a particular speciality is essential for the treatment of the patient. Any advances in knowledge and technique must be disseminated and thus the patient is assured of the most up-to-date treatment.

Sir Robert Jones met and instructed many of the surgeons of the world who came to work with him during the 1914–1918 Great War. During and after the war he travelled extensively to America, Canada, Australia, New Zealand, India, France, Switzerland, Portugal and Italy. From his meetings and travels many of the Orthopaedic Associations over the world were formed. These are established and have branches in many countries but all communicate through meetings and publications such as the *Journal of Bone and Joint Surgery*.

Orthopaedic services

The work of the surgeon must be supported by many ancillary services. Many orthopaedic patients require prolonged treatment and follow-up. The infant born with club feet, for example, must be treated at birth and treatment must be continued until the child is walking well, on reliable feet. This form of treatment and follow-up can only be maintained in a community when it is served by an orthopaedic team of doctors, nurses, physiotherapists, radiographers, occupational therapists, social caseworkers, splint makers, pharmacists, pathology technicians, stenographers and clerical records staff —and many others who, though not directly concerned with the treatment of the patient are essential for efficient orthopaedic care. Absence of orthopaedic services in a country can seriously impair the health and efficiency of a nation; in the United Kingdom they arose from the challenge of beggardom and crippling that existed because of a lack of orthopaedic facilities.

The orthopaedic services are usually centred on hospitals which must be suitably equipped. Additionally there must be after-care services to ensure the continuation of treatment. If the patient is unable to reach hospital or lives far away, such services may take the form of peripheral clinics and a domiciliary service for visiting patients in their homes.

Accident services. An important aspect of a modern orthopaedic service is the provision of an accident service integrated with a multiple injuries unit (see Chapter 7, p. 63. This requires a comprehensive integration of ambulance, police, fire and air transport service with the hospital service to ensure the rapid transfer of the injured to hospital.

Splint and limb making and fitting. An important (if expensive) part of an orthopaedic service is the provision of accurately fitted and properly made splints and other appliances. Originally splints were made on the premises of orthopaedic hospitals, but this era has passed and production is now mainly in the hands of commercial enterprises. Without adequate appliance-making services, however, the orthopaedic services may be seriously handicapped.

Research and the development of new appliances is, however, still the duty of hospitals and related university departments.

Clinical examination and diagnosis. Orthopaedic diagnosis is primarily based on careful history taking, accurate observation and painstaking examination. There is still a case for the observation of the many other factors which point to the patient's pathological state. Such tests were devised long before radiographs were taken (the earliest known use of radiography in orthopaedics in the United Kingdom was by Sir Robert Jones at the Royal Southern Hospital, Liverpool in 1896) when other more empirical forms of observation had to be used. Advances in radiographic and photographic techniques have made diagnosis more accurate and simple, both for the patient and medical staff. Reliable radiographs of consistent quality are now an everyday part of the hospital scene.

Another diagnostic department where great progress has been made in recent years is the pathological laboratory. Useful detailed and specific reports are supplied which greatly assist the doctor.

Observation of gait and posture, the history of the patient's condition, measurement of limb circumference to note wasting of muscles, measurement of the minimal and maximal range of movement at a joint using a goniometer, measurement of the height of the patient and length of the limbs are all used by the orthopaedic surgeon and nurse to assist diagnosis and compare progress during treatment.

Methods of measurement. To produce standard results in measuring patients for either diagnostic purposes or fitting splints and appliances, certain constant rules must be followed; the only accurate way to measure the patient is when he is unclothed.

(a) *To measure the patient in the standing position.* To measure the upright patient it is necessary to note posture and any deformity, adjusting the stance of the patient accordingly. For example, if the patient has one leg shorter than the other, blocks of wood of varying thickness must be used to equalize the height of the foot on the short leg so that the pelvis is horizontal; the two anterior superior iliac spines should be clearly defined with a wax pencil and they should then appear to be on the same horizontal plane. This enables the nurse or doctor to record:

1   The difference in length between the long and short legs. The height of the blocks used will indicate the precise amount.

2   That one limb is shorter than the normal or, one limb is longer than the normal.

3   The true standing height of the patient, assuming there is no spinal deformity.

4   If there is a curvature of the patient's spine before the blocks were placed under his foot and it disappears after they were inserted, this indicates that the curve in the spine was mainly caused by a pelvic tilt rather than by an intrinsic spinal deformity.

There are other devices for measurement and the recording of spinal deformities on the standing patient, but the correct use of radiographs and photographs of the nude patient against a background of horizontal and vertical lines of known distance apart is probably the best method of estimation and recording the degree of deformity. Posterior, lateral and forward and sideways bending views of the patient must all be taken. A simple plumb line is an asset in defining faults of spinal posture.

For Trendelenberg's test see p. 305.

(b) *To measure the patient in the horizontal position.* A tape measure and wax marking pencil are necessary for measurement in this case. The patient must lie on a firm base such as a plinth or bed with a firm mattress on a rigid base. The following measurements are taken:

1   *Measurement of the length of the spine.* Such measurement may be required for the purpose of supplying a saddle for a spinal frame or a posterior

spinal support (see Chapter 29, p. 505). The patient is placed in the prone position with his arms by his side; there are no pillows or other accessories on the bed. Two points are marked on his body with the wax pencil:

(i) The spinous process of the seventh cervical vertebra (vertebra prominens) which is the first spinous process to be felt at the base of the neck and top of the thorax.

(ii) The tip of the coccyx which is between the gluteal folds.

The tape measure is laid loosely along the length of the spine following its curves. Measurement is recorded in centimetres.

2   *Measurement of the leg lengths.* For calipers, the following points are defined with the wax pencil:

(i)   The great trochanter of the femur.

(ii) The adductor tendon in the groin.

(iii) The external malleolus of the ankle.

(iv) The internal malleolus of the ankle.

The external measurement, from great trochanter to external malleolus, and then the internal measurement, from the adductor tendon to the internal malleolus are both recorded.

3   *Measurement for* TRUE *shortening.* The patient lies supine on the bed as straight as possible, without pillows, and with the arms by his side. The anterior superior spines of the pelvis and apices of the internal malleoli are marked with a wax skin pencil. The distance between the anterior superior spine and internal malleolus on each side is measured and recorded. If there is a difference between these measurements, this is *true* shortening.

4   *Measurement for* APPARENT *shortening.* One leg may appear to be short in a patient even when it is not. This may be because the leg is in fixed adduction; the pelvis is tilted so that, as the patient lies supine with the legs parallel, one foot appears raised and the other lowered.

To test for apparent shortening, the apex of the internal malleolus on each leg is marked. A tape measure is used to measure the distance between the umbilicus and the internal malleolus. If the apparent shortening is greater than the real, this indicates that the hip is adducted, or that the pelvis is asymmetrical, or that the lumbar spine is curved.

5   *The Thomas' hip flexion test.* This is to test for a decreased range of extension or fixed flexion deformity in the hip joint.

The patient lies unclothed and supine on a firm plinth. The examiner places one hand under the lumbar curve of the patient's back. With the other hand he grasps the patient's ankle and flexes the hip and knee. At the expiry of the range of flexion of the hip joint the pelvis will tilt and the concavity of the lumbar spine will flatten; as the examiner feels the pressure of the patient's lumbar spine on his hand he knows that the lumbar spine is now straight. The angle which the femur on the affected limb makes with the horizontal can be measured with a goniometer and recorded in the case notes. The rationale behind this test is that many patients compensate for a fixed flexion deformity of the hip by hyperextending their lumbar spine.

6   *The straight leg raising test.* This is used to test the presence of irritative lesions affecting the roots of the sciatic nerve as they leave the neural canal and pass into the intervertebral foraminae.

The patient lies supine on a firm plinth. The surgeon grasps the patient's foot and lifts the leg gradually, i.e. the hip is flexed with the knee straight. If there is no pain as the limb is elevated, the test gives a negative result. If there is pain between 30 degrees and 70 degrees of elevation, this indicates irritation of the roots of the sciatic nerve.

7   *Trendelenburg's test.* This test is positive when the hip joint is dislocated; when the gluteus medius is paralysed; when there is gross coxa vara; permanent adduction of the hip joint, or in non-union of the neck of the femur. It can only be used on the patient old enough to stand upright. The patient is asked to stand first on one lower limb, he lowers it and then he stands on the other.

In normal people, i.e. when the test is negative, the patient's pelvis tilts in transferring the weight of the body on to the leg on which he stands. In other words, the iliac crest on the side of the limb which is lifted off the ground is also elevated and that on the weight-bearing side remains about the same level.

If the test is positive, the pelvis remains horizontal and the opposite side drops to a lower position when the patient stands on the side of the affected hip joint. On the affected side the gluteal fold will increase in depth and will also drop in height.

8   (i) *The hip clicking test.* This is performed on newly born infants in order to test for abnormal laxity of the hip joint. There are a number of similar procedures—the von Rosen test, Ortolani's sign, and the Barlow's test.

(ii) *Barlow's test.* The baby is placed supine without diapers or napkins. The examiner grasps the front of the infants thigh with one hand and steadies the pelvis with the other; the thumb is placed over the patella with the index finger on the great trochanter. The hips and knees of the baby are then flexed upwards towards the abdomen.

The legs are now gradually abducted and, if the test is negative, the surgeon carries the flexed legs laterally into the abducted position and there is a smooth uninterrupted action in abducting the legs. When the test is positive, a jerk is felt and a click is heard as the head of the femur slips out of the acetabulum. Feeling a jerk is the most reliable part of a positive test, indicating a lax hip joint.

9   *Babinski's sign.* This is used in examination for neurological disorders. It is positive in most upper motor neurone lesions (see Chapter 16, p. 247). The patient may be supine or sitting with his feet hanging clear of the floor.

A blunt point is passed firmly over the plantar surface of the foot. As this is done, the toes of the patient will move—this is most evident on the great toe. A negative Babinski sign is seen when the toes flex towards the sole of the foot. It is positive when the toes extend towards the head and separate fan-wise.

10   *Gastrocnemius pinch test.* Normally, if the patient kneels or lies with his feet dangling loosely over the side of the couch, then pinching his calf muscle causes it to contract and the foot to plantarflex. If there is a rupture of the tendo Achillis, the foot will not plantarflex.

There are many other tests which are used in clinical examinations but these are the tests in most common use in orthopaedic practice.

Radiographic examination of the orthopaedic patient

Preparation of the patient. (a) As the patient must be still during radiographic exposure, adequate reassurance and an explanation of what is about to happen should be given to him before he goes to the radiography department. This is particularly important when the patient must be examined in a darkened room.

During the actual exposure of the radiograph it is important that hospital personnel should not be exposed to radiation so it is customary that nurses and radiographers shelter behind a radio-opaque screen.

In the case of children a parent may stay with the child. If a nurse, doctor, or radiographer must be with the patient, e.g. to hold a certain position, he or she should wear protective clothing.

(b) When a limb is to be X-rayed for bone position only, the plaster splint may be left in position and the radiographs taken through it. Should a more sensitive examination be required, such as, of bone structure in osteomyelitis, or of soft tissues in myositis ossificans, or changes in arterial structure, the plaster splint will impede the passage of the rays through the limb and must therefore be bivalved. The limb is then carefully lifted out of the splint and cleaned before radiography. Traction materials, particularly those with a diachylon lead based adhesive, have a similar effect and must be temporarily removed. Gutter splinting made of sheet steel also impedes the passage of rays and should not be used as permanent splintage on patients who must be repeatedly X-rayed. Aluminium or plaster is more suitable.

(c) As repetitive films of a fracture are necessary it is always an asset to the radiographer to have previous radiographs brought to the department with the patient for comparison. The X-ray films should be numbered and arranged in correct sequence.

(d) When radiographs are to be made of the vertebral column below the level of the diaphragm, the abdomen is also included. Gas and faeces will impede the passage of the rays and will appear on the film. It is necessary to check that the patient is not constipated or distended with flatus. A flatus tube may be passed into the rectum and descending colon, or an enema given before radiography when the image required on the film is of bone or soft tissue structure. This is particularly important when the patient has, for example, been fixed on a plaster bed.

(e) Radiography using portable equipment in the ward or accident unit is more exacting because of the low-powered output of the equipment used. Ward staff should co-operate fully in positioning the patient accurately and removing impedimenta from around the patient.

(f) The recently injured patient must be transferred from the ambulance on to a special trolley with a top which is translucent to X-rays. The same trolley can also serve as an emergency operating table. It should also have a polyfoam mattress.

(g) When special investigations such as tomography, intravenous pyelography, retrograde pyelography, cystography, myelography, arthrography, sinography, arteriography, venography, encephalography or ventriculography are to be performed, the special instructions of the radiologist and doctor in charge of the patient must be sought.

(h) Repeated and frequent radiography causes a cumulative absorption of the rays and is harmful. Unnecessary pictures must be avoided.

The orthopaedic patient
The basic management of a patient with an orthopaedic condition is no different from that of any patient. He requires the same physical sustenance which any other human being needs; he must be maintained in a clean and comfortable condition with adequate balanced nutrition and psychological support. There are, however, some special aspects of care which are applicable to orthopaedic patients.

(a) *Intensive care*. Pre- and post-operatively or after injury, he may require the concentrated attention of specialized staff. This is usually given in the intensive care or accident unit where the best facilities exist for this form of therapy.

(i) *Blood and fluid replacement.* Severe shock from blood loss is treated by adequate transfusion of blood. Any large operation, for example on the spine or hip joint, will cause loss of blood; this loss must be measured and replaced during and immediately after the operation. If the patient is not adequately transfused he will become anaemic which will retard recovery, including the formation of callus in the healing of broken or cut bones and efficient healing of wounds.

Where a considerable amount of bone has been exposed at operation, considerable post-operative oozing of blood is likely to occur. The use of suction drainage enables this to be measured and a corresponding amount of blood restored to the patient.

(ii) *Respiratory management.* Crushing injuries of the thoracic walls, injuries to the face, nose and throat, penetrating wounds of the chest, bleeding into the thoracic cavity, paralysis of the thoracic muscles, operations on the thoracic spine or thoracic walls will all create severe respiratory problems. The patient may require special treatment in an oxygen tent or attached to an intermittent positive pressure ventilation machine. Tracheostomy may be required and most certainly the patient will require constant special nursing and observation.

Wounds of the thorax may require special underwater seal drainage.

(iii) *Urinary management.* Injuries of the pelvis and trunk, trauma involving the kidneys and ureters, paralysis of the urinary bladder, or operations on the hips and pelvis may create urinary problems which again require intensive nursing, involving the use of special equipment, for example, peritoneal dialysis or haemodialysis.

(iv) *Spinal trauma.* In the initial stages of treatment of the paralysed patient, the turning and positioning of the patient must be established as part of intensive care. Much time and effort have also been devoted to devise appliances which will lift and move weak or paralysed patients. Nurses often find that inserting the lifting canvas under the patient takes too much time so that appliances are not as used as they ought to be. One suggestion to overcome this is that the mattress should be partially divided vertically by furrows along which lifting straps can be passed. It is then easy to place a sling under the patient so that when the different slings are attached to the lifting machine the patient can be lifted or turned with the minimum of trouble. Previously it was necessary to turn the patient from one side to the other in order to insert the slings under the patient. In the case of a paralysed patient this requires a team comprising at least two nurses. As a considerable amount of nursing time is spent either avoiding bed sores or moving patients any new developments which could make this easier are of the greatest possible importance.

(v) *Special observations*. Taking and recording blood pressure, observation of levels of consciousness, fluid intake and output, respiratory rate and volume, as well as the pulse rate, are some of the commoner observations which can best be made in an intensive care unit. There are, of course, many other examples of intensive care in an orthopaedic unit. Acute infections and head injuries are other obvious examples.

(b) *Recovery*. Once the intensive phase of treatment has passed, patients require varying lengths of time of rest and recovery in the orthopaedic unit.

In the early days of orthopaedics this often meant that the patient was fixed for a long period of time in a plaster bed or on a spinal frame. This attitude to patient care has passed and there is less need to immobilize the body completely because of improved knowledge, better surgery with internal fixation of more effective drugs and antibiotics. Most bone lesions still require the 'rest, prolonged, enforced and uninterrupted' advocated by Hugh Owen Thomas as an orthopaedic principle; it is only the length of the rest and method of achieving it which has altered.

Patients with orthopaedic conditions often require more prolonged treatment than other patients and the atmosphere of an orthopaedic ward must be suited to such patients. Fixation in bed with inability to leave the bed for any purpose is frustrating and inevitably intensely boring and tedious.

Part of this tedium can be relieved by bed mobility. Orthopaedic units are often equipped with beds with large wheels which enable the staff to move the patient easily about the ward to day rooms, dressing rooms or out of the ward and into the open air. It is an asset also to be able to take the patient to the radiography, physiotherapy or occupational therapy department without transferring him to a trolley.

The attitude of the staff to the patients is inevitably different when the patients feel well and are in hospital for a longer period of time. The orthopaedic ward usually has a relaxed atmosphere, although the regime of treatment must be strictly maintained.

Particular features of management at this stage are:

1 *Cleanliness*. The morale of the patient is enhanced by absolute cleanliness. A daily blanket bath or shower is necessary, as is washing of the genitalia, perineum and gluteal fold after excretion. Changing the bed, bathing and other forms of attention tend to create landmarks in the patient's day and break the monotony.

2   *Grooming.* When possible, high standards of dress and appearance should be encouraged and a slovenly, untidy, unshaven look should merit disapproval. When the patient leaves his bed he should dress himself properly; good shoes should be worn rather than soft slippers, as these are better for walking when a disability affects the legs. Cosmetics and attention to hairstyling help the morale of the female patient and a hospital hairdresser is an asset in the management of the patients.

3   *Diet and nutrition.* The formation of a callus at the site of a fracture requires an adequate intake of food. Protein, and mineral elements, such as calcium, phosphorus, sodium and potassium, vitamins—particularly vitamins A and D, are necessary items in the diet and must be profusely supplied. Dairy produce such as milk, eggs, cheese and butter are important, but so are cereals and animal protein such as fish, meat and chicken. In a patient who is restricted in exercise and activity, roughage such as vegetable cellulose is also important to prevent constipation.

The same problems of ensuring that the patient eats enough when he is particular or unwell which exist on a medical or general surgical unit are also found on an orthopaedic ward. A full range of therapeutic diets are required, for example, fluid, light, high protein, diabetic and gastric. The therapeutic dietician is as important in an orthopaedic unit as elsewhere in a hospital. The patient with a bone lesion who is not taking enough nutrition or the right kind of food will take longer to form callus: in extreme cases the bone will not unite and non-union or fibrous union only will occur.

4   *Obesity.* There is a danger that the patient who must remain in bed without exercise may become overweight through overfeeding, particularly if he has no other interests except the frequent arrival of meals. There is a strong case for reducing the quantity of fats and carbohydrates in the diet in such patients. Hunger may still be satisfied by the use of low calorie foods and the therapeutic dietician will help in providing a suitable diet. Generally the instructions to the patient will be:

To eat plenty of:

Lean meat	Eggs
Fish	Fruit
Game	Vegetables (other than potatoes)
Poultry	Clear soups
Cheese	Green salads

Not to eat:

Bread (in all forms)	Chocolate
Biscuits	Cakes
Toast	Pastries

Sugar   Puddings
Sweets   Potatoes

Generally when a patient is in hospital for a long time it is difficult to avoid monotony in the diet and the use of several alternatives on the daily menu is desirable. Chewing helps to give the feeling of having had a satisfactory meal. Raw carrot or similar vegetables and fresh fruit, when chewed, serve to relieve hunger and promote good oral hygiene.

5   *Physiotherapy*. This is the use of exercises and other physical methods to rehabilitate and maintain the physique of the patient. The physiotherapist provides a graduated programme of training for the individual patient in order to prevent stiffness of joints, muscle wasting and poor posture. This training, for the orthopaedic patient particularly, commences as early as possible after his admission and continues through to full recovery.

When the range of movement in a joint has been reduced by recent injury or acute inflammation, careful repetitive exercises are given, but force is never applied.

Weakness of muscles is improved by exercises graduated in strength and duration. When improvement is noted, it is recorded. Pulleys and weights may be used to create resistance to the muscles, as muscles working against a force or resistance increase more quickly in strength.

During the time that the patient's limb is in splintage it is difficult to exercise the limb and the physiotherapist will give muscle training by the use of static exercises; that is, the patient will be asked to exert muscle pull across a joint without moving it. An example of this is quadriceps drill; the patient is trained to pull up the patella of the knee with the muscles on the front of the thigh; he then practises this exercise for a specific five minutes in every hour during which he is awake.

A useful adjunct to a physiotherapy department is a pool of warmed water for hydrotherapy. The warmth and buoyancy created by the water enable the patient to exercise with less fatigue.

Another important function of the physiotherapist is to improve the respiratory function of the patient, particularly in those with poor respiratory volume.

6   *Occupational therapy*. The occupational therapists of a hospital serve the orthopaedic patient in many ways, but these can be classified into the following main activities:

(i) To complement the work of the physiotherapist by causing the patient to exercise relevant joints to prevent and overcome stiffness. Related to this is the use of muscles against increasing resistance to prevent wasting and increase strength. The use of equipment which is creative and productive to

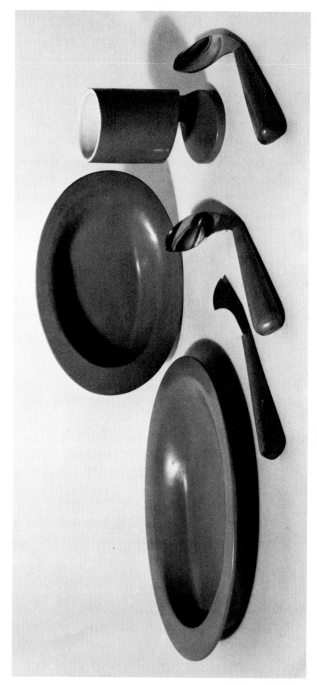

Fig. 27.1   Eating aids for the disabled. (By courtesy of Melaware.)

maintain the interest of the patient whilst exercising is part of occupational therapy.

(ii) To re-educate a disabled patient in the use of any function that remains. Thus, for example, the patient with paralysis of the upper limb will be trained in trick movements using special devices (Fig. 27.1) to transfer food from plate to mouth, etc. These are called 'Activities of Daily Living'.

(iii) To collaborate with the Disablement Resettlement Officer in directing the patient who must find an alternative occupation, towards the abilities of which he was unaware and which can be developed even though he is disabled.

(iv) To introduce diversional activities. Being confined to bed in hospital for long periods is intensely boring. In addition to books, television and games, a diversionary handicraft is of great value—model making, leather work, crochet, embroidery, macramé, etc.

7 *The dental officer.* An important member of the orthopaedic team; the dental surgeon contributes to the recovery of the patient by treating dental caries, found in many patients, thus improving the patient's morale and enabling him to eat and digest food more efficiently, and eradicating a probable source of infection.

The dental officer also serves as the maxillo-facial consultant in the treatment of patients requiring reconstructive treatment for fractures of the jaw.

8 *Records office and clinical photography.* The records of an orthopaedic patient can extend from birth to death. There is a need in all such patients to be aware of any variations, whether improvement or retardation. Both efficiently recorded notes and repeated photographs are useful aids to the surgeon in deciding the future course of action on the patient's behalf.

9 *Radiology.* An orthopaedic unit could not function without a well organised radiography department. The radiography team are involved in most activities affecting the patient from the diagnosis in the casualty department to surgery in the operating theatre. All plaster work and traction requires check radiography to ensure that the fracture or dislocation is suitably positioned in the splint.

(c) *Rehabilitation.* The aim of any hospital must be the return of the patient to his home and occupation or previous way of life. The worst form of existence for any individual is to become 'institutionalized'; that is, dependent upon others than members of his family for all his needs, whether physical, financial or psychological. Society today accepts that large institutions such as prisons or county mental institutions can destroy the initiative of an individual

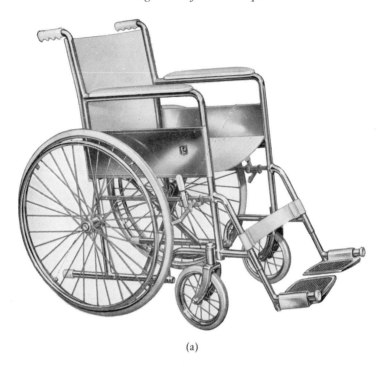

(a)

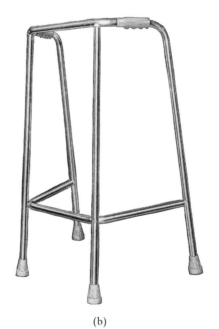

(b)

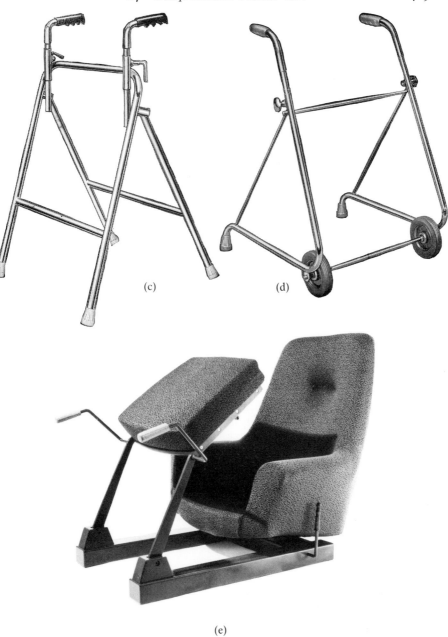

(c)

(d)

(e)

Fig. 27.2 Special appliances for the disabled. (a) Wheelchair. (b) Walking Aid. (c) Folding Walking Aid. (d) 'Rolling' Walking Aid. (e) Adjustable chair to assist in standing up.

(By courtesy of G. Morse-Brown & Co.)

and ultimately make him fear independence. An orthopaedic unit that retains a patient longer than is necessary also does this. Whenever possible the patient must be encouraged to return to his home and family, even though he must return for further treatment some time later.

1   *Social casework.* From the day of his admission to hospital to his discharge the social caseworker should be helping the patient where necessary, to live as normal a way of life as is possible. This involves the social caseworker in many activities:

(i) *Financial.* Admission to hospital may have created a serious financial crisis for the patient and his family. Often resolution of such a crisis is a matter of knowing how to obtain money to which the patient is entitled by law; many people are surprisingly ignorant of such matters and benefit from advice. The function of a caseworker is to give such advice.

(ii) *Residential.* Disability, senility or involvement in a catastrophe such

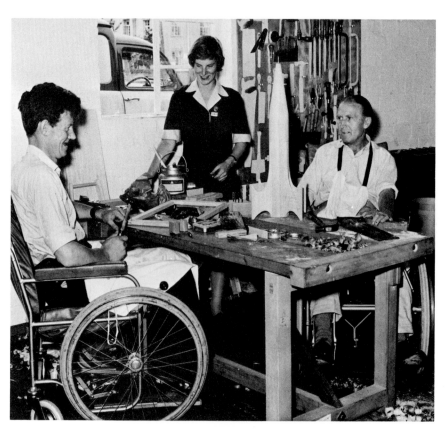

Fig. 27.3   Retraining the disabled for alternative occupations.

as a car crash often means that the previous dwelling of the patient is unsuitable or no longer available. The aged patient who has lived alone may be no longer fit to care for himself and must be admitted as an inmate of a special hostel. The chairbound patient may require some modifications to his present home or rehousing with his family in a bungalow with ramps instead of steps. Communication with local authorities may be required and the caseworker does this on behalf of the patient.

(iii) *Special appliances.* Even moderate disability may require the use of an appliance such as a modified shoe or back support; severe disability such as paraplegia calls for the provision of many appliances such as urinals, calipers, wheelchairs, crutches, special clothing, motorized transport, etc. All these items are costly, and few patients can afford large sums of money. The social caseworker undertakes action for the provision of these and their continued repair, maintenance and replacement. A child using an appliance can outgrow it rapidly, and frequent replacements related to increasing height and weight are required.

(iv) *Re-employment.* Close liaison with the Government Disablement Resettlement Officer and, through him, the patient's employer, may ensure that work is waiting for the patient when he is ready to return. If he is unable to continue his previous job his employer may be able to provide alternative work, especially if he has been a loyal and useful employee in the past.

If employment in his previous occupation is not feasible, retraining in an entirely new skill by admission to an Industrial Rehabilitation Unit may be undertaken.

2   *Education.* If a child is to spend any period in hospital it is important that his education should be continued without any lapse. Admission to hospital for a long period may seriously affect the whole future of the patient if his education is not maintained. The hospital special school which is established on the wards by the local authority tries to prevent this unfortunate happening, although education is not always possible in the face of major surgery or treatment which must come before lessons.

Relevant long-term pre-operative preparation of the orthopaedic patient

Infection in bones or joints can cause permanent irrevocable damage in addition to toxaemia, malaise and pain of the acute infection. Infection can manifest itself as:
Acute osteomyelitis.

Chronic osteomyelitis.

Acute suppurative arthritis.

Osteoarthritis in later years.

Non-union of a fracture, through interference with callus formation.

Amyloid disease—a serious generalized disease due to long-standing chronic infection.   Special care has always been considered necessary in operations on the skeleton. Antibiotics can be used prophylactically in the prevention of infections, and therapeutically for their treatment, but there is no case for relaxation of the rules of aseptic technique because of the existence of antibiotics.

Many of the operations performed by orthopaedic surgeons are elective or cosmetic procedures: in other words, they are performed to correct deformity or impaired function. Operations should only be performed in ideal conditions with suitably designed buildings, correctly ventilated and cleaned.

Orientation and psychological preparation of the patient

All patients fear the unknown, particularly when surgery is to be performed. With all patients and their next of kin, a full explanation of that which is to be done, plus the effects of the surgical treatment must be given, preferably by the surgeon who is to perform the operation. A relaxed co-operative patient is preferable to one who is tense and afraid.

When major surgery is to be carried out, e.g. spinal fusion, or joint replacement, a longer period of orientation to the ward, the staff who will deal with him and to the equipment he will use, is needed than if a small operation is performed. Such a period could be as long as two weeks in a child who is to be nursed on a plaster bed for example. During this time the plaster bed is made, dried, mounted on a stand and lined; the patient learns to sleep, consume food and drink and excrete, using the plaster bed in the pre-operative period; after the operation the patient is already an expert in the management of these vital activities and the stress of recovery from surgery is thus reduced.

During the pre-operative phase also, the patient meets the physiotherapist and learns the exercises which he will have to carry out post-operatively; the nurses who care for him also learn his foibles and quirks and can do much to support him during the period when he most needs help.

The previous history of the patient. An important aspect of the patient's history is to know his drug regime before admission. Many patients with painful orthopaedic conditions have a previous history of corticosteroid therapy (see p. 224) and special arrangements for anaesthesia must be made. Patients who are on prolonged barbiturate and tranquillizer therapy must also be given special consideration as these drugs require an extensive period—as much as ten days to three weeks—to be excreted and to cease their effect on the patient. Anti-depressive and anti-hypertensive drugs may also pose problems for the anaesthetist. Some of these must be stopped some days before operation.

Clinical examination. This must always be thorough; although the patient may be admitted with an obviously orthopaedic condition, this may only be secondary to another medical condition, such as diabetes, cardiac or pulmonary conditions, or malnutrition. Ample time must be permitted when possible for pathological and radiographic investigations.

The anaesthetist has many techniques and drugs in his armementarium but he must be fully aware of the condition of the patient if he is to use them effectively and safely.

Haemoglobin estimation and blood replacement. A major factor in the recovery of the patient after an operation is the level of haemoglobin in his bloodstream and the absence of anaemia. If the chemical constitution of his blood is within normal limits:

1 His rate of recovery from shock and the anaesthetic is faster.
2 The rate of healing of the tissues which have been damaged as a result of surgery is increased.
3 Callus formation at the site of a fracture or osteotomy is quicker.
4 The patient's resistance to infection is increased.
5 The morale of the patient is improved, he quickly recovers his appetite and feels less apathetic.

The blood chemistry of the patient should be estimated on arrival at the hospital and action taken to correct any abnormality shown by such tests. The physician may order the appropriate drugs or vitamins if there is marked anaemia, blood transfusion may be the most rapid and efficient method of correcting this and will also give the patient a reserve of red blood cells for the operation. Cross matching of a sufficient quantity of blood to balance any blood loss during and after the operation must be carried out.

Excretion. (a) *Faeces.* The routine practice of giving every patient an enema before operation has been discarded by many hospitals. This is justified, as this form of treatment is unpleasant for the patient. It is essential, however, to know that the regularity of bowel evacuation is maintained in the patient up to the day of operation for the following reasons:

(i)   The danger of soiling the operating table during the anaesthetic.

(ii) The possibility of constipation in the post-operative phase.

(iii) The problems of a patient fixed in recumbency, for example, on a plaster bed or frame, are enough without the added worry of being unable to evacuate a loaded bowel.

If the patient has had no bowel action on the day before operation an evacuant suppository or a micro-enema should be given.

(b) *Urine.* When the fluid intake and output of the patient are adequate there is no further reason for action unless the operation is on the pelvic basin or sacrum, when a full bladder may be a hazard to the patient and an impedance to the surgeon's field of vision. In such cases an indwelling catheter is inserted and connected to a sterile plastic urine sac so as to permit the urine to drain from the bladder as soon as it enters the bladder, i.e. the bladder is kept completely empty, even though the kidneys continue to form urine.

(c) *Dental care.* In pre-operative preparation examination of the mouth and teeth is necessary. The patient may have loose carious teeth which may dislodge and be inhaled into the trachea and lungs; carious teeth may also provide a focus of micro-organisms which can infect the site of operation via the blood stream.

Small dental plates and complete dentures are removed from the mouth and carefully stored just prior to departure for the operating theatre.

The dental officer in the hospital usually assists in the management of patients with injuries affecting the mouth and jaw (maxillo-facial injuries).

(d) *Prophylactic drugs.* Many patients have medical conditions which are secondary to the treatment of the orthopaedic condition but which are just as important. The recovery of the patient with a chest infection, for example, may be retarded by respiratory inadequacy and defective oxygenation of the tissues.

The doctor may order suitable prophylactic coverage for any such condition. Examples of this coverage would be:

(i)   Antibiotic or chemotherapy for chronic chest or upper respiratory tract infections.

(ii) An increase in corticosteroids for patients on such a therapy.

(iii) Conversion to a soluble insulin for diabetic patients.

(e) *Improving vital capacity.* Some patients may have an impaired volume of respiration because of deformity and/or inefficient action of the thoracic cage or diaphragm, or because of relentless chain smoking. The physiotherapist may be required to help by estimating the vital capacity of the patient, using a spirometer, before instituting a regime of breathing exercises. At intervals, estimation of the vital capacity is repeated. For the heavy smoker a process of weaning from the quantity of tobacco smoked, or better still, cessation of smoking is recommended.

Although the anaesthetist can deal with most situations, if he is aware of them, a poor vital capacity makes matters more difficult for him.

In conditions such as scoliosis, kyphosis, or the rigid spine and thorax of ankylosing spondylitis, the vital capacity and respiratory volume of the patient are greatly decreased. It is essential that the surgical team, including the anaesthetist and physical therapist, meet in sufficient time before operation in order to decide on the best plan of preparation for the anaesthetic and operation, as well as the regime of treatment which will best assist the recovery of the patient after anaesthesia and surgery.

(f) *Planning and preparation of post-operative splintage and traction.* 'Experience teaches'. In the field of orthopaedic nursing, this is particularly true. The ward sister who has cared for the patients of an orthopaedic surgeon for many years will know his methods and requirements for his patients who have had a particular operation, and she will ensure that all is ready both in the operating theatre and in the ward on the return of the patient from operation. Methods and people can change, however, and it is unwise to assume that every surgeon will require exactly the same equipment for every patient who has a particular operation. Experience also teaches one to be ready for variations on a theme. It is wisdom to inquire from the surgeon beforehand so that all is ready and the patient is not kept waiting under prolonged anaesthesia whilst a particular size of splint or other equipment is sought.

Preparation of the patient immediately prior to operation

Personal hygiene
In the days prior to the day of operation, bathing of the patient once or twice daily to reduce the numbers of micro-organisms which are the normal denizens of the human skin is carried out. The usual rules of personal hygiene are followed to ensure good oral hygiene and care of the hands, feet and hair.

Preparation of the skin
Traditionally, any surgery on bones or joints has called for extreme precautions in order to prevent infection with its disastrous results—e.g. osteomyelitis or pyogenic arthritis.

Many orthopaedic surgeons retain the 'three day' method of skin preparation. Others have now modified and prefer preparation of the skin only on the day prior to operation and on the day of operation. Some do not wish the skin to be shaved. Nurses must follow the local rules of the hospital and it is therefore only possible to lay down principles in these pages. It is *most* important that the skin is free of infective lesions such as boils or abscesses.

Prior to preparing the skin for surgery
1   The nurse should examine the area for any unusual manifestations. If any unusual conditions are present, this should be reported to the surgeon.
2   Make the patient comfortable, reassure him and provide for privacy.
3   Skin preparation should be done as close to the scheduled time of surgical operation as possible in order to minimize the re-growth of bacteria or hair. For some surgical procedures it may be necessary to prepare the skin after the patient has been anaesthetized. In any case, the patient must be completely prepared for surgery when the surgeon is ready to start the procedure.

1   *Shaving*. It is difficult to cleanse hair adequately. Each hair is a capillary, inside which micro-organisms such as staphylococcus albus can live. The removal of hair is the simplest approach to the elimination of micro-organisms. Shaving the skin, however, is likely to drag out the hairs and leave open follicles in which the micro-organisms continue to multiply. Shaving is also unpleasant for the patient and the stubble that remains, particularly after shaving in the genital area, can be prickly and uncomfortable. Long hair must be clipped however.

If shaving is necessary, the following procedures should be followed. Where individual kits containing sterile equipment are available, these are disposable.
(a) Apply Povidone-Iodine surgical scrub preparation to the skin area to be prepared, work up a lather using a sponge moistened with water.
(b) Begin washing the skin using circular motions from the proposed site of incision and rotate outwards to the most distant part of the area. As sponges become soiled, discard them and continue with a fresh sponge.
(c) Using a sterile, sharp razor, shave hair from the area. In soft areas, the skin should be held taut with your free hand to reduce the chance of nicking the skin as this increases the chances of infection.
   After shaving:
(i) Scrub the area again—the length of time required is usually about 2–3 minutes. The same technique used for the pre-shave scrub (described in

(b) above) is repeated for this procedure.

(ii) Rinse with water and blot dry with sterile towel.

(iii) All disposable items are discarded and re-usable items should be sent for sterilization.

2 *Removal of grease and ingrained dirt*. When clean skin is rubbed with a swab soaked in ether, ether soap or detergent, a film of black material is seen on a white swab. It is therefore of value to cleanse the site of operation in this fashion using a warmed medical detergent solution.

3 *The application of a lotion*. The range of lotions which can be applied is wide and variable. Some are of more value than others. An example of a commonly used preparation at the time of writing is 0·5 per cent chlorhexidine in 70 per cent alcohol. Others are (a) hexachlorophane, (b) a solution of picloxydine digluconate, and (c) povidone-iodine.

All four preparations named have patent trade names and are commercially produced. Some are supplied as aerosol sprays.

4 *Special skin preparation*. Certain patients have a high risk of infection of their wounds with Clostridium Welchii (the micro-organism of gas gangrene) and Clostridium tetani (the micro-organism of tetanus). Such patients would be those with a poor blood supply to the affected limb caused by an avascular disorder such as Reynaud's disease or diabetic gangrene, or those whose skin and wound have been badly soiled with mud and ordure from farm-land.

A special skin preparation is used on such patients, particularly when they are to have amputation of a limb. This is iodophor povidone-iodine, which is supplied by the makers with all accessories and instructions for use (see Chapter 32, p. 588).

5 *Towelling*. Sterile towels to exclude air and dust from the prepared area are commonly used. The efficacy of sterile towelling prior to operation is traditional but unproven. Nevertheless it imprints on the patient's mind the idea that the area should be kept clean.

6 *Final pre-operative skin preparation*. This procedure is carried out in the operating theatre or in a room next to the operating theatre immediately prior to surgery.

(a) Examine the skin area and report any unusual condition to the Operating Theatre Sister and/or the Surgeon.

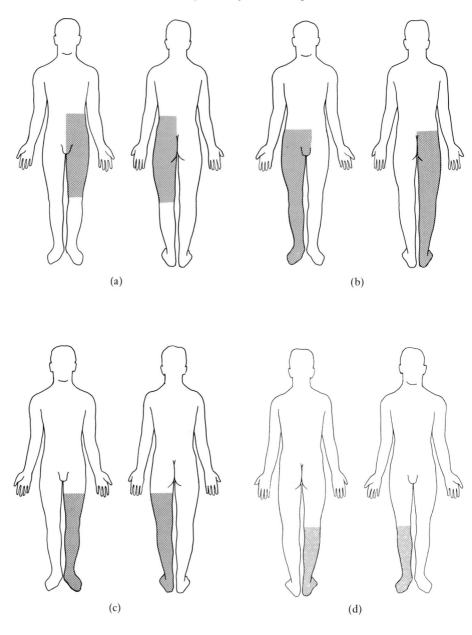

Fig. 27.4 Areas to be prepared for (a) unilateral hip surgery, (b) unilateral thigh and leg surgery, (c) lower leg and foot surgery, and (d) ankle, foot or toe surgery.

(b) The operative site (Fig. 27.4a–d) is cleansed with Povidone-Iodine Surgical Scrub followed by the application of Povidone-Iodine Antiseptic Solution.

The following procedure is recommended:

(i) Dilute 5–10 cc of Povidone-Iodine Surgical Scrub with approximately 2 oz of water.

(ii) Apply this solution to the operative site using standard surgical preparation techniques and rub thoroughly for approximately 5 minutes.

(iii) Wipe off all Povidone-Iodine Surgical Scrub with a sterile towel.

(iv) Apply Povidone-Iodine Antiseptic Solution to the operative site.

(v) Pat excess Povidone-Iodine Antiseptic solution dry with sterile towel. If you wish to hasten drying, the entire area may be patted dry so that some brown coloration remains on the skin.

(vi) If self-adhering plastic drapes are to be used, you may apply these directly over the dried Povidone-Iodine Solution.

(c) The Povidone-Iodine Antiseptic Solution is applied with a saturated gauze sponge held in forceps. The used sponges are discarded as they become soiled.

7 *Skin treatment in the operating theatre.* Within the operating theatre the skin of the limb for operation is re-painted with the skin lotion. Sterile stockinette or transparent polythene may be used to envelope a limb and the incision is made through the stockinette or polythene.

8 *Marking the correct site of operation.* Mistakes can easily be made and, in particular, a patient may have the correct operation performed on the wrong side of the body or on the wrong digit. The members of the surgical team must be ever conscious of such a possibility and must work constantly to prevent such a happening. Careful marking of the correct side and site when the patient is fully awake and can respond to questioning; checking and double-checking of radiographs and notes, and loud and vocal reporting by doctor or nurse if there is a doubt in the mind about the site of operation being the correct one.

The site of operation should be marked with indelible ink preferably in the ward the previous day.

It is essential that all the relevant radiographs and notes should accompany the patient to the operating theatre.

The reader is referred to the Medical Defence Union and Royal College of Nursing Memorandum entitled 'Steps that might be taken to obviate the risks of a surgeon performing an operation on the wrong patient, side, limb, or digit' shown as Appendix of this book.

9   Other aspects of preparation of the patient for operation are the same as for any surgical operation.

(i)   A properly signed and witnessed permission form for operation must be completed by the patient; or the parent or guardian in the case of a minor.

(ii)   The patient is clad in garments which give adequate warmth but access to the site of operation. The hair must be enclosed in a suitable cap or cloth.

(iii) The dentures and any other personal items such as watches and jewellery, should be carefully stored with the name of the patient attached.

(iv) The pre-operative drugs ordered by the anaesthetist must be given in ample time for them to be effective before the patient is taken to the operating theatre.

(v)   The urinary bladder and bowel must be empty before the patient is anaesthetized; the anaesthetics will cause the sphincters of the patient to relax and evacuation of excreta to occur.

(vi) The complete set of notes and radiographs for the patient must accompany him to the operation.

Exsanguination of a limb

The orthopaedic surgeon usually operates on the elbow, wrist, hand, fingers, knee, ankle, foot and toes in a bloodless field. When the patient has been anaesthetized the appropriate limb is elevated above the level of the trunk and a rubber bandage is tightly stretched and wound around the limb from the toes (or fingers) to the thigh (or upper arm). A constricting pneumatic tourniquet is then applied at the upper limit of the bandage and is then inflated so as to occlude the flow of blood into the limb after the rubber bandage has been taken off. The tourniquet must be maintained at an adequate pressure throughout the operation.

The time of the application of the tourniquet is recorded and the surgeon is kept informed of the duration of time for which the tourniquet has been inflated. Although it is the primary responsibility of the surgeon to ensure that the tourniquet has been removed, it is possible that a tourniquet may be left on in error. Therefore, both when the patient leaves the operating theatre and on putting him back into bed, the nurse in charge of the patient and the ward team must always check that the tourniquet has been removed and that there is a good circulation in the limb.

Notes on the relevant post-operative care of the orthopaedic patient

The orthopaedic patient's post-operative management is basically similar to that of any patient recovering from anaesthetic drugs and surgical intervention; there are however some variations:

1 *Position.* Some patients must be kept in the recumbent position; those who have had spinal operations for example, may be lying in a plaster bed. This creates problems should vomiting occur, as the vomitus cannot be cleared easily from the mouth and there is a danger of the patient inhaling the material into the respiratory passages. The anaesthetist will try to adjust the level of anaesthesia in order to prevent vomiting, but careful observation of the unconscious patient—as of any comatose patient—is needed.

2 *Observations.* (a) *General.* Full nursing observation and charting are necessary. When the patient has had an operation on a large joint such as the hip, the tissues around the joint can absorb a large quantity of blood which is stagnant and out of circulation. The surgeon will overcome the reduction in blood volume by giving blood transfusions. Recording of blood pressure every fifteen minutes during the unconscious period is necessary in order to detect such 'internal bleeding' at an early stage.

(b) *Local.* The wound is observed for bleeding. For larger deep wounds affecting muscle and other soft tissues, aspiration by a vacuum drainage bottle through a stab drainage (Fig. 13.4) is usual, and the quantity of blood lost must be recorded. A limb in plaster must be observed for constriction (see p. 523). A patient in a plaster jacket or hip spica must have the plaster exposed to a warm atmosphere so as to enable the plaster to dry. During this procedure the patient will feel cold and uncomfortable. The post-operative drugs for sedation and analgesics are necessary both to give comfort and sleep to the patient and to relieve the pain of operation.

3 *Post-operative sedation and analgesia.* Surgery of bone and joint can be more painful than surgery on other forms of tissue. The post-operative drugs must be adequate to relieve pain and maintain euphoria until the patient has rested and recovered from the pain. Inadequate sedation, or too long an interval between administrations of the drug can only cause the patient suffering.

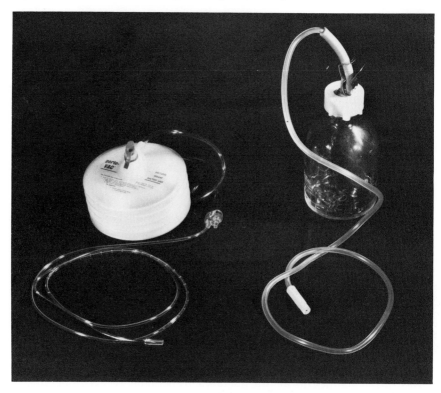

Fig. 27.5   A vacuum drainage bottle.

4 *Micturition*. The usual position for passing urine is either in the upright position or squatting. The patient who is fixed in recumbency cannot adopt either position and may have extreme difficulty in micturating. This, added to the urinary difficulties that may exist in any patient, can cause him much distress.

The usual nursing methods of encouraging the patient to micturate are tried but if unsuccessful, then the drug carbachol or, alternatively catheterization must be used to give the patient relief from a full and painfully distended bladder.

Venous obstruction by thrombosis

This may be called either phlebothrombosis or thrombophlebitis. The former is not accompanied by general and local inflammatory changes but the latter is; this is how the two are distinguished.

Either condition is a serious hazard to the patient as the blood in the large veins (usually in the leg or pelvis) may clot and then dislodge to form a large loose body moving around the circulatory system until it meets a smaller vessel in which it becomes lodged; it then obstructs the flow of blood. This obstruction may occur in a vessel supplying the brain, heart, lungs or intestine, resulting in a sudden and sometimes final catastrophe for the patient.

Pulmonary embolism

Commonly the embolism lodges in a pulmonary artery or one of its branches. This may be rapidly fatal or there may be recurrent obstructions, this can lead to permanent impairment of lung function. Lesser degrees of obstruction may mimic pneumonia. The condition is always serious.

Aetiology and prevention

There are many obscure features in the aetiology of thrombophlebitis. It is very rare in Asia or Africa or in vegetarians. Both constipation and toxic products from protein decomposition in the bowel have been blamed. Many authorities advocate a high residue diet, e.g. bran. Others give repeated small doses of heparin. It is also suggested that stasis during the operation is important and some surgeons use intermittent pressure on the legs to increase blood flow. Whatever the cause, early diagnosis and vigorous treatment with anti thrombotic agents is important.

Early diagnosis

In addition to the clinical features the diagnosis may be confirmed by:
1   Ultra sonic scanning,
2   The injection of activated protein,
3   Phlebography.
Active leg raising should be encouraged as soon as the patient recovers consciousness. Tight bed clothes must be removed!

There are predisposing factors to the possibility of thrombosis and if the doctor is aware of their existence in the patient, he can take action to prevent embolus formation. Pre-existing factors are:

1   Varicosed veins   6   Surgery
2   Obesity   7   Infection
3   Anaemia   8   Sluggish circulation
4   Heart disease   9   Pre-existing vascular abnormalities
5   Trauma   10   Age

Patients who are kept static and immobile in bed for a prolonged period with external pressure on the tissues of the legs, and the patients with injuries to large blood vessels are also liable to suffer this hazard.

Nursing staff should always be alert for the signs and symptoms of the condition in the patient and should report *at once* any of the following:

Phlebothrombosis. Pain in the calf and tenderness of the deep veins of the leg. This may be demonstrated by Holman's sign, which is positive if dorsiflexion of the foot causes pain in the calf.

Thrombophlebitis. Sudden, severe, throbbing pain in the veins. In the superficial veins it may be felt as a tender cord. Oedema and cyanosis of the limb may be present.

Any of these symptoms or signs must be reported immediately. As soon as they are noticed the patient should be returned to bed if he has been an up-patient, and the affected limb slightly raised. He must remain in bed until his temperature and pulse are normal. Absolute bed rest must not be prolonged as this will only increase the further risk of clotting. Passive and later, active movements of the limb are necessary to recover the muscle tone. The doctor will order the relevant drugs such as anticoagulants or antibiotics.

Prevention by nursing measures

Stasis must be avoided in every patient so as to prevent its many complications, and one of these is venous thrombosis. Pillows and pads which compress the lower limbs should be avoided. If they must be used, they should be removed several times a day. Frequent turning of the patient and flexion and extension exercises of the hips, ankles and knees will improve the venous circulation of the lower limbs if these exercises are possible. As soon as possible after an operation the patient should be helped to sit out of bed and standing and walking should be encouraged.

Excessive dehydration and anaemia must also be prevented.

The medical prophylaxis of the condition is the use of anticoagulant therapy in the form of Heparin and Phenindrone.

The care of the recumbent patient

There are various reasons why a patient must be nursed flat in bed or with the foot of the bed elevated, without being permitted to sit up. This section deals with the principles of the nursing care of such patients whether they are fixed to a frame, lying in a plaster bed, or with traction on the legs or pelvis.

1   *The patient's orientation to the horizontal plane.* The psychology of each patient is different. Some will accept positioning in the horizontal plane quickly and without complaint; others will take a day or two; a few will require much longer. All need help and understanding.

If the patient can be given a few days before fixation (in a plaster bed for example) when she can rise from the bed and return to it, thus learning to use it; this is a help to her in establishing herself in prolonged recumbency.

2   *Situation of the bed.* Part of the patient's distress when first placed in recumbency, may be a feeling of nausea and claustrophobia. This may be increased if the bed-head is up against a wall, or worse, in a corner. It is preferable to have space between the bed-head and wall or, alternatively, the bed-head should be placed near a window. This same claustrophobic effect may also be caused by pillows encroaching on the line of vision of the patient. A head mirror, correctly positioned, can help.

3   *'Frame' sickness.* This sometimes occurs when a patient is fastened securely down in a plaster bed or on an orthopaedic frame with the abdominal muscles stretched and the hips in extension. There is a feeling of nausea which goes on to headache and vomiting. Once the patient is settled into the recumbent position the problem passes. However, help related to the orthopaedic condition of the patient may be given in extreme cases by:

(a) Temporarily releasing the patient's legs so that some flexion of the hips is possible and the abdominal muscles can be relaxed.

(b) Temporarily releasing the shoulders and head so that the patient can flex the spine and again relieve the stretching of the abdominal muscles.

(c) Elevating the upper end of a plaster bed or frame.

(d) The use of relevant drugs.

(e) An explanation of the reason for the fixation and the co-operation required from the patient.

(f) Passing an intragastric tube and aspirating the stomach contents intermittently. In severe cases, gastric suction may need to be combined with intravenous infusion.

4   *Micturition and defaecation.* In normal circumstances most individuals seek privacy for excretion; this is a characteristic imbued into those raised in

a community which has bathrooms and closed lavatories. This privacy may be denied the patient fixed in bed.

Additionally, the position for defaecation and micturition required of the recumbent patient is unnatural to her and she may have extreme difficulty in expelling the contents of the bowel or urinary bladder when horizontal. There is usually no alternative to the position in bed and the patient must learn to adapt to the problem.

The nursing staff can help by ensuring that the patient does have privacy and is warm and comfortable; adequate screening is necessary when the unit has other patients adjacent; if the patient is in a single room there should be an indication that visitors must not enter when the patient is using the bedpan or urinal. Given reasonable conditions, the patient will learn to manage.

(a) *Constipation.* When additional help is needed an evacuant suppository inserted into the rectum will help. Important considerations, however, must be the dietary and fluid intake of the patient. If the patient can consume a normal meal there should be ample roughage in the diet to help him avoid constipation; the roughage intake should, in fact, be increased to counter the absence of exercise and reduced pressure from the abdominal musculature.

(b) *Fluid intake and bowel function.* All patients confined to bed must have a large amount of fluid; every nurse, as she attends the patient, should ensure that he drinks some fluid before she goes away from his bedside; efficient recording of fluid balance is essential for the safe knowledge that the patient is drinking sufficiently.

A problem when the patient is in a plaster bed or turning case, or hip spica, or abduction frame, is the possibility of soiling the plaster of Paris or splintage. It should be a matter of pride to the staff of an orthopaedic unit that the equipment is *not* soiled by urine or faeces. This is achieved in several ways:

(a) By ensuring that the genital area on a plaster of Paris bed or spica is clear of the vulva of the female and the gluteal cleft in both male and female patients. The opening on the plaster bed or spica must not be too large or the tissues of the patient will tend to protrude through and the edges of the genital opening of the plaster bed will cut and excoriate the patient's skin. There should be sufficient abduction on a frame or spica to allow sufficient space for bedpans and urinals.

(b) By using suitable equipment for the orthopaedic patient on a frame or plaster bed. For micturition in both male and female patients, a urinal should be provided. There is a urinal designed to fit the shape of the female vulva and, with practice, the patient can manage to micturate into this without soiling her bed. For defaecation, a flat dish placed beneath the gluteal cleft may be more satisfactory than the conventional bedpan.

(c) By thorough washing and cleaning of the patient. Although paper tissues are necessary, they are not as effective as soap and water.

If the plaster of Paris or the leather of the saddle should become soiled, it must be made thoroughly clean again. It is demoralizing for the patient to know that her splintage is malodourous and unpleasant to see.

5 *Eructation and vomiting.* The abdominal muscles contribute to all processes of expulsion of products from the abdominal cavity. Defaecation, discarding flatus, micturition, eructation and vomiting all require inward compression from the abdominal walls, pelvic floor and diaphragm. If the patient cannot effectively compress inwards, these functions are impaired and the patient has difficulties.

Micturition and defaecation have already been discussed. Vomiting and the expulsion of gas from the stomach are now considered. If the patient is usually a sufferer from gastric disorders she will still have these problems and an unsuitable diet may distress her. A diet containing much seasoning and spice will cause the production of much gas which must be expelled, or the patient will feel distended and uncomfortable and will be unable to settle until the gas has been raised; such items in the diet should be avoided. The use of carminatives such as Aqua Menth. Pip. or peppermint cordials may help; assisting with firm pressure on the anterior abdominal wall of the patient may also be of value.

Vomiting may occur for one of many various reasons. If the patient cannot stand or turn onto his side in bed, or raise his head, shoulders or neck, he may be in serious difficulties. If the vomit cannot be effectively expelled from the mouth it may be inhaled which will cause coughing and choking. To help the patient lying flat during vomiting, a receiver with a concave edge should be held against the cheek. A cloth is an asset. After vomiting, a mouth rinse should be supplied and facilities given to clean the teeth.

When vomiting is anticipated, and if there is time, an intragastric tube may be passed and the contents of the stomach aspirated before the vomiting commences.

6 *Feeding.* Even though the patient lies recumbent, she must eat sufficient food not only for daily physiological requirements, but also to aid the recovery of the tissues of her lesion. A high protein diet is necessary for this.

The horizontal position is a difficult one in which to transfer food from plate to mouth, but if the patient is physically able, she must learn to feed herself and not be dependent upon the nursing staff.

(a) *Self-feeding*. A diet-cloth, large enough to cover the clothing on the thorax is placed on the patient after her hands and face have been washed and dried. The plate of food is placed on the diet cloth in as stable a position as possible, and near to the mouth. The overhead vision mirror is adjusted so that the patient can see the plate and her mouth; she now transfers the food from plate to mouth.

This procedure is soon learned and many patients can use a knife and fork to chop the food into a reasonable size when lying flat. If this cannot be achieved, then it must be done for the patient.

When the patient is lying flat, drinking is achieved by the use of flexible straws or bent glass tubes or polythene tubing.

(b) *Assisted feeding*. When the patient must be fed by the nursing staff, it can be a pleasant or unpleasant experience for her, depending upon the attitude and method of the nurse engaged in giving the food. The occasion should be properly prepared and must be felt to be a 'proper' meal by the patient. She must feel clean and comfortable, having had the opportunity

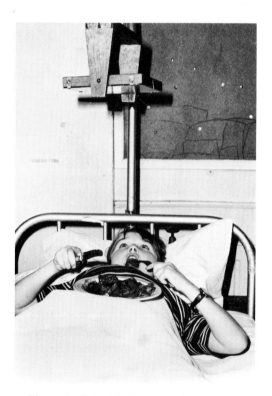

Fig. 27.6   Patient feeding in horizontal position.

previously to empty the bowel and bladder; the patient's hands and face are washed and the bed tidied; a clean diet cloth is placed to protect the bedding and clothing.

The tray is brought to the bedside and laid correctly and attractively; the meal is neatly arranged on the plate.

During the meal the nurse must create a pleasant and unhurried atmosphere. If the level of the bed warrants it, the nurse will sit down during the process of feeding. The patient is given small amounts of food and is allowed sufficient time to chew and swallow.

Meal times become interval marks in the course of the day for every patient; they should be served punctually and with the highest standard of presentation possible.

7 *Dress.* Suitable clothing for the patient on a frame or plaster bed, or on complete rest requires special consideration. Garments which must be put over the head and pulled down the body, or pyjama trousers will not do. The most useful garment is one which is divided down the back and fastens only at the neck level; it should be long enough to reach the level of the patient's knees. Briefs which are divided for fastening at each side are also necessary.

As the patient cannot rub the feet together or move them about, the lower extremities tend to get cold. If the room is centrally heated to a temperature of 22°C the patient will probably be warm enough, but some prefer bedsocks.

Clothing is important to the morale of the patient even though fixed flat in bed. Personal and individual modifications to dress and appearance should be encouraged. Garments which are institutional and worn by all other patients may depress the patient. This also applies to the use of cosmetics, scents, and coiffure by the female patient.

8 *The hair.* For most patients in an orthopaedic unit, management of the hair is no more of a problem than for patients confined to bed in any other unit. If the patient is fixed in some device which covers the head, special problems exist. Such devices could be a minerva jacket, or a head piece on a plaster bed. If the hair cannot be reached for effective attention, there is little that can be done until the patient is turned or released from the head piece. Inevitably, the hair will become sweaty, matted and long. It is essential to ensure that there are no head lice in other patients in the ward as these may infest the patient in the head piece and cause severe problems in disinfecting the head. Before putting a patient in a Minerva jacket or on a frame a thorough hair wash is desirable.

9   *Oral hygiene.* Teeth cleaning requires some special management. The method is as follows:

(a) A mouth rinse is first given.

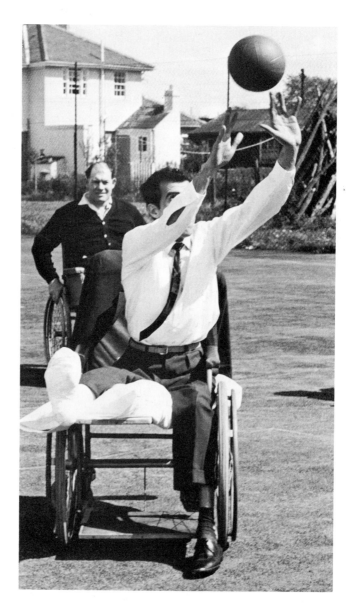

Fig. 27.7   'A successful try' wheelchair netball.

(b) The toothbrush is loaded with toothpaste by the nurse. Alternatively the toothpaste is smeared onto the front teeth of the patient. The toothbrush is used to clean the teeth in the usual manner.

(c) Using a polythene or bent glass tube or a drinking straw, the patient fills the mouth with water. A receiver or vomit bowl with a concave or straight edge is held against the patient's cheek and the mouth rinse is ejected into it from the side of the mouth.

A dental chip syringe may be useful in rinsing the mouth for the patient who is unable to co-operate.

10   *Sleep.* As the patient is unable to turn into his normal sleep posture, and is unused to lying in bed all day, his normal sleeping habits are deranged. For the first few nights after fixation a hypnotic drug may be ordered to assist sleeping, but soon the patient should reorientate his sleeping pattern to the change.

Long-continued medication, apart from specific reasons, is undesirable.

On the first day the patient should be fixed onto the bed or frame as early in the day as possible to help him to be used to the position by night time.

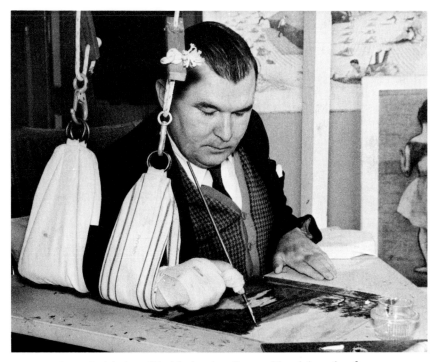

Fig. 27.8 'Artist at Work', showing slings and brush bound to finger.

11   *Avoiding boredom.* Special equipment is necessary to enable the patient to write, type, draw, read or undertake any other activity. An overhead angled mirror which the patient can move is essential to keep him in constant touch with all that goes on around him and to enable him to watch television. An adjustable easel mounted over the bed and patient will aid the patient to fix writing paper and reading material into a convenient position.

Suitable diversionary occupational therapy is also necessary. For children, school work is a must.

The principles of nursing management in joint-replacement surgery

Although joint-replacement surgery has been practised for many years new developments are constantly occurring. The management of the patients depends upon many factors such as the bio-mechanical form of the operation and the attitude of the surgeon.

Patient selection
As these are elective operations, careful assessment and selection of patients is necessary.

(a) *Psychological factors*
Not every patient who requests such an operation is a suitable subject. Sometimes when an operation result is obviously excellent the patient receives no benefit because of psychological depression and pessimism. Factors which would contribute to such a state must be taken into account. Such personal and emotional problems as financial or marital insecurity, severe solitary loneliness and absence of affection must be considered. When there are 'borderline' cases and doubt exists about the suitability of the patient for an operation the assistance of a psychiatrist may be sought.

The very success of joint replacement and the attendant publicity leads patients with relatively minor symptoms to ask for it. Even now the operation has risks and complications particularly in men. It is essential that the patient's symptoms are sufficiently severe, e.g. he cannot sleep at night or his walking distance is severely restricted.

(b) *Physical factors*
The surgeon must eliminate skeletal, muscular, neurological problems which might militate against success. Gross skeletal deformity, ineffective

musculature, or inefficient muscle co-ordination of neurological origin must be assessed against the probable effects of the operation.

Previous infection in or around the joint may also be a contra-indication.

(c) *Pathological factors*

An arthroplasty usually requires the cementing of an implant such as vitallium to bone; it must have a strong, efficient attachment to good quality bone. Osteoporotic bone or bone which is fragile and erodible will not serve as a suitable fixation for the implant. Infection at the site or a generalized anaemia are also adverse factors.

Patient assessment

The patient must be given a comprehensive assessment before the operation. A full survey of all relevant joints, the opposite limb, erythrocyte sedimentation rate, haemoglobin, blood-chemistry and blood-pressure, renal function and previous history of illness must all be considered.

The occupational-therapy staff must assess the 'Activities of Daily Living' function of the patient; this is of use in assessing the effectiveness of the operation.

Communication with the patient

As this form of surgery is still being developed it is essential that the patient is fully informed of the anticipated results. He must be aware of the limitations of the operation as he may have pre-conceived ideas of his own which may go beyond the effects the surgeon hopes to achieve. The results are often excellent and the patient is given relief from pain and greatly improved function; frequently patients return for an operation on the opposite limb because they are so pleased with results of the first operation.

At the time of signing the 'consent for operation' form the patient must have ample opportunity to ask questions and receive frank and complete answers.

Some aspects of pre-operative preparation

Additional to the routine pre-operative preparation for any operation the following must be considered.

1   *Skin.* Elective operations demand the highest standard of aseptic technique. The method of skin preparation for the particular operation is usually the choice of the surgeon and this must be discussed with him. An example of a pre-operative preparation is the three-day physiological

hexachlorophane bath method. There must be total absence of infective lesions on the skin and an operation may have to be deferred if there is the slightest sign of pustules on the skin. Povidone-iodine is often used to locally prepare the skin.

2 *Drugs.* Frequently the patients who come into hospital for an arthroplasty have been established, for a long period of time, on a regime of drugs relevant to their joint damage. Phenylbutazone, aspirin or indomethacin are examples of such drugs but the range of possibilities is wide. It is essential to notify the surgeon and anaesthetist of the pre-admission drug therapy and to arrange to continue it as instructed. Additionally there must be consideration of the drug regime related to the prolonged anaesthetic which will be necessary.

3 *Blood-grouping and cross-matching.* The operation may cause minimal blood-loss or a large amount may inevitably be lost. This depends upon the site of the operation. An operation involving a large joint with heavy musculature around it will create greater blood-loss than a joint which is superficial to the skin with little muscle surrounding it.

In either case it is wisdom to ensure that the blood of the patient is grouped and cross-matched with three pints of donor blood prior to the day of operation.

4 *Physiotherapy.* An essential part of the pre-operative preparation is the training of the patient to carry out the post-operative regime of exercises. In the immediate post-anaesthetic phase the patient will not be in a fit state to understand the instructions given. If, however, the patient has been fully instructed in the reason for, and method of doing the post-operative physiotherapy in the days prior to surgery the exercises will be performed with good grace no matter how feeble the patient may feel.

The physiotherapy regime has many different functions:

(a) Prevention of post-operative coughs and respiratory problems caused by anaesthesia and the restricted post-operative breathing of the patient who may be tense and afraid to inhale sufficiently.

(b) Prevention of stasis due to lack of movement in bed.

(c) Prevention of stiffness in joints adjacent to the operation site.

(d) Maintenance of muscle quality and function at the joint which has been replaced. This is an essential aspect of the operation and neglect of this can result in the failure of the arthroplasty.

(e) Prevention of thrombo-embolytic and phlebo-thrombotic problems in the limbs.

(f) Improvement of the morale of the patient who is soon made aware that his limb can function normally.

(g) Prevention of dislocation of the joint because of non-function of the rotator cuff muscles of a ball and socket joint.

As soon as feasible after the return of the patient from the operating theatre the physiotherapist commences treatment. In lower limb joint replacement, the quadriceps femaris group of muscles particularly *must* be maintained in full function. Straight-leg raising exercises are usually commenced on the day of operation.

Some aspects of early post-operative management

Additional to the routine post-operative care for any operation the following must be considered.

1   *The bed.* The base of the bed to which the patient is returned must be firm and stable. Most orthopaedic wards are equipped with beds which have a metal base for the mattress but if the bed has a sprung base then fracture-boards must be used to support the mattress. There must be no drooping or sagging of the mattress.

2   *Soft-tissue drainage.* Prevention of haematoma formation and any stagnation of blood in the tissues adjacent to the joint must be avoided. Normally every pocket or compartment which could retain static blood is drained by a polythene tube drain connected to a vacuum pump (see Fig. 27.5). Two drains and two pumps may commonly be used. These are left in for four or five days or until there is no further exudate from the wound.

3   *Elevation of the foot of the bed.* For lower limb joint-replacement 15 cm blocks are used to elevate the foot of the bed to aid venous return from the limb and avoid swelling. A bed cradle is also used to avoid the weight of the bedding compressing the limb.

4   *Post-operative drugs.* Bone surgery is painful but no patient need suffer pain. An analgesic and sedative drug regime should allay pain and is necessary to enable the physiotherapist to commence the post-operative exercises.

5   *Prophylactic antibiotics.* A five day post-operative anti-infection course of antibiotics may be ordered. An example of such a regime could be:

Ampicillin 250 mg ⎫
Flucocloxacillin 250 mg ⎬ every six hours.

Relevant post-operative management for arthroplasty of the hip

Additional to the routine post-operative care for any patient the following matters are particularly applicable to the management of the patient who has had a total hip-replacement.

1   *Preparation of the site*

The hip is so near to the gluteal cleft and perineum that extra consideration must be given to the preparation of the patient's skin prior to the operation. The micro-organisms which are the normal denizens of the animal bowel can be disastrously pathogenic if they gain entrance to an open wound at operation. Therefore extremes of hygiene and cleanliness are sought in an attempt to avoid wound infection. Pre-operative bathing must be frequent and physiological hexachlorophane in the bath on each of the three days prior to the operation is often used. A povidone-iodine preparation is used to prepare the area.

2   *The bed and equipment for post-operative care*

The bed used is the standard orthopaedic bed with a firm base. Additional equipment in the post-operative phase includes devices to prevent the lateral rotation of the femurs at the hips before the muscles supporting the hip have recovered sufficiently to allow control by the patient. These may be polyurethane troughs, with a flat base, in which each leg rests. The additional advantage of these is that they maintain the knees in 5 degrees of flexion and prevent the heels from pressing into the mattress—a severe problem in nursing these patients. Special heel troughs may also be needed to prevent soreness but frequent movement and attention must not be overlooked.

Sometimes undulating ripple beds are used but not every surgeon would agree to their use.

3   *Position of the patient*

The patient is nursed recumbent for the first twenty-four hours. On the second day the patient is raised to the sitting posture. Some surgeons require the patient to be stood out of bed on the second day. A most important aspect of the care of the patient in the first days after operation is the maintenance of the legs in the abducted position. This may be achieved by the use of the triangular mattresses fixed between the thighs. These are only removed on the instructions of the surgeon; the programme of post-operative management varies according to the patient's condition and must be discussed with the surgeon. After the tenth day the patient should spend some time each day in the prone position to encourage full extension of the hips and prevent flexion contractures of the joints.

The positioning, maintenance of the position, and the prevention of the problem of decubitus and friction sores on the heels and other parts is a major aspect of the nursing management of the patient.

4   *Wound care*

(a)   *Drainage.* The wound may be on the lateral or anterior aspect of the thigh. The patient will be returned to the nursing unit with two or three polythene tubes draining the adjacent tissues and attached to vacuum pumps. Removal of these relates to the amount of fluid they are draining. As the quantity decreases they are gradually withdrawn from the tissues and totally removed when there is no longer any fluid passing along the tube.

(b)   *Tension sutures.* As the tissues are loose and adipose in this area it is common for the surgeon to use tension sutures with supporting buttons to prevent the wound gaping and tearing out the skin sutures. These are removed four or five days after operation.

(c)   *Dressings.* The volume of the dressings applied in the operating theatre is large enough to absorb the drainage from the large wound. This is normally left untouched for forty-eight hours and then reduced to a lightweight dressing held in place with microporous tape or a crêpe bandage to facilitate adequate movement during physiotherapy.

There is, of course, a regime of wound observation related to consistent recording of the temperature, pulse and respiration to note the presence of any infection.

5   *Parenteral infusion*

Post-operatively a five-day regime of intravenous dextran is continued; between 250 and 500 ml per day may be ordered.

Relevant post-operative management for arthroplasty of the knee

Additional to the routine post-operative care of any patient the following aspects are relevant.

1   *Skin cleanliness.* As high a standard of pre-operative cleanliness of the skin as it is possible to attain is necessary. A three bath method using physiological hexachlorophane is recommended.

2   *Compression bandaging.* This operation is performed in a bloodless field after exsanguination of the limb with a rubber bandage and inflatable tourniquet. Before the tourniquet is removed a Robert Jones compression bandage is applied over the surgical dressing.

3   *Wound drainage.* As for arthroplasty of the hip, two drainage tubes and vacuum drainage pumps are used to prevent haematoma formation in pockets within the wound.

4   *Mobilization.* On the fourth day after operation the dressing is changed and the drainage tubes and pumps are removed. If feasible, the wound is covered with a light dressing and a simple crêpe bandage for the purpose of exercising the limb. The patient is got out of bed and walks a few steps with help. The instruction is to walk with the knee held stiff to help the maintenance of the quadriceps muscles. The patient walks like this as much as possible and is discouraged from flexing the knee. After the tenth day the patient is *encouraged* to flex the knee as much as possible. 70 degrees of flexion is possible at first and this is increased later to 90 degrees of flexion. Stair-climbing exercises are particularly encouraged.

Before discharge the occupational therapist assesses the activities of daily living of the patient to estimate if these have improved.

The patient may be discharged from hospital about two weeks after operation.

28

Traction

Hugh Owen Thomas (see Chapter 1) designed and made a variety of splints but constantly stressed the importance of *principles* rather than methods. In a chapter such as this it is essential to describe both the basic principles and the various methods of applying traction; the principles laid down in the early part of the chapter are maintained throughout but it is always necessary to modify the method of traction to the needs of a particular person. No patient should be in distress through discomfort or pain due to slavishly following what is said 'in the book'. In an age of ingenious gadgets there is a danger that we do not profit from a vast store of experience of the pioneers. The principles of applied traction are simple and definite; they must be borne in mind whenever traction is applied to a patient.

The dictionary defines traction as, 'the drawing of a body along a surface'. This is what is mainly done in the orthopaedic application of traction, but an opposing force known as counter-traction is necessary (Fig. 28.1), as the aim of the treatment is to draw apart two portions of the body.

Fixed traction
In this form of traction no weights or pulleys are used. The patient is fixed to a device at one point and the limb is pulled away from the point of fixation by extensions and cords which are tied to the device. Thus, the fixation point is 'counter-traction' and the pulling extensions are 'traction'. Examples of this are seen:

(a) When a Thomas' splint is applied to a leg using skin extensions tied to the end of the splint (Fig. 28.2).

(b) When a patient is fixed to an abduction frame and the leg or legs are extended and attached to the bows on the frame (Fig. 28.3). Thus the frame serves as *counter-traction* and the pulling extensions as *traction*.

The advantage of fixed traction is that the force required is small. It can be used to overcome muscle spasm when spasmodic muscles are causing either pain or deformity. As the muscles relax the traction can readily be adjusted and the process repeated until the 'normal' length is reached.

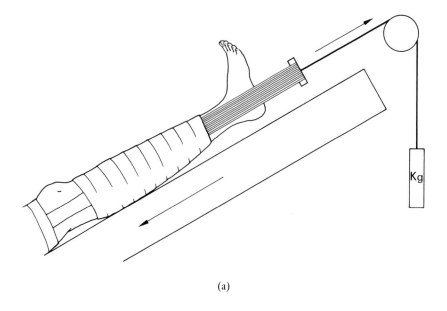

(a)

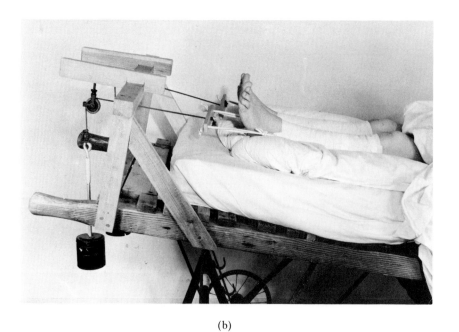

(b)

Fig. 28.1	(a) and (b) The opposing forces used in traction.

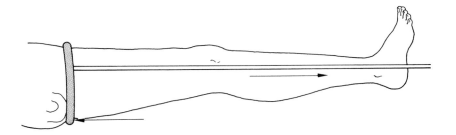

Fig. 28.2   (a) The principles of fixed traction using a Thomas' splint.

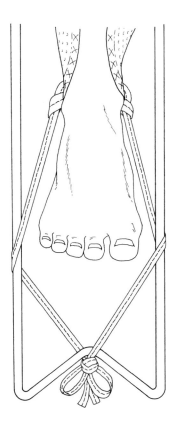

Fig. 28.2   (b) A traction kit showing sewn-on lampwicks.

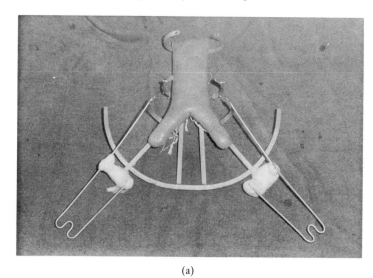

(a)

(b)

Fig. 28.3   Double abduction frame with (a) c-shaped bar and saddle,
(b) c-shaped bar no saddle.

Sliding traction

This makes use of the same principles of traction opposed by counter-traction as in fixed traction, but in this case the directions are reversed. The extensions and cords are applied to the legs of the patient and fixed to the foot end of the bed. If the foot of the bed is then elevated, an inclined plane is

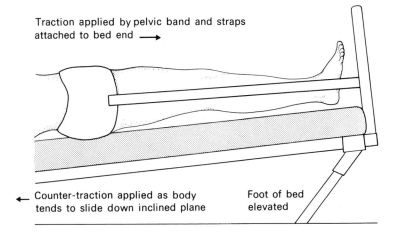

Traction applied by pelvic band and straps
attached to bed end ——►

← Counter-traction applied as body   Foot of bed
tends to slide down inclined plane   elevated

Fig. 28.3   (c) Pelvic traction used for low back pain.

made, down which the body of the patient will slide away from the point of
fixation. Thus the extensions serve as counter-traction and the sliding body
of the patient forms the traction. This form of traction is used in:

(a) *Pugh's traction* (Fig. 28.13b).

(b) *Pelvic traction*, this is modified as the extensions are applied to the
pelvic sling and not the legs.

(c) *Sliding bed traction* (Fig. 28.13a). The principles of traction versus
counter-traction are enhanced by placing the body of the patient on a board
arranged on runners or castors. This method overcomes the friction which
must exist between the patient's body and the underlying mattress in
methods (a) and (b), therefore the force is greater.

Weight and pulley traction

This method uses the same principles of traction opposed by counter-
traction, but in this example pulleys and weights are used. The system
may be simple using a single pulley to alter the direction of the force so
that weights can be conveniently suspended (Fig. 28.1), or a compound
system when a number of pulleys are used in combination to increase the
efficiency of the force applied as well as alter its direction. An example of this
is Hamilton-Russell traction (Fig. 28.4). In all weighted traction the weights
must hang freely and not touch the floor or the side of the bed.

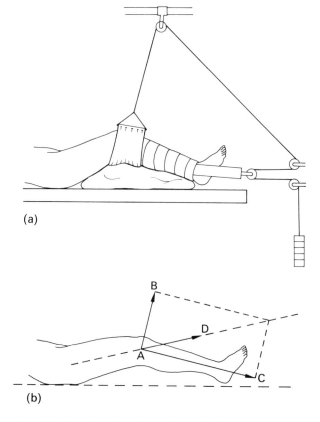

(a)

(b)

Fig. 28.4   (a) Hamilton-Russell traction. (b) Compound pulley system doubles the pull on the leg. By construction of a parallelogram of forces, with side AC twice as long as AB: direction of resultant D can be obtained.

The pulley

A pulley is a wheel with a grooved edge suspended on an axle, around which it rotates in a framework or block. In orthopaedic suspension or traction they may be used either as single fixed pulleys or as pairs of pulley blocks.

Single fixed pulleys. A single fixed pulley used in traction offers no mechanical advantage, as the force (the weight) applied at one end of the cord is equal to the load (Fig. 28.5). The advantages of using a single fixed pulley in traction or suspension is that traction cords can be passed in any convenient direction to reach a hanging weight, that is, a single fixed pulley serves to direct the force in a particular direction.

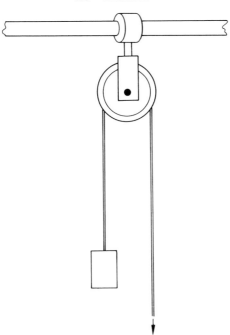

Fig. 28.5   A single fixed pulley used in traction.

Pairs of pulley blocks. A pulley block is a grouping of two or three pulleys on a single common axle in a frame. Two such pulley blocks are required at each point of suspension; they are used in orthopaedic treatment to suspend plaster beds from overhead beams (Fig. 28.6). The bed can easily be tilted in any direction by the patient and thus give him a range of mobility that would not exist if the bed were fixed on a base. Using such pairs of blocks it is possible to use the mechanical advantage thus gained to balance the heavy weight of the patient plus his plaster bed against a number of small weights suspended at the bed end.

Combinations of single pulleys. In Hamilton-Russell traction an arrangement of four single pulleys arranged as in Fig. 28.7 offers the advantage of the pulley-block system to suspend the leg of the patient and the direction of the traction force can be altered according to the principles of the parallelogram of forces (see Fig. 28.4).

The efficiency of any pulley system is related to the condition of the pulleys. They must be in good condition and revolve easily around the axis.

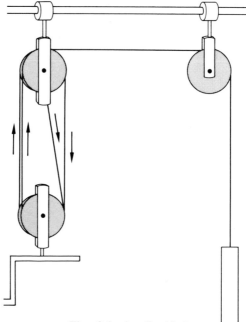

Fig. 28.6   A pulley block.

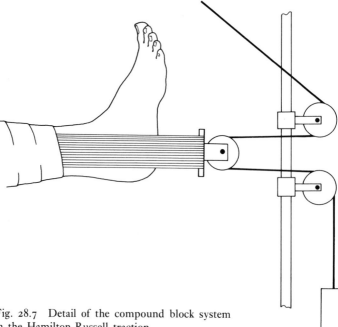

Fig. 28.7   Detail of the compound block system
in the Hamilton-Russell traction.

In a hospital ward any squeak of wheels serves to irritate both patients and staff. An oil can is a useful accessory in overcoming both noise and friction.

Sets of yacht pulleys which are arranged in compound systems and have frames with openings and fastenings to allow traction cord to be slipped in at the side are used in suspending plaster beds. They also have composition wheels which make less noise as they turn.

Traction force may be applied to the body in any of five ways:

1   *Skin traction.* In this method adhesive materials are fastened to the skin and the traction cord is attached to this material.

2   *Skeletal traction.* This requires the drilling of a bone and passing of a strong metal pin through the bone. A special stirrup is attached to the pin and the cord is fixed to this.

3   *Pulp traction.* A metal pin is passed through soft tissues such as the pad of the fingers or toes. A small stirrup is attached to this pin and traction is then applied.

4   *Pelvic traction.* A specially fitted harness made of canvas is fastened around the patient's pelvic area. The harness is attached to the foot of the bed by cords or straps. When the foot of the bed is elevated the body of the patient tends to slide down the inclined plane away from the foot of the bed.

5   *Head traction.* This may be applied by:
(a) A harness (Glisson's sling) or a Criles head tractor (Fig. 28.18a and b).
(b) Skull calipers (see Fig. 28.18c).
(c) Halo splint (see Fig. 28.20a–e).

The functions of traction

Traction may be used:

(a) To restore the length of a bone or limb if, because of trauma or disease, the length of the limb is reduced.

(b) To maintain the length of a fractured limb when the fracture is un-stable, for example, when the line of the fracture is oblique. The traction should overcome the spasm of the longitudinal muscles which cause over-lapping of the broken fragments and consequent shortening.

(c) To reduce a dislocated joint.

(d) To correct joint deformity.

(e) To diminish painful muscle spasm; in particular the spasm caused by irritation of a joint due to infective arthritis, or when the derangement of an intervertebral disc sets up spasm in muscles.

(f) As a post-operative measure to rest the parts involved in surgery and contribute to healing.

(g) As a pre-operative measure prior to internal fixation.

The disadvantages of traction

Like other forms of orthopaedic treatment, traction has its function but it also has limitations and dangers and these must be realized:

1   Traction may be too great. At the site of a fracture this could result in the complete separation of the broken surfaces with subsequent delayed union.

2   Traction at a joint may cause too great a separation of the joint surfaces and stretching of the capsule of the joint with resultant instability or stiffness of the joint.

3   Continuous traction reduces the activity of the muscles adjacent to the lesion. These muscles then waste with the need for considerable effort in physiotherapy to rehabilitate the wasted muscles.

4   The stretching process may be applied to arteries or nerves with vascular or neurological problems as a result.

5   Traction and disuse of the limbs may result in osteoporosis of the bones involved.

6   Traction may lead to skin sores.

7   Skin traction may lead to occlusion of the circulation or pressure on nerves.

8   Bone traction may lead to infection.

9   Pressure of a splint, e.g. the ring of a Thomas' splint, may lead to skin sores or, if the ring is too tight, to circulatory obstruction.

10   In the presence of a large haematoma, traction may cause a dangerous increase of pressure inside the limb.

Skin traction classifications

Adhesive types

(a) *Self-adhesive.* These are prepared by the manufacturers by spreading a self-adhesive medium in a thin layer upon a supporting material. The medium consists of agents which should be innocuous to the skin. The most common of these is zinc-oxide. The supporting material may be:

(i)   unstretchable perforated cloth in the form of zinc-oxide plaster;

(ii)   cross-wise elastic fabric which may be perforated for ventilation.

Self-adhesive extension materials adhere closely to the skin at body temperature and do not require warming before application. The skin should be thoroughly dry and free from hair before application. They are supplied commercially either as rolls of material which must be measured and prepared by sewing on lampwick loops before application (Fig. 28.8) or as prepared traction kits using latex foam strips to protect the malleoli of the ankle from friction (Fig. 28.9). Such kits are offered by the makers in either adult or child sizes.

A disadvantage of the zinc-oxide preparation is that some patients develop

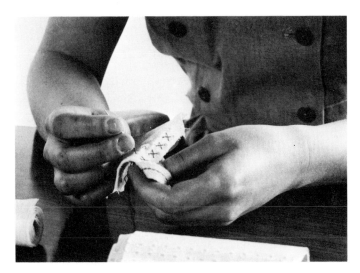

Fig. 28.8   Sewing on lampwick loops.

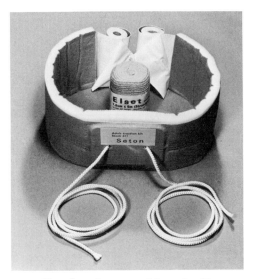

Fig. 28.9   A commercial traction kit.

a reaction to them in the form of contact dermatitis, and it is then necessary to seek an alternative form of application.

(b) *Diachylon adhesive*. This is a lead base adhesive material spread on various supporting materials. The adhesive is commonly prepared from the reaction products of lead monoxide and vegetable oils. The supporting material may be:

(i) *Holland cloth*. This is supplied in 10 inch wide rolls. The material is inelastic and must be measured and prepared with lampwick extension loops (see Fig. 28.8) before application. Usually holland cloth should be warmed before application, although this is not necessary with some of the more recent adhesive materials.

(ii) *Ventilated elastic cloth*. This has a cross-wise stretch and the adhesive arranged in bands along the length of the cloth to permit ventilation. This material is supplied commercially as a complete traction kit with all requirements for extensions. The makers provide either adult or child sizes.

Diachylon adhesives will adhere to the skin as they are warmed by the heat of the body and the bandage should be held in position until it sticks. Alternatively, they may be warmed before application. An advantage of this form of adhesive over the zinc-oxide type is that they can be re-applied after temporary removal. They are also less likely to create a contact dermatitis reaction.

A disadvantage is that the lead monoxide may slightly impede the passage of the rays in radiography and the diachylon material will show on the film. If they are used it may be necessary to temporarily remove the extensions during radiography.

(c) *Unna's paste*. The formula of Unna's paste is 15 per cent zinc-oxide in gelatin, glycerin and water. It is a gelatinous paste which is stored in airtight jars, and it is melted for use by standing the jar in water and heating until it becomes fluid. In the fluid state it is painted onto prepared calico extensions before application to the limb for which the extensions were prepared. Two layers of calico, attached to the one extension loop, are coated with the warmed Unna's paste and applied separately one on top of the other. As the paste cools it sets and fastens the extension to the skin. Setting takes some hours so that traction must not be applied until the paste has completely set. Another disadvantage is that the extensions tend to slip down the limb and form a hard mass around the ankle, with the danger of causing pressure sores.

Non-adhesive extensions

(a) *Latex-foam pads or bandages.* These may either be improvised extensions or commercially supplied extension packs. They have the disadvantages that to serve as extensions they must be firmly bandaged to the skin, using either roller or tubular bandages with the danger of constriction of the limb. If not firmly bandaged on they will slip down the limb when traction is applied, and must constantly be checked and re-applied. They may serve as temporary extensions, however, when light traction or short-term traction is required.

(b) *Gamgee tissue under a clove hitch.* An anklet of gamgee padding with a calico bandage arranged as a clove hitch attaching the limb to the foot of an elevated bed may sometimes be used as a temporary extension whilst permanent extensions are being replaced or Unna's paste extensions are setting. This practice is dangerous, however, as there is a possibility of constricting the limb and impairing the blood supply to the foot. It should therefore only be used:

(i) with thick padding,

(ii) for a limited period of time,

(iii) with constant observation of the foot to check for changes in colour or temperature which would indicate an impairment of the blood supply,

(iv) on a limb that is not paralysed or has loss of sensation so that the patient is unaware of changes in the limb,

(v) on a patient whose condition does not indicate a poor blood supply to the limbs.

These classifications are given to show the alternatives which are available; when one form cannot be used because of idiosyncrasy and reaction to the material, another may be tried.

Contact dermatitis. Some of the products used in the manufacture of the adhesives for use in skin extensions may cause a reaction on the skin of the patient at the sites where they are applied. This is very distressing for the patient; it may mean that the extensions must be removed and his orthopaedic treatment discontinued. The help of a dermatologist is useful in caring for such patients who often give a history of allergy to certain materials and de-sensitization may have been used in their earlier treatment.

The immediate aim is to seek an alternative method of applying skin extensions or even to apply skeletal traction, if this is feasible. The patient's complaints must never be ignored; they usually indicate that a modification of treatment is desirable.

The application of extensions

A limb to which extensions are being applied may be painful—so painful that an anaesthetic is often necessary when extension is first applied. Conversely, in replacing existing skin extensions, or in conditions such as Perthes' disease of the hip, the patient is not in pain and no anaesthetic is needed. In either case, skill and gentleness are required in handling the limb, maintaining manual traction, and applying the extensions with speed and dexterity.

Manual traction. Two persons are required for this part of the procedure, the first to maintain a constant pull along the length of the limb, the second to apply firm pressure at the site of the lesion with one hand above and one below. Another person is needed to apply the extensions and handle the splint; once traction is commenced it must not be interrupted.

The person applying the pull along the limb should sit comfortably at the end of the bed; it should not be necessary for her to work at arms length or to stand and be bending forwards. The reasons for this are (1) that discomfort means that the arm muscles become fatigued and, as a result, lowering of the hands or trembling begins, which is transmitted to the patient's limb, and (2) the limb is probably heavy and support must be maintained for a long time with resultant back strain to a standing, bending worker. This helper places her hands as shown in Fig. 28.10 with one hand behing the ankle with the index finger resting along the tendo Achillis and the second hand across the top of the forefoot. A firm pull is maintained and not relaxed until extensions are applied and traction continued through these.

The helper supporting the site of the lesion should also sit. Both should apply firm but slow and gentle movements in handling the limb.

Sandbags. Small bags of various shapes and sizes, made of strong canvas or bed ticking, filled with sand which is then sewn in, with the whole covered with waterproof material are essential equipment in an orthopaedic unit. Until all is ready for the application of splints and extensions, the painful limb may be held still with a number of such sandbags.

Measuring for extensions
Commercially produced traction kits (see p. 469) are now commonly used. As the use of such kits saves the nursing staff time-consuming measuring and sewing, their usage will increase; the cost of a traction kit is offset by the cost of the time of staff who sew the extensions.

The length of an extension is related to its purpose. It may be classified as

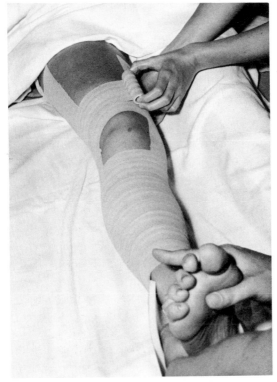

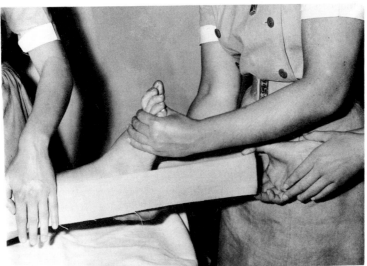

Fig. 28.10   Applying extensions.

(a) an above-knee extension (for femoral or hip lesions), or (b) a below-knee extension (for knee or tibial lesions). The principles involved are that if below-knee extensions are applied to a hip or femoral lesion, the knee joint is strained by the traction being applied *through* the joint; if above-knee extensions are used the knee joint is supported.

Skin preparation. The skin of the patient is prepared for the application of extensions. To shave the limb or not to shave the limb depends upon the quantity of hairs which cover it. On a limb profusely covered by thick tough hairs, the adhesive will stick to the hair, not to the skin, and soon the extensions will come off; the limb will be sore as the traction is applied only to the hair follicles. If the limb is covered only by a thin covering of fine hairs, shaving is unnecessary but may be preferred. In either case, the hairs will grow underneath the extensions.

Painting the limb with tincture benzoin compound is a good practice; it serves several purposes: to reduce moisture through perspiration; to harden the skin; to give greater attachment for the adhesive; to act as a barrier to the adhesive in the event of the patient being sensitive to the adhesive on the extensions.

Applying the extensions

The extensions must be applied without folds or creases, otherwise a sore may form under the material (Fig. 28.10). They should mould well to the limb. The bony points on the limb must not be covered by the extension. The malleoli should be protected from friction as the extensions pass over them; this protection can be with pieces of adhesive felt or adhesive latex foam. Another way to protect the malleoli is to pass two turns of soft open-wove or crêpe bandage around the ankle, just above the malleoli; this same bandage is then continued up the limb over the adhesive extensions.

The crest of the tibia can also be protected from friction of the bandage or slings with lint or felt, or latex foam strips when considered necessary.

A soft bandage is applied over the extensions. The turns of this bandage should not overlap more than is needed to cover the limb and the extensions. The patella is left exposed. The bandage is then fixed by sewing the end to its previous turn rather than using a safety-pin.

Spreaders. These are pieces of wood, plastic or metal which serve to maintain the pull of the extensions along parallel lines as they are attached to the traction cord (Fig. 28.11). The width of the spreader should be the same as the width between the apex of the internal and external malleoli on the limb.

The traction cord is passed through the spreader and the weights or force applied to the cord, so that the spreader receives the full force of the traction and should be strong. In practice a single central hole in the spreader is not always the best as it may tend to pivot at this point; two holes at points away from the centre are better.

The distance between the sole of the foot and the spreader should be adequate to allow the foot to pass through a full range of plantarflexion and dorsiflexion; the patient should be made to carry out a drill by moving the foot up and down repeatedly for a set period of time in each hour of the day.

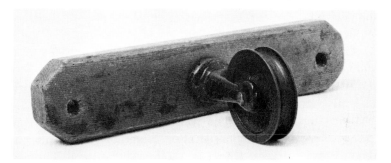

Fig. 28.11   A traction spreader.

Observation of skin extensions

Once the weights or force are applied to extensions they are subject to stresses, as is the skin of the patient underneath them. Careful frequent checking and observation of the limbs is needed. These observations should include:

(a) The efficiency of the extension; it must be capable of receiving the force or weight applied to it without slipping down the limb. An increase in the distance between the sole of the foot and the spreader would show that the extensions were slipping.

(b) The tension of the bandage passing around the limb which may be either too loose or too tight. Constant checking of the temperature and colour of the foot is required. Removal and re-application of bandages may be required.

(c) Attention to the complaints of discomfort by the patient. Any complaint of pain, 'pins and needles', joint pain, coldness of the feet or irritation of the skin should be investigated and positive action should be taken in seeking and treating the cause.

(d) The position of the leg and foot; the limb should, unless a deformity is present, be in the 'anatomical position'—that is, with the feet and patellae pointing upwards when the patient is in the supine position. The ankle joint should be free to allow full plantarflexion and dorsiflexion of the foot. The knee should be ten to fifteen degrees off full extension.

Skeletal traction

Skin extensions are not always the best means of applying traction to a limb and the orthopaedic surgeon may prefer the use of strong pins which are passed surgically through the bone under anaesthesia. This must be done with full aseptic surgical technique. Great traction can be applied by this method. The pins used to pass through the bone are of three varieties:

    (i)   Steinmann's pins,

    (ii) Kirschner wires,

    (iii) Denham's pins.

    Various implements are required for their insertion and stirrups are used to attach the traction cord to the pin.

    When pins are used to provide skeletal traction, the nursing care and observations are modified. The site of entry and exit of the pin must be treated as any other surgical wound so as to prevent infection. The temperature, pulse and respirations are recorded, and any changes in the appearance or demeanour of the patient that would indicate the presence of infection must be reported to the surgeon at once.

The problems of skeletal traction

1   A low grade osteomyelitis, due to micro-organisms tracking along the pin.

2   Necrosis of the bone adjacent to the pin, due to impaired blood supply.

3   When used on children, the pin may cut through the bone; skeletal traction is only used in special circumstances for children.

Traction beds

It is desirable when a patient is on traction that the line of traction is constant. If the mattress and base of the bed is soft and malleable, the limb or part under traction may tend to sink into the bed and alter the direction of the force. The bed used for orthopaedic patients therefore has a hard base and a firm mattress. When a conventional bed must be used, boards called fracture boards are placed under the mattress to give firm support. It is unlikely that patients will come to harm by being nursed on a firm bed, but the transition from his usual soft bed to the firm orthopaedic bed may be an unhappy one. Much can be done to gain the co-operation of the patient and acceptance of the hard bed if the reasons for its use are explained to him.

Particular forms of traction

The Thomas' splint

Hugh Owen Thomas (see Chapter 1) devised this splint for a particular purpose. This was for the treatment of lesions of the lower limb in patients who needed transport from his surgery to home and home to surgery. His free Sunday clinics were attended by patients who were taken to the clinic on makeshift box-carts and perambulators. After consultation and treatment, often with a Thomas' splint or other apparatus he had devised, the patient would be taken home to return the following week.

The essence of the splint is in its simplicity. A patient's leg can be suitably adjusted in it and fixed traction can be applied. In the original method, the patient was not attached to the bed or beam by cords, weights and pulleys. However, the splint is such a useful piece of equipment that many modifications to its original use have been made.

The splint consists of a ring, made of cylindrical bar metal, with parallel longitudinal bars welded to it. The bars are bent at the distal end to form a 'bow'. The ring is carefully padded with felt and soft leather is sewn in position over the felt (Fig. 28.12).

Ideally the splint should fit accurately and should conform to the circumference of the highest point on the patient's thigh; the bows should extend beyond the malleoli for six inches on a child and ten inches on an adult. The

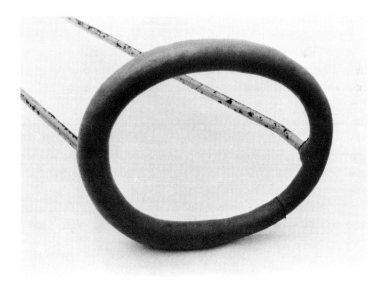

Fig. 28.12   A Thomas' splint ring.

circumference of the thigh is measured with a tape measure; from the great trochanter, passing around the thigh to the starting point. The total length of the lateral bar is measured from the great trochanter and the length of the medial bar from the abductor tendon at the groin. A well-equipped splint room will have a large collection of classified Thomas' splints.

When considerable swelling develops around the site of a fracture of the femur it may not be feasible to slide a close-fitting ring over the leg and a looser fit will have to be accepted, or a splint selected which has a divided ring with a hinge at the bow ends.

The leather of the ring of the splint must be soft and should be treated with saddle soap for maintenance and cleaning.

1   *Fixed traction on a Thomas' splint.* This is used:

    (a) For conservative treatment for a fracture of the shaft of the femur;

    (b) For ensuring immobilization and complete rest for some lesions of the knee;

    (c) For correcting deformity of the leg in some instances;

    (d) Temporarily for fractures at either the upper or lower end of the femur which will ultimately require intervention;

    (e) In some forms of hip disease with marked spasm as an alternative to Pugh's traction;

    (f) After operative correction of genu varum or valgum—usually combined with lateral pressure on the knee.

After fixing the skin extensions with traction cord in position on the skin, the ring of the Thomas' splint is threaded along the leg until it fits snugly against the top of the thigh. The cords are then tied off on the bows as shown in Fig. 28.2b. The tying of these cords influences the degree of rotation of the foot. The cords are tied with the strongest tension that can be produced manually.

A number of slings are then placed between the bars of the Thomas' splint to support a padded gutter splint on which the leg rests. The surgeon may wish a pad of splint wool to be placed behind the knee to create five degrees of flexion. The whole limb, including the splint, is then bandaged, leaving the patella exposed.

The end of the splint may be fastened to the bed end with a special clamp or else rest on a block in the bed. Alternatively, the limb in its splint may be suspended with traction cords, pulleys and weights to relieve the patient of the weight of the splint.

The foot and heel must be free of encumbrance so that the full range of ankle movement is possible. Some surgeons prefer to support the foot against a footpiece. This is necessary if the foot dorsiflexor muscles are paralysed or the patient does not co-operate in ankle exercises.

2   *Traction using a Thomas' splint and Pearson knee flexion piece*. This is used:
   (a) In supracondylar fractures of the femur with posterior displacement of the proximal end of the distal fragment.
   (b) To overcome flexion contractures of the knee.
This method calls for the use of skeletal traction with the pin through the upper end of the tibia. The knee is bent to 55 degrees of flexion and the traction cords are aligned with the traction force passing along the length of the femur. The limb below the knee is adjusted in the flexion piece with slings and bandages.
   By reducing the angulation of the flexion piece with the Thomas' splint it is possible to correct flexion contractures of the knee (see Fig. 28.14).

Pugh's traction
This is an example of sliding traction. The feet and legs are attached by extensions and traction cords to a bar at the foot of the bed which is then elevated on to blocks. The body of the patient tends to slide down the inclined plane towards the head of the bed and away from the point of fixation (Fig. 28.13). Pugh's traction is used:
   (a) As temporary traction whilst awaiting delivery of a hip abduction frame and saddle.
   (b) By some surgeons as part of the treatment for a patient with low back pain.
   (c) In treating patients with conditions where a more rigid form of traction is not required.
   Pugh's traction may be modified by the use of back splints padded with splint wool and bandaged to the legs of the patient with the knees in 5 degrees of flexion.
   It is important to ensure that the posture of the patient in the bed is good; so that the traction on each leg is equal and the pelvis is in good alignment.
   Although Pugh's traction appears to be simple, careful observation is required to ensure efficiency. The extensions must be checked daily and the skin of the patient cared for in order to prevent pressure sores occurring.
   Many patients cannot tolerate the position of the body when this form of traction is used as the head is lower than the rest of the body. This can cause headache, difficulty in swallowing and gastric distress. Using urinal bottles or bedpans are procedures that require practice and skill by the patient. Even

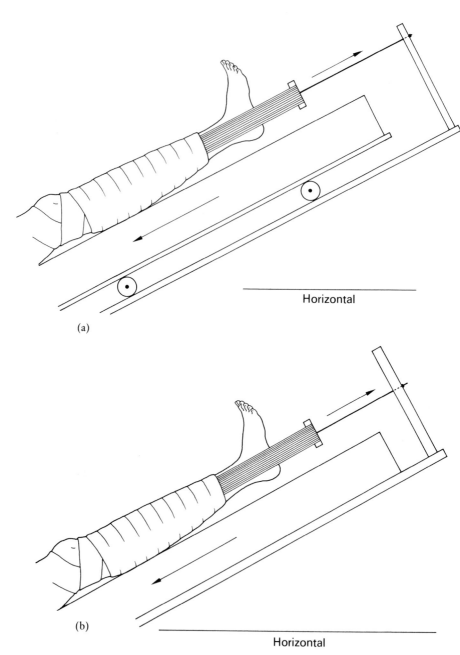

Fig. 28.13 (a) Sliding-bed traction (note rollers). (b) Pugh's traction.

leisure activities, such as reading, writing or sewing call for experience and are difficult when the feet are higher than the head.

After a day or so on this form of traction the patient accepts and tolerates it but much sympathy and help from the nursing staff are required in the adjustment period (see also Chapter 27, p. 421, *et seq.*).

Weight and pulley traction

This is a modification of Pugh's traction. Instead of attaching the cords to the bed end, weights are hung from them and they are passed over pulleys on the foot of the bed. The foot of the bed must still be elevated (Fig. 28.1a and b).

The Hodgen splint with Pearson knee flexion piece. The Hodgen splint consists of an anterior half of a ring with side bars which terminate below the knee where they are connected by a similar half-ring. The upper half-ring is not padded by the makers and must be covered with splint wool and soft bandages before application. The Hodgen splint is combined with a Pearson knee flexion piece as in Fig. 28.14a. Slings of flannel or other material are used to suspend the limb in the splint. The knee is arranged in flexion.

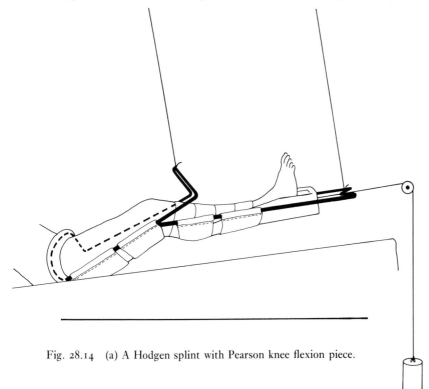

Fig. 28.14 (a) A Hodgen splint with Pearson knee flexion piece.

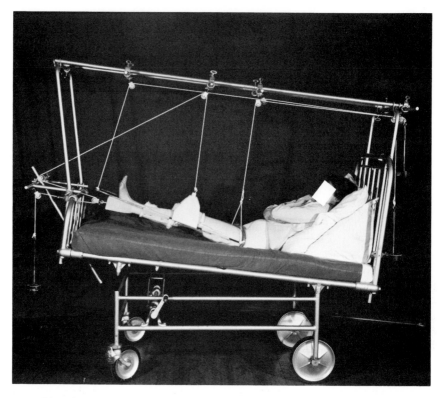

Fig. 28.14 (b) Patient in Thomas' splint with Pearson knee flexion piece. Knee extended.

As the groin ring is incomplete this cannot be used as counter pressure for fixed traction. It serves to align the limb whilst weight and pulley traction is applied. This may be either skin or skeletal traction.

It is commonly used after arthroplasty of the hip joint to maintain the limb in abduction and internal rotation in combination with longitudinal traction. It may also serve to correct flexion contractures of the knee by gradually decreasing the angulation of the splints.

Bohler-Braun splint

This is normally used with skeletal traction (see Fig. 9.12). The splint serves to elevate and support the leg while traction is applied. This may be either in the line of the femur when treating low femoral fractures, or in the line of the tibia for tibial fractures; in this case the leg may also be placed in plaster of Paris. The limb is suspended on slings of unstretchable soft cloth which are

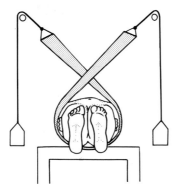

Fig. 28.15   Suspension for fracture of pelvis (see page 119).

attached to the upper bars of the splint. The splint is tied to the foot of the
bed which is then elevated.

It is an excellent and safe method of treating severe fractures of the tibia
initially, particularly if they are compound and there is a risk of limb
ischaemia or delayed skin healing.

Smillie's traction (Fig. 28.16a)
This is a method of treating and preventing flexion contractures of the knee.
The direction of the pressure exerted by the sling at the level of the knee
tends to push it backwards into extension. It is sometimes used in treatment
of rheumatoid arthritis and after synovectomy of the knee-joint.

Hamilton-Russell traction (Fig. 28.4)
This type of traction was described by Hamilton-Russell, an orthopaedic
surgeon, in 1923 and was used by him in the treatment of fractures of the
shaft of the femur. He tried to reproduce the action of the surgeon in applying manual traction to a fractured shaft of femur by using slings, cords and
pulleys; by applying a sling support behind the patient's knee to represent one
hand, and skin traction on the lower leg to represent the other hand of the
surgeon in pulling the limb. The leg was supported on pillows to prevent
backward displacement of the fragments.

Today it is rarely used for treatment of fractures of the shaft of the femur;
it is more commonly used in the treatment of lesions of the hip and in fractures of the upper end of the femur. It is often used as a temporary measure
before operation in such fractures. It can be used for correction of flexion
contractures of the knee particularly if there is posterior subluxation of the
tibia.

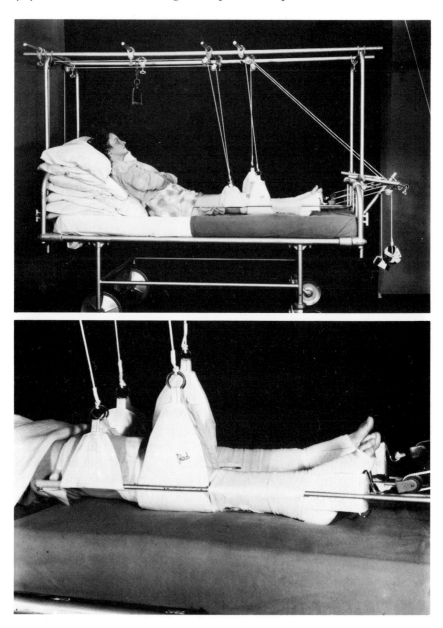

Fig. 28.16 (a) Smillies' traction.

The method. A balkan beam is required and three single pulleys are attached to it as indicated in Fig. 28.7. A fourth single pulley is attached to the spreader used in applying skin traction to the patient.

The sling behind the knee is important. This must be unstretchable but of soft material to avoid cutting into the patient. It must not ruck up easily and is best kept from creasing with bars of wood incorporated into channels at each end (Fig. 28.7). The cord is knotted to this sling before passing up to the pulley on the cross-beam. This pulley is arranged so that it is lower down the beam than the level of the patient's knee. The cord is then threaded through the remaining pulleys as shown in Fig. 28.7. The heel of the patient must not rub on the bed and there should be ample distance between the patient's foot and the bed end for the pulleys to be effective.

The weight to be applied is about 3·5 kg for an adult and 0·25 to 2 kg for a child. In theory, the two single pulleys at the foot of the bed double the pull on the leg, but this is modified by many factors such as friction at the pulleys and the angulation of the inclined plane that is formed when the foot of the bed is raised.

The theory of Hamilton-Russell traction utilizes the parallelogram of forces (Fig. 28.4 and legend).

The principles behind its use are that a relatively small weight will provide great traction which is constant and comfortable.

Modified Hamilton-Russell traction using a compound pulley sling with traction. This is a modification of Hamilton-Russell traction using a separate compound pulley block system to support the knee sling. This form of pulley runs more smoothly than a single pulley arrangement.

Modified Hamilton-Russell traction using skeletal traction with a Tulloch-Brown or nissen 'U' loop. This is never used with children.

A Steinmann pin is passed through the upper end of the tibia to which pin are now attached two other metal devices: (1) a stirrup for suspending the limb to pulleys on the balkan beam and (2) a light metal 'U' loop which passes down each side of the leg and joins beyond the patient's foot. A traction cord is attached to the 'U' loop to provide longitudinal weighted traction over a pulley at the foot of the bed. The limb is supported in a sling attached to this 'U' loop.

The weights attached to each of the traction cords varies with the size of the patient. Two kilograms will be enough for most patients but three kilograms will be required for heavier patients; the amount to be used is decided by the surgeon. The knee should usually be in about ten degrees of flexion, and the foot of the bed is elevated. In all forms of Hamilton-Russell traction, care should be taken to avoid excessive pressure on the popliteal vessels and nerves which are behind the knee and on the lateral side of the leg.

Pelvic traction

This is a modification of Pugh's traction. A specially fitted wide pelvic band is fixed to the patient's pelvis. This has long straps attached which are secured to the foot of the bed, which is then elevated.

This form of traction is preferred by some surgeons in the treatment of lesions of the lumbar region of the vertebral column.

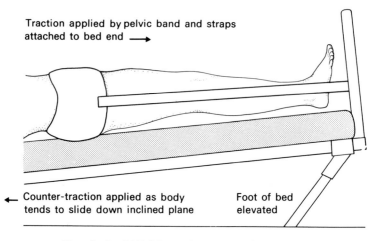

Fig. 28.16   (b) Pelvic traction used for low back pain.

Gallows traction

This is of value in treating infants and very young children with fractures of the femur.

Skin extensions are applied to the legs of the child with spreaders, to which traction cord is attached. The traction cords are then fastened to an overhead beam fixed across the patient's cot at the level of the buttocks so that the hips are flexed to right angles with the legs raised from the bed. The buttocks should be clear of the mattress. If the buttocks are supported, the traction ceases to be effective.

Alvik traction (Fig. 28.17a)

This was devised in Oslo, Norway, for the treatment of young children with congenital dislocation of the hip. It is a means of reducing the dislocation by

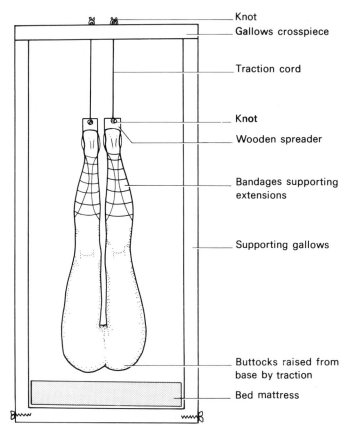

Knot

Gallows crosspiece

Traction cord

Knot

Wooden spreader

Bandages supporting
extensions

Supporting gallows

Buttocks raised from
base by traction

Bed mattress

Fig. 28.16   (c) Gallows traction.

applying traction along the length of the legs with an accompanying rotation
medial traction of the thighs.

Above-knee skin extensions are applied to the legs. To these are attached
spreaders and traction cords which pass over pulleys to weights. The position
of the pulleys is such that the thighs are in wide abduction. Two kilogram
weights will usually serve but sometimes three kilograms may be needed
according to the instructions of the surgeon.

Rotatory traction to cause medial rotation and medial pressure on the
upper end of the femur on the affected side is then applied. Latex foam extensions attached to strong calico bandages are used. These are applied in the
directions shown in Fig. 28.17b, so that the extension at the back of the thigh
pulls laterally and that at the front pulls medially. Each skin extension of the
rotatory traction is attached to a cord passing over a pulley situated on the

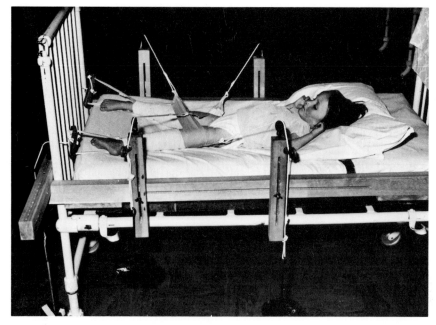

Fig. 28.17   (a) Alvik traction.

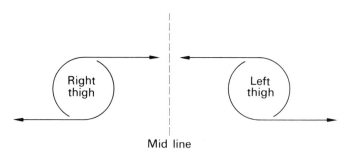

Fig. 28.17   (b) Rotating forces in Alvik traction.

edge of the bed at the optimum position for applying the correct force. Each traction cord is loaded with a half, to one and a half kilogram weight.

The foot of the bed is elevated.

Cervical traction
This is used in the treatment of patients with lesions affecting the cervical vertebrae. It may be applied in one of several ways:

(a) Using a Glisson's sling. This is a head harness which passes under the chin, in front and around the occiput at the back (Fig. 28.18a, b).

(b) Using Criles head tractor. A patent device which fits around the forehead and occiput of the patient but leaves the chin free.

(c) Using skull calipers, that is, a form of skeletal traction (Fig. 28.18c). These calipers are inserted surgically into the vault of the cranium.

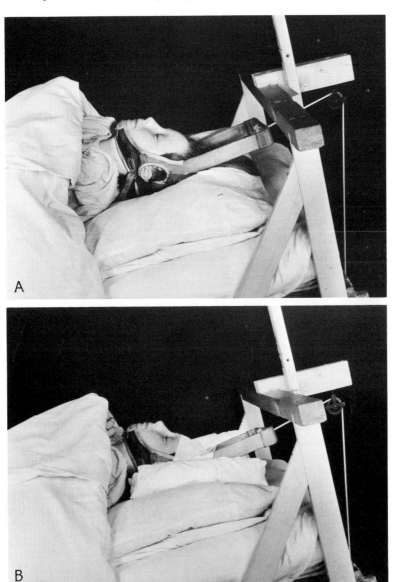

Fig. 28.18(a) and (b)   Cervical traction with a Glisson sling.

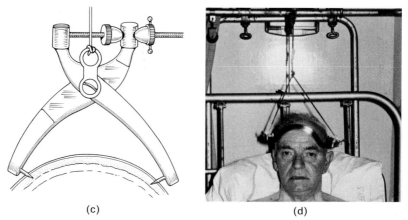

(c)   (d)

Fig. 28.18   Instruments for cervical traction (c) skull calipers and (d) halo-splint.

(d) Halo Traction (Fig. 28.20). The 'halo' is a metal circle through which four screws are passed and these are then inserted into the outer table of the skull. It is a very effective method which gives firm fixation and is less likely to slip than other methods.

Of the three methods listed above the last is most commonly used when prolonged and heavy traction must be maintained. Whatever method is used, the halter or calipers are attached to a traction cord which passes over a pulley at the head of the bed to a suspended weight. The height of the pulley is adjusted so that the traction can be applied in varying degrees of extension and flexion. The head of the bed is elevated to provide an inclined plane and thus the body weight of the patient provides counter-traction.

Traction can be increased by incorporating a handle as well as a weight at the end of the cord beyond the pulley. The patient pulls on the handle himself and thus increases the traction.

Skull calipers may also be used in conjunction with a Stryker frame for turning the patient (see Fig. 10.17). This is one way of managing a paralysed patient (see also Chapter 31).

Suspending plaster beds

This may be used for a patient who must be nursed on a plaster bed for a prolonged period of time. It makes fixation more tolerable for him if the bed can be inclined in any chosen direction, under his control. He can thus cope with eating and drinking or diversions such as reading, or watching television more easily.

When the plaster bed is being completed in the plaster room, strong transverse bars with holes at each end are incorporated into the plaster at three
points: firstly, at the central balancing point of the bed; then at
shoulder level, and thirdly at ankle level.

When the plaster bed is lined and finished, suspension may be arranged as
follows:

(a) Six double yacht pulleys are arranged on a double balkan beam over a
hospital bed. These should be the same distance from each other as are the
holes in the bars on the plaster bed.

(b) A further six double yacht pulleys are attached to each end of the bars
on the plaster bed.

(c) Long lengths of traction cord are then first tied to each of the double
pulleys on the balkan beam, carried down to the double pulleys on the plaster
bed and threaded around a pulley wheel. A system of pairs of pulley blocks is
arranged at each point of suspension of the plaster bed (see Fig. 28.6).

(d) The traction cords are carried over six single pulleys mounted on a bar
at the head of the bed.

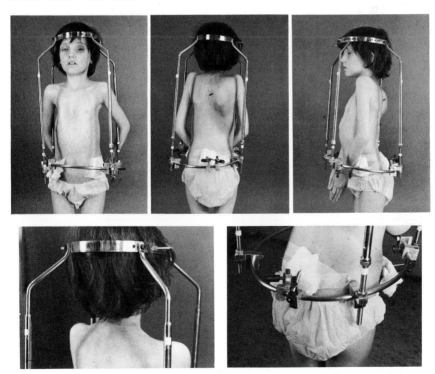

Fig. 28.19   Halo–pelvic traction apparatus in position.

(e) Six separate weights are attached to the ends of the suspension cords. These should all be equal in amount. The correct weight for each patient in a plaster bed can only be found by trial and error. The bed should remain fixed and balanced at any position of choice.

Halo-pelvic traction (Figs. 28.19 and 28.20 a–e)

This is a form of traction used, as an adjunct to surgery on the vertebral column, by some orthopaedic surgeons.

Both the pelvic-band and halo-band are surgically fixed and the four connecting bars are used to distract the pelvis and cranium away from each other. This extends and immobilizes the vertebral column. Bone-grafting with callus formation, and other surgical procedures, may be performed with the halo-pelvic traction in position.

Such procedures would be carried out in stages. The halo-pelvic traction is applied first; when the patient has recovered from this procedure and accepted the problems it presents in activities of daily living, further stages of the operation are performed.

The halo can be used as an alternative to skull calipers (see Fig. 28.18 d).

As with any other form of spinal correction there is a risk of kinking or stretching the blood vessels supplying the spinal cord and thus causing paraplegia. During correction of a spinal deformity by conservative means and particularly by traction the patient's leg function must be examined daily and recorded daily. Any difficulty with micturition or incontinence of urine must be reported at once by the nurse to the doctor responsible.

Frame fixation

The needs for complete and prolonged immobilization of patients are decreasing. There are many reasons for this; apart from the obvious reason of progress in medical science and knowledge, there are many known physiological disadvantages to fixing a patient in recumbency for many months. Fixing patients to frames and saddles or in plaster beds is fast losing favour as a method of treatment.

Unless frame fixation is frequently used in a ward it is better not to try to use it occasionally.

The observation and care of patients on traction

The application of traction to a patient usually serves to relieve him of pain and to increase his comfort. However, no traction should be left unchecked or without maintenance for very long. In the supervision of a patient, the following points should be borne in mind.

General observations

The position of the patient. If the patient must adopt a position which is unnatural to him, there must be a period of orientation to this position. This may be a period of distress for the patient. The obvious example of this is when the patient is placed head down on an inclined plane. There are many problems of managing everyday functions such as eating, drinking, washing, shaving, reading, or applying cosmetics, and a large amount of relearning of these skills is needed. Probably the patient's greatest distress and problem will be in using bedpans or urinals. If the patient is new to hospital, his problems are great enough; if in addition, he must lie with his head lower than his feet, his problems are enormous. A great deal of help and sympathy is required from the nursing staff until he has developed new ways of dealing with the situation.

The head down position may create headache and even a feeling of claustrophobia in some people; the doctor should be informed, but often it is best to encourage the patient to adapt to his position as quickly as possible, but mild sedation may be required (see also Chapter 27, p. 421, *et seq.*).

Stasis. The traction may fix the patient in one position without the ability to alter his position. This is undesirable, but there may not be an alternative method of treatment available. Complete immobilization may lead to various forms of stagnation which are always undesirable. Examples of these are:

1   *Pressure sores.* The skin and underlying tissues in direct contact with the bed may become sore, the skin may break down and allow infection to enter. Eventually necrosis of the tissues may occur. This process is most likely to happen in the aged, the very ill or anaemic, and the incontinent patient. Frequent cleansing of the parts in contact with the bed is essential and repeated minor alterations in the position of the patient are necessary so that continuous pressure on the area is avoided. The doctor will take all measures to improve the general health of the patient and overcome any anaemia.

A great deal of nursing effort is directed to avoiding pressure sores. In addition to frequently changing the patient's position it is important that bed-ridden or anaesthetic patients should not have any area of their skin subjected to a pressure of more than 20 millimetres of mercury for any length of time. One method of trying to avoid excessive local pressure is the use of materials for mattresses and cushions which conform to the patient's shape. In this respect sorbo-rubber has certain virtues but tends to be rather

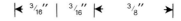

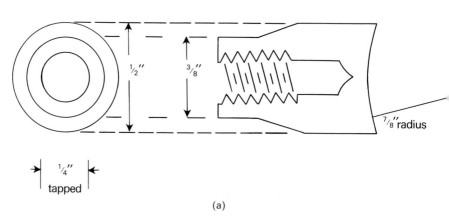

(a)

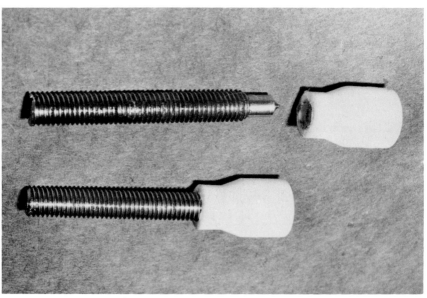

(b)

Fig. 28.20a, b, c, d, e   Details of the halo-bound fittings.

hot and sweaty and may lead to maceration of the skin. Alternative materials are sheep skin, certain plastics, e.g. plastozote or bags filled with fine particles or small balls. These are often referred to as 'solid fluid' cushions and mattresses.

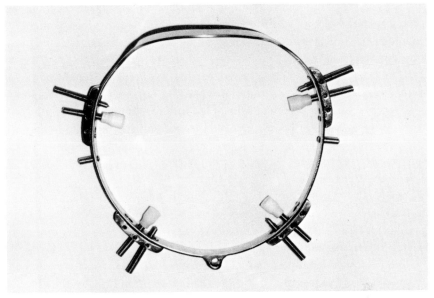

(c)

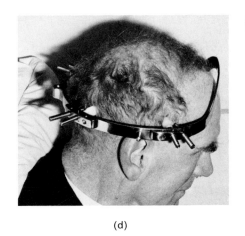

(d)

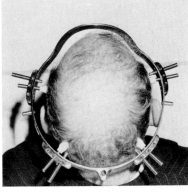

(e)

Ideally if a mattress or cushion forms to the patient's shape no area of skin is subjected to excessive pressure.

2   *Kidneys*. Stasis of urine in the kidneys may result in the formation of stones in the kidney with resultant anuria, oliguria or haematuria. An increase in the fluid intake of any patient who is immobilized is a good nursing measure. Regular urine testing and a fluid balance chart are also useful.

3   *Bowel.* Loss of the usual amount of exercise and a decrease in the intake of roughage in the diet may lead to constipation. A diet with a high content of cellulose and fluid is necessary. It may be necessary to use laxatives and even evacuant suppositories.

4   *Thorax.* The chest will be affected, particularly in aged patients and those with a previous history of chronic bronchitis or heavy smoking. This stasis may take the form of oedema of the lungs with respiratory distress. Physiotherapy, supervision of breathing exercises and suitable medication may all be required.

Local observations

The limb. The constriction of a limb with bandages and other forms of pressure may reduce the efficiency of: (a) the circulatory system; (b) the muscles; (c) the joints; and (d) the nerve supply, and these all require constant observation and supervision.

The colour and temperature of the skin of the foot must be checked frequently. Any complaint of either tingling or numbness by the patient should be investigated at once. Complaints of this sort are usually related to constriction because the bandages around the limb are too tight.

There must never be a constriction or pressure upon the area of the leg below the knee on the lateral side. This is where the lateral popliteal nerve winds around the neck of the fibula. Continuous unrelieved pressure here would cause tingling and numbness of the foot and later paralysis of the muscles on the front and side of the leg, resulting in 'foot-drop'—a condition in which the patient is unable to dorsiflex the foot and toes.

Complete absence of movement at the knee and ankle joints will cause stiffness of the joint and severe wasting of the muscles serving the joint. This may lead to months of disability after the traction is discontinued. It can be prevented by consistent daily physiotherapy. Every joint which can be safely moved is put through its full range of movement; joints which cannot be moved are treated by static muscle contraction; an immobilized knee is treated by quadriceps contractions and patella movements. The patient is taught an exercise drill which he can practise at times of the day when he is not supervised by the physiotherapist. The most obvious example of this is quadriceps drill; the patient is taught to pull his knee cap upwards repeatedly for five minutes in every hour throughout his waking day. If he is conscientious in maintaining this regime, he will have little trouble in walking and standing when he leaves his bed.

Skin traction. This must be examined for (a) slipping, (b) contact dermatitis of the skin or other sores and (c) constriction by tight bandages.

It is the normal practice of an orthopaedic unit to unwind the bandages, examine the skin extensions and rewind the bandages daily. If there is any deterioration in the efficiency of the extensions, they may require replacement. Whilst this is being done, temporary extensions will be necessary.

Skeletal traction. This must be examined for:

(a) *Pin slipping.* This may take the form of (i) slipping through from one side to the other carrying an area of non-sterile pin into the bone or (ii) rotatory slipping indicating that the pin is loose in the bone and that there may be an area of necrotic or osteoporotic bone around the pin. Either of these should be reported to the surgeon.

(b) *Signs of infection.* Some seepage of serum due to irritation by the pin is common, this provides an ideal culture medium for bacteria and can lead to infection, therefore strict cleanliness and asepsis are essential. The presence of pus, pain, redness, heat or swelling adjacent to the pin indicate the presence of pathogenic micro-organisms. This should at once be reported to the surgeon who may order a suitable antibiotic therapy.

(c) *Signs of venous thrombosis.* Swelling, oedema, pain and discolouration below the site of insertion of the pin are ominous signs and must be reported at once.

The presence of a metal pin in the bone requires the same surgical nursing care as any wound. The points of entry and exit of the pin must be treated as wounds and kept covered with a surgical dressing which is changed as often as required by the surgeon.

29

External Splintage

External splintage means the application of a mechanical device to the exterior surface of the body so as to serve one of the following functions:

1 To immobilize a fracture temporarily so that the patient can be transferred to hospital with less pain. Correct splinting also reduces blood loss at the site of the fracture and, as a result of this, 'shock' is diminished. This form of splintage may be improvised from materials locally available.

2 To immobilize a fracture for the duration of treatment until callus formation at the site of the fracture has advanced sufficiently to unite the bones; included in this is the provision of the means of traction and counter-traction, as when using a Thomas' splint for a fracture of the femur.

3 To immobilize a painful joint.

4 To take the weight of the body off a limb or joint.

5 To rest an infected joint until antibiotics have overcome the infection: in addition the splint prevents deformity and reduces the damage to the joint surfaces.

6 To stabilize a joint when the controlling muscles are paralysed. This enables the patient to make use of the affected limb. Calipers worn by paraplegic patients are examples of this use of splintage.

7 To support the vertebral column so as to enable a patient with paralysed trunk muscles to sit or stand.

8 To counterbalance the action of active or hypertonic muscles, when the opposing group of muscles is paralysed or hypotonic; the splint simulates the action of the weak or defective muscles. Working splints (see Chapter 11, p. 117) are examples.

9 To prevent compression on nerves when a disability exists. A cervical collar may be effective in relieving pains in the arms when the roots of the nerves to the arm are being compressed (see Figs. 10.11 and 29.2).

10 To prevent or maintain correction of a deformity. For example, splintage in the treatment of talipes equinovarus.

11 To stabilize a limb when there is an ununited fracture.

12   For comfort after an operation.

13   As an adjunct to intravenous therapy.

Materials used for splintage

The materials which can be used are many and varied.

(a) *Metal.* Steel has its place where strength is required but it is radio opaque; lightness is often also a necessary feature and aluminium has many uses in modern splints where strength is not too important and radio translucency is desirable.

(b) *Leather.* Many different qualities and varieties of leather are used, for example, a heavy quality is required for making block leather splints, and soft kid or chamois leather is used for linings and on surfaces in contact with the skin. Strap-leather is required for fastenings.

(c) *Plastics and resins.* These are the man-made materials that are being increasingly used in splintage. They have many advantages, not the least of

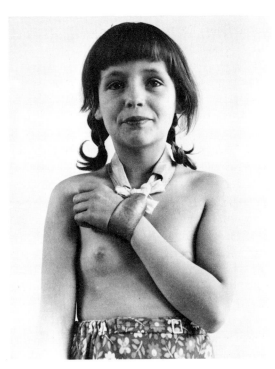

Fig. 29.1   Collar and cuff sling.

these being that efficient, permanent splints can be made on the premises of a hospital. The plastics available fall into two main varieties:

(i) Sheeting which softens when heated in a special oven and can be moulded around a plaster of Paris cast that is a model of the patient's limb, neck or trunk. When cooled the plastic becomes firm and gives effective support.

Some plastics only become ductile at a high temperature but are very stiff and strong when cool. Others become soft at relatively low temperatures, these can be moulded directly onto a thin layer of padding applied to the patient's skin, but they are not so rigid and strong.

(ii) Powder which can be poured and moulded to almost any permanent shape when mixed with an activator (the epoxy-resins).

(d) *Padding.* A wide variety of material can be used for padding according to the purpose for which it is required. Grey wadding, various thicknesses of felt and soft animal wools all have their uses. Grey felt is specially treated and may be hardened in acetone to make a splint.

(e) *Plaster of Paris* (see Chapter 30).

(f) *Wood.* Wood is now rarely used for splinting but it can serve to make temporary improvised splints.

(g) *Inflatable splints.* These are used for first-aid purposes. They are radio translucent and allow wounds to be inspected without being removed. They must not be over inflated, however, or the circulation may be obstructed. If inflated by mouth they are safe; a pump should not be used.

Splint storage and maintenance

An orthopaedic unit must carry a large stock of Thomas' splints, gutter splints and other impedimenta. A room must be set aside for this purpose and the contents of the room carefully graded and labelled and the splints placed neatly on racks and hooks. It must be possible to select a splint of the relevant size quickly.

After each use, a splint requires cleaning and overhaul; often painting and re-padding are also necessary. The leather on a splint can be a means of cross infection as it is difficult to sterilize leather. There must be a routine for over-hauling each splint as soon as it is returned after use; a suitable technician is usually charged with this responsibility.

Ordering splints and appliances

Hugh Owen Thomas made his splints in his own workshop. Orthopaedic hospitals which traditionally employ appliance makers and have workshops on the premises are fortunate in that the service given to the surgeon and patient is speedy, efficient and personal. This state of affairs appears to be ending, however, and most splint making and fitting has passed into the hands of commercial enterprises. Most splint making firms are conscientious in ensuring that the patient receives his appliances quickly and that it fits accurately. They often employ representatives who attend clinics and under-take the whole task of measuring, supplying and fitting splints.

The supply for such equipment for a patient is expensive. The majority of splints must be made for an individual and there is a limited field for supply-ing mass produced items. Nevertheless, adjustable cervical collars and lumbar supports are available and can provide relatively inexpensive temporary supports 'on demand'.

The splint must fit accurately, be comfortable, unobtrusive, durable and efficient. Mistakes in measuring the patient, or errors caused by ordering a wrongly named item are very costly.

Measuring for an appliance

(See also Chapter 28, p. 459 and Chapter 30, p. 516.)

(a) *Making a cast*. The most practical method of ensuring that a patient will have an accurate fit, when an item is specially made for him, is to supply a plaster of Paris model of that part of the patient which is to be splinted or supported. Thus, when a spinal support or belt is required, a plaster jacket is made on the patient (the skin of the patient is coated with oil first), cut off and the cut repaired; one end of the completed jacket is closed off; the inside of the jacket is smeared with petroleum jelly; the jacket is then filled with plaster cream which is allowed to set. When the negative jacket is removed from the positive filling, an accurate model of the patient exists. The splint maker can now use this model on which to make a spinal support or any other device required. The finished appliance must be an accurate fit (Fig. 30.3).

The same method can be used to provide a caliper, particularly one with a bucket top, by supplying a model of the patient's thigh, with other measure-ments. It can also be used to make a block leather or plastic support for the forearm and wrist by supplying a model of these.

(b) *Supplying measurements*. The experienced orthopaedic nurse takes pride in her ability to measure with accuracy and record her findings on the order form. If any doubts exist in her mind she must re-measure; the progression of the patient is retarded if he must wait for a splint to be re-made.

The patient must be unclothed and placed in the position which the splint or support is intended to maintain. Using a wax skin pencil, the points of measurement are indicated on the patient and a linen tape-measure is used to record the distance between the two points. There are some instances when a goniometer (a form of protractor) is used to indicate degrees of flexion at a joint, but if an irregular deformity exists then the plaster cast method is the best. In some circumstances—e.g. for a Thomas' back support, a malleable lead strip is used to record the shape of the patient's back.

Supplying artificial limbs

(See also Chapter 32.) The measuring, assessing requirements, fitting and training in the management of artificial limbs is a complex process requiring the efforts of a team, all of whom are experts in this work. It is usual to arrange for the patient to attend a limb fitting centre.

In parts of the world where limb makers are not available and the supply of limbs from abroad is too costly, it is possible to make artificial limbs from epoxy resin.

Plastazote technique*

Plastazote is a material which has recently been introduced for making splints which can be applied directly to the patient in the clinic (Fig. 29.2). It consists of foamed polyethylene of closed cell construction, cross linked to ensure extreme lightness and improve resistance to the temperature required for mouldability. It is non-toxic. Flammability is of low order—it melts and burns slowly—comparable with 'polythene' sheet. Chemical resistance is excellent since it is unaffected by all common acids, alkalis and solvents.

Spinal supports

(a) *Rationale of spinal supports.* Spinal supports should not be supplied without due consideration of the needs of the patient. There are conditions where improved spinal and abdominal musculature is preferable to dependence upon corsetry or other devices. Some patients with a chronic or

---

* Plastazote is a registered trade mark of Bakelite Xylonite Ltd. and is obtainable from Smith & Nephew Ltd., Bessemer Road, Welwyn Garden City, Herts. The reader is referred to the manufacturer's current literature about the product.

residual back lesion, however, must have a spinal support at any rate for a time, if not for the rest of life. In others it may be supplied to aid the healing of a treated lesion and it can then be discarded when the condition has improved.

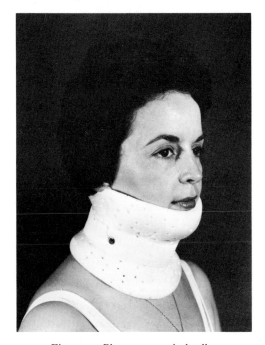

Fig. 29.2 Plastazote cervical collar.

A spinal support does not give complete rest to the back; it is preferable that it should not be provided to serve as a 'second best' to complete bed rest if the patient really needs this latter and tries to avoid it. It is used only to give partial support to a local lesion by restricting movements of the spine. It should therefore extend for some distance in each direction beyond the site of the spinal lesion in order to be effective. It must be designed and supplied to fit the individual; because of this it is an expensive item to manufacture. Stock adjustable supports can, however, play a useful palliative role if they are well made and the hospital has an adequate variety.

(b) *Classification.*

   (i)   Jones posterior spinal support.

   (ii) Goldthwait belt and other belts.

   (iii) Plaster jackets (Chapter 30, p. 525).

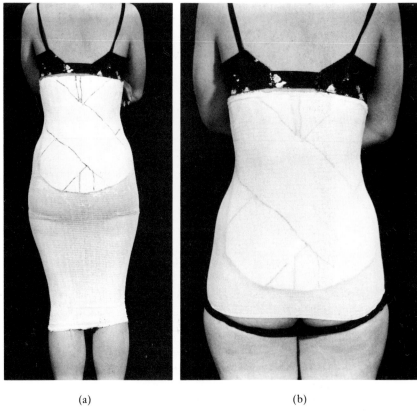

(a)   (b)

Fig. 29.3 (a) and (b) Posterior spinal support, held in position with tubigrip.

  (iv) Plaster posterior spinal support with tubular supporting bandage (Chapter 30, p. 525).

  (v) Plastazote spinal support (p. 525).

Jones posterior spinal support. The Jones posterior spinal support (Fig. 10.12) is a rigid structure which gives extensive support from the sacrum to high up in the thoracic region of the vertebral column. It was primarily devised for convalescent ambulant patients with healing spinal tuberculosis.

  It consists of a shaped metal frame covered in felt which fits accurately against the curves of the patient's spine. The frame is encased in smooth leather into which it is strongly sewn; the leather is perforated for ventilation of the under-skin. Buckles are incorporated into the edges of the leather for the attachment of the retaining straps. The retaining straps are arranged as follows:

(i)   a pelvic band,

(ii) axillary straps, one on each side,

(iii) groin straps, one on each side, attaching at the front to the pelvic band,

(iv) a waist band.

The axillary and groin straps are padded and curve-shaped; they must not be straightened or the leather will crack; careful maintenance treatment of all leather with saddle soap is essential.

Ordering the Jones posterior spinal support. The patient is unclothed and carefully placed prone with the curves of the spine arranged in the position in which they must be supported. A negative cast is made of the patient's back and from this a positive cast is prepared (Chapter 30, p. 525). This is marked with the name and personal reference number of the patient; it is then sent to the splint-making firm who use it to produce the Jones posterior spinal support, shaping the support on the model of the patient's back. Alternatively the shape of the patient's spine is reproduced on a lead 'stick' and a record of the shape is then transferred from the lead 'stick' to a large piece of paper.

Measurements of the girth, the axillae and thigh are also needed.

Fitting the support to the patient. A patient who has a spinal lesion and has been treated by complete immobilization on a plaster bed or frame for a long period has wasted, inefficient spinal muscles. This is recognized as a serious disadvantage of complete immobilization in a plaster bed or on a frame. The transition from the supine position to the sitting or standing position, and then to walking, requires a firm support until the physiotherapist can help the patient to improve his musculature; the function of the back muscles improves with use and exercise. When the appliance has been fitted the patient wears it constantly for some days whilst still remaining bed fast. He then gradually attempts sitting and eventually standing, under the supervision of the physiotherapist. The posterior spinal support is only removed for short periods with the patient on his bed in the prone position; it is taken off for washing and powdering of the back, axillae and groins and for physiotherapy.

Method of fitting. The patient is carefully turned into the prone position from his bed or spinal frame and onto a number of pillows. Whilst the patient is in this position the back is washed and any loose scales of epidermis are removed; it may be necessary to use a lanolin cream to soften the scales for removal. The back, axillae and groins are then powdered.

The posterior support is now laid upon the patient's back and examined for accuracy of fit; when pressure is applied to the lower end of the support against the sacrum, the upper end should stand three centimetres away from the shoulders, as its function is to hold the spine in an extended position. The retaining straps and bands are now firmly applied and adjusted in the following order:

    (i)   pelvic band,

    (ii) axillary straps,

    (iii) groin straps,

    (iv) waist band.

Until the musculature of the patient is sufficiently developed for him to be able to turn himself the patient must be turned regularly by a nursing team; however, the patient must soon be encouraged to turn himself.

The Goldthwait belt. This was first devised by the well-known American surgeon, Dr. Joel E. Goldthwait of Boston, United States of America. He

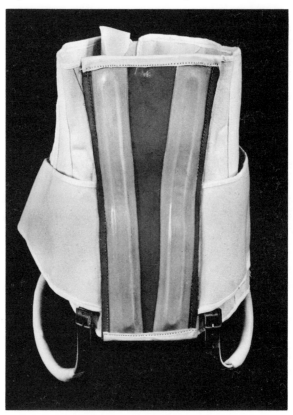

Fig. 29.4   A Goldthwait belt.

was the friend of Sir Robert Jones who cemented the many ties which exist to this day between the British and American Orthopaedic Associations. From the Goldthwait belt pattern many others have been fashioned and there are many names given to different supporting belts which serve the same function as the Goldthwait belt (Fig. 29.4) here described (see also Fig. 24.4).

It consists of a stiff leather spinal support reinforced by two long studded flat steel bars joined at their upper and lower ends (the Goldthwait plate). There is one longitudinal bar on each side of the patient's vertebral column to which they are accurately moulded. It is used to support the lumbo-sacral region and must therefore extend upwards from the level of the tip of the coccyx to the mid-thoracic region of the vertebral column. The leather support is incorporated in a sailcloth belt of the same depth; this belt may also be reinforced with flat steel bars. The belt is prevented from riding up by groin straps for male patients and stocking suspenders for females.

Similar belts and corsets are made to support the sacral, the sacroiliac and the thoraco-lumbar regions.

The Goldthwait plate may be incorporated in a canvas belt—i.e. by omitting the leather casing or two or more unconnected strips of metal or 'whale bone' may be substituted for the Goldthwait plate. As a general rule the lighter and more flexible the material the less effective the mechanical support of the belt will be.

General management of a patient wearing a splint

The supply of a caliper or other device may be a temporary matter, but in addition there are many people who must wear such splints for the remainder of their lives.

In either case the patient tolerates the wearing of the splint as a necessary evil. Being dependent on a splint may distress a patient, or she may object to its appearance. The design and manufacture of a splint must be excellent if it is not to be seen by others; even when it is not visible, the patient is aware of its presence and worries about the cosmetic effect. This is particularly so in young people, whether male or female, and may cause them to withdraw from the society of their friends. Most disabled people, however, cheerfully accept and ignore their problem. Occasionally there are those who would wish to be seen with splintage or a walking stick as a means of gaining attention and sympathy. The child with a residual disability, who will grow to be an adult with a permanent physical problem, must be educated to make full use of all the faculties that remain in order to compete against the undisabled and enjoy as full a life as possible.

Careful observation of the splint must be made if it is supplied for a child. The rapid growth of children requires frequent replacement of splints in order that its size corresponds with the child's growth.

A splint which is too small will constrict a limb and may cause ischaemia and venous obstruction, or nerve pressure and paralysis; it will certainly defeat its purpose, and may cause a secondary deformity. An adult may also alter in size during the life of the splint; obesity or emaciation may mean that the splint is no longer suitable and must be replaced.

Ischaemia

This is a condition caused by impairment of the blood supply to a part; it may be caused when a splint is too small for a limb. Its presence will be indicated by:

(a) Coldness of the extremity of the limb.

(b) Loss of sensation in the limb.

(c) Discolouration; either pallor or blueness.

(d) Sluggish return of circulation after thumb pressure on the hand or foot. Both limbs should be equal in response; if there is a delay on one side it indicates circulatory impairment.

(e) Swelling and loss of movement.

(f) Pain in the limb, particularly with a feeling of distension.

Any of these are significant and require immediate action to remove the constriction.

Nerve pressure

There are many main nerves which between them serve the whole of the body but those which are most likely to be compressed by splints or appliances are those which are closely related to a bone with only a thin layer of intervening tissue. The best example is the common peroneal (lateral popliteal) nerve which passes around the neck of the fibula on its route to the front of the leg and the foot. A tight band below the knee at this level will compress the nerve and cause a 'drop foot' deformity. Other examples in the lower extremity are the lateral cutaneous nerve of thigh at the side of the hip, the terminal branch of the anterior tibial nerve on the top of the foot, and the digital nerves of the toes.

In the upper extremity the radial (musculo-spiral) nerve as it spirals around the lateral side of the humerus, the ulnar, median and radial nerves around the elbow and the wrist, and the digital nerves to the fingers are other examples.

Nerve pressure results at first in temperature changes—the part is cold and discoloured, then a 'pins and needles' sensation occurs; then anaesthesia and paralysis, and finally, wasting of the muscles.

Decubitus ulcers

Any prolonged local pressure will cause diminished blood supply to the area under pressure. If this local pressure is maintained for too long, the skin will break and a sore will form; this may progress to a deep craterous ulcer which requires surgical repair.

It is more likely to happen to patients who are frail, weak and anaemic with an absence of tone in their tissues. Children or patients with paralysis will also be prone to pressure sores.

Any comment of pain or pressure by any patient wearing a splint or plaster must be investigated *immediately*; it is never safe to 'wait and see what happens'. Once an ulcer has formed it is often painless so that the disappearance of pain does not signify that all is well. A disagreeable odour from a plaster often indicates that a painless sore has developed.

If an ulcer does occur, the pressure on its site must be relieved, even though this entails the removal of the appliance or replacement with an alternative form of splintage. The sore must be dressed using an aseptic technique. If healing does not readily occur, a surgical toilet of the wound may be necessary and perhaps skin grafting.

The general physical condition of the patient must also be investigated and anaemia or malnutrition treated so as to improve the rate of healing.

The care of the skin

When a splint is worn the area of skin in contact with the material of the splint will perspire and may become sore. This possibility is increased if crumbs or other particles of material lodge between the skin and the splint. Children frequently insert toys, coins and other objects under splints or plaster.

Frequent washing of the skin, followed by drying and the use of methylated spirits to retard the production of perspiration is necessary. During this procedure the tissues are moved about to increase the flow of blood to the area; the patient is also trained to do this.

Whilst the patient is in hospital, treatment of the skin is repeated every four hours. After discharge from hospital, if the patient must continue to wear the appliance, he must also continue the above routine. When the skin under the leather has hardened, the frequency of the routine can be decreased but the cleanliness of the area must be constantly maintained.

Care of the splint

The splint must be carefully maintained. Particular attention must be paid to the leatherwork. This is liable to perish and crack if it is not properly cared for; methylated spirits should not be allowed to toughen it. Urine and perspiration also make leather hard, rough and abrasive. To keep it soft and pliable, the leather is treated with saddle soap; this is the preparation used on the harness of horses; it is a soft paste which is rubbed into the leatherwork so as to keep it supple and soft. The leather is rubbed over with a soft cloth after saddle soaping to remove excess.

The quality and fit of a splint should always be excellent. It is safer to discard and replace a splint than to make do with one which is damaged or of a wrong size.

Various splints are discussed where relevant elsewhere in the book, the reader is referred to the index for particular splints.

30

Plaster of Paris Techniques

Introduction

Efficiently used, plaster of Paris is a useful adaptable material. The plaster bandages and other requirements can be packed into a small space and require only a bucket of water: this gives plaster of Paris a major advantage over metal, wood and leather which require heavy and ponderous equipment to produce them. Splints for most patients are only temporary supports so that the commercial manufacture of a metal and leather splint made to fit a patient accurately is expensive. A splint of plaster of Paris costs less and is quickly made; when no longer required it can be discarded.

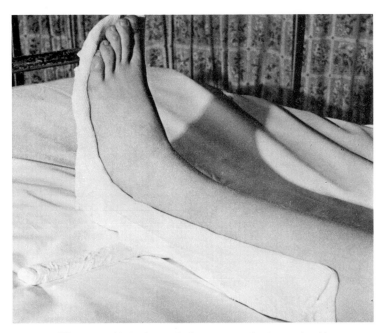

Fig. 30.1   (a) A plaster shell to support the foot and ankle.

Functions of plaster of Paris in orthopaedics

1   The immobilization of fractured bones as a temporary emergency measure in a first-aid situation.

2   The immobilization after reduction of fractured bones and dislocated joints as a long-term measure until the damaged tissues have healed.

3   The production of night splints, back splints or shells for resting and supporting a part during intermittent periods only; these are taken off and replaced as desired. They are used, for example, in the correction of the deformities of rheumatoid arthritis; after physiotherapy the splint is bandaged into position to maintain any correction which has been achieved (Fig. 30.1a and b).

4   To rest and prevent movement in the joints of patients with tendo-synovitis when passage of the tendon in its sheath results in severe pain.

5   To correct deformity; for example, in children with congenital talipes and patients with contractures of joints (see 'wedging', Fig. 30.4).

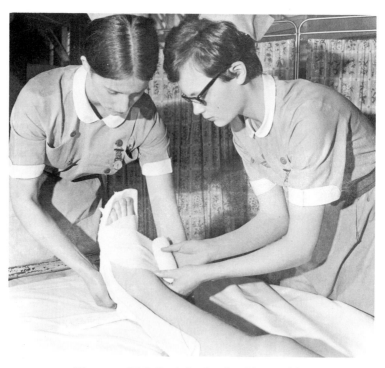

Fig. 30.1   (b) Splint being bandaged into position.

6   The production of exact models of parts of patients for sending to the splintmaker who then uses the plaster models to make a splint which fits accurately (Fig. 30.3).

7   To support and rest a part after surgical intervention, until healing occurs.

The chemistry of plaster of Paris

The material is so called because it was originally made from large deposits of natural mineral in Montmartre in Paris. Gypsum, the mineral element of plaster of Paris is available in large quantities in the United Kingdom and other countries, however.

It consists of a dehydrate of calcium sulphate ($CaSO_4 . 2H_2O$). When heat is applied to this material in manufacture it loses some of its water content to convert it from a crystalline form. When water is mixed with this hemihydrate form, it is reconverted to a crystalline interlocking mass which forms the plaster of Paris splint.

Because of its deliquescent properties it must always be stored in airtight waterproof conditions. If it is allowed to become damp through the humidity of the atmosphere it is useless.

The special property of plaster of Paris which makes it so useful is that the original powder, when wet, forms a paste; when this paste dries it forms a firm continuous mass or sheet. If this is combined with an open weave bandage it is much stronger.

The plaster is used with open weave bandages which are impregnated with it usually by manufacturers. It is also possible to make plaster bandages locally by hand. Plaster without the bandage material may be used as a cream, into which sheets of muslin are dipped to make plaster beds, or the cream may be poured into a mould to make positive casts.

The temperature of the water affects the setting time of the plaster. The warmer the water, the more rapid the setting of the plaster. Too high a temperature may result in a weak cast.

As with all chemical changes, heat is given off as the plaster sets. Once setting is completed, however, the moisture contained in it becomes as cool as the atmosphere to which it is exposed; the excess water then evaporates which lowers the temperature; in a cold room the limb encased in plaster becomes very cold and the heat regulating mechanisms of the patient must work harder to keep his body warm.

The objectives in the application of a
plaster of Paris splint

The application of plaster of Paris is a skill which can only be acquired by practical experience. There is a tendency to give this task to a technician in many hospitals and thus the nursing staff do not gain this ability. The application of plaster of Paris must not be regarded as a mystical rite which can only be performed by the chosen few. A competent nurse with the ability to apply a good plaster splint is an asset in any unit which receives casualties and multiple injuries.

The objectives should be:

1   To apply the splint with the minimum of fuss, mess and distress to the patient. Although special rooms or departments are used in most hospitals, there are many occasions where plaster may have to be applied in the ward, operating theatre or other situations. The use of adequate protective sheeting and the minimal amount of water (after squeezing out the plaster bandage), means that the least time is wasted in cleaning the floor, furniture and clothing afterwards.

2   The production of a neat splint which has been polished, trimmed and finished. The patient may have to wear it for many weeks.

3   The splint must fit accurately, being neither too slack nor too tight. The former will both be inefficient and cause irritation at the edges as the splint rubs the skin, and the latter will constrict the part.

4   The splint must only be as heavy as is necessary for its effectiveness. In many situations a thin light splint will suffice. If extra strength is required for a particular reason, the splint must be made stronger by making it thicker where necessary. A strong splint with extra layers of plaster bandage is tiring to wear and carry.

5   The padding within the splint has a specific purpose and its thickness is related to need. When a part is unlikely to swell, a thin layer of either wool roll or stockinette is adequate. If swelling is anticipated, extra padding is required to permit this increase without constriction of the limb within the splint. Extra padding is also needed on bony projections and in thin patients.

Requirements for plastering

(a) The department

A plaster department is important to the efficient functioning of an orthopaedic unit. The following areas are required:

A storage unit. The impedimenta of such a unit is extensive and bulky;

storage facilities for the plaster bandages must serve to prevent humidity in the unit atmosphere from affecting them.

Changing rooms or cubicles. When patients are required to strip, a warm cubicle with dressing gowns and briefs should be provided.

Drying rooms. Plaster beds, negative casts and other plasters require a warm room with convected currents of air for efficient drying. This room may also serve as a storage area for plasters.

Plastering rooms. The plastering room must be large, warm and well ventilated. Good access doors for patients on beds or trolleys are necessary. Flooring and walls must be tiled or terrazzo for easy removal of plaster. Plenty of tables and working surfaces with radiography viewing boxes are required.

The annexe. This is the room for emptying buckets of water used in plastering and for storage of enamel ware and buckets. The sink is of a special design with a wide drainage throat and a sump for the reception of plaster residue; this is essential in order to avoid blocking the drains. The sink should be at a low level to make it easier to empty the buckets of water. A large flat surface for washing down mackintosh and plastic sheeting and hanging racks for these items are assets. Positive casts are also made here.

(b) **The equipment**

(i) *Positioning equipment.* An orthopaedic operating table is useful but not essential. An Abbot's or Risser frame is useful for correction of spinal deformities with jackets of plaster of Paris. A long narrow plinth. Hip props. Shoulder supports and props. Knee bending supports. Stools. Chairs. Suspension gallows. Double pulleys. Single pulleys. Nylon rope. Cross bar or gambrel. Equipment for elevating one end of the plinth on which the patient is treated.

(ii) *Plastering equipment.* Pails and bowls. Protective sheeting. Plastic covered pillows. Plastic covered sandbags. Plastic aprons and overalls for staff. Rubber boots for staff. Trimming knives. Copying pencils. Vaseline gauze. Oil and a brush. Rulers. Wires for making cutting lines in casts.

(iii) *Removal equipment.* Plaster knives. Electric saw. Plaster saws and tenon saws. Plaster scissors. Plaster shears. Plaster openers.

(iv) *Surgical equipment.* Packs containing equipment for giving injections. Packs of suture removal equipment. Dressing packs.

(v)   *Anaesthetic equipment.* This will probably be brought from another department as needed.

The method of applying casts

The patient. It is always advisable and ethical to explain to the patient what is to be done and why. Before commencing it is as well to tell him how the cast will appear when finished and how it will affect him.

As the patient will be at any rate partly and often completely undressed, the room must be warm enough for his comfort; at least 22°C is desirable.

Children will be frightened of the unknown. A kind word of explanation must be given; a nurse from the ward should be present.

Positioning. The position in which the patient is to be fixed must be held until the cast is in position and drying. The holder has a difficult task if the position is awkward and the limb or plaster is heavy. Therefore, supports, sandbags, props, and pillows which will help to take the weight of the limb and maintain a constant and stable position must be used. If necessary an orthopaedic table to fix the limb or part should be used. Slings for the holder to support are useful. The holder should be provided with a chair or stool related to his height and the height of the part he is supporting. The responsibility for the correct position in the cast is normally taken by the surgeon in charge of the patient (Fig. 30.6).

Padded casts. Padding of wool roll must be evenly and firmly applied. It must not constrict or be creased. Wool roll may also be used to protect bony prominences and crests over a stockinette sheath.

Padded casts are used:
1   In all recent injury.
2   After operation on a part when swelling may occur.
3   After forcible manipulation under anaesthesia.
4   In correcting a deformity with a plaster splint.
5   On patients who are thin and bony.

Various thicknesses of felt may also be used but this is not necessarily adhesive. It must be bevelled at the edges to prevent the felt pad cutting into the skin.

Unpadded casts. Unpadded casts are applied over a sheath of stockinette when a firm and accurate fit is desired. The stockinette is supplied in various widths and the correct width is used to avoid looseness of fit or creasing. An electric cutter is never used to remove such a cast.

Wetting the bandages. Plenty of water in large pails is needed which must be changed frequently during the procedure. A high concentration of plaster residue in the water delays soaking.

The bandage must be allowed to saturate through to the centre core and is kept in the water until the bubbles cease to rise. It should then be used at once. The soaked bandage is handed to the operator with the first few inches unwound (Fig. 30.2a), after lightly squeezing to remove excess water.

Plaster slabs are folded in order to reduce their size. Two hands must be used to hold them while soaking (Fig. 30.2b). A fold and an end to the slab is held in each hand; the end between index finger and thumb and the fold between the index finger and the next finger. A slab is a multi-layer length of bandage measured to the required length for the patient; it may be cut from a boxed commercial slab pack or else made from a folded plaster bandage.

Applying the bandages. These are rolled on. To fit the bandage accurately, a pleat or fold is made in each turn as is required to make it conform to the irregular shape of the patient. At each stage the hands are dipped into the water and the cast is 'polished' and smoothed. The hands must be kept flat in smoothing and there must be no point pressure with fingers gripping the cast in holding. In holding the cast, the hands must be constantly moved to avoid digging in. Two thirds of the previous turn are covered by each subsequent turn.

Moulding the cast to the shape of the part must be done rapidly once the bandage is put on to the cast. The malleoli and other bony prominences must be included in the moulding; skilful use of the hands so as to make the cast conform to the shape of the part is essential.

The cast should give a neat polished appearance when finished, but even more important is its internal surface which should be smooth and conform to the contours of the patient's body.

Trimming. A sharp carbon-steel knife with a short blade is used to trim the cast. In a plaster which includes the foot, trimming should expose the toes so that movement can occur. On a jacket, trimming of the lower edges to allow the patient to sit down in comfort is needed; the patient is asked to sit so that the amount of trimming needed can be estimated. Care is needed to ensure that over-trimming does not reduce the efficiency of the cast.

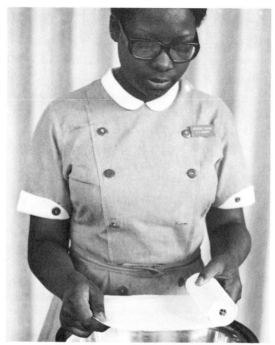

(a)

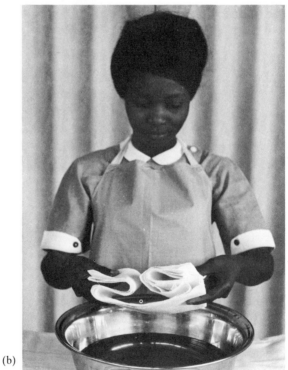

(b)

Fig. 30.2   Holding (a) a plaster bandage and (b) a plaster slab prior to soaking.

Finishing. When stockinette is used it is turned back over the edges of the cast and fastened neatly down with either rubber upholstery adhesive or cellulose wallpaper adhesive. Some operators fasten the edges down with the last turn of the plaster bandage.

Posterior and anterior removable splints

Such splints consist of slabs of the desired length which are moulded over stockinette to the shape of the part they are to support. Wrist-support splints or right angle foot shells (Fig. 30.1) are made in this way. When the plaster is dry the stockinette is slit along its length and the slab is taken off for finishing. The stockinette is turned back onto the splint and fastened down. The finished splint is then left to dry. It is bandaged into place as a night splint or temporary support.

Drying plaster splints and jackets. As in the drying of any garment or wet surface, the moisture in a plaster splint must be allowed to evaporate. This means that the limb or part encased in a plaster splint must be exposed to the atmosphere or to a current of warmed air for sufficient time for all the excess water to be converted to vapour and leave the splint hard and dry. Contamination of a setting cast by blood, may weaken the cast.

This process may take a long time; the larger the splint, particularly in thickness, the longer it will take to dry. At least two days is required for most splints and jackets to dry and five days must be allowed when stress is to be applied to it, for instance when a lower limb cast is to be used as a walking splint.

The jacket, cast or splint must be left uncovered for the first twenty-four hours. It must not be covered during the drying period with materials such as plastic sheeting which will prevent evaporation of moisture. All surfaces of large plasters must be exposed in turn and regular turning of patients (who are conscious) wearing plaster jackets or hip spicas, must be carried out. When such patients cannot be turned, the cast should be supported in such a way that air can reach most of its surface.

The completed cast should be supported on pillows on a firm base. Small projections such as the heel in a leg plaster must not be allowed to rest on hard surfaces or they will flatten and press inwards on the skin.

Direct radiant heat to the cast is not the best way to dry it and a patient can burn through the plaster if items such as hot water bottles or electric elements are placed near it. Convected warm currents of air are the most suitable means of drying large plasters. Small and large casts will all dry well in time if left exposed in a warm ventilated room.

The out-patient's problems

The nurse who sends the patient away from the casualty department to his home with a plaster splint on his limb may not be aware of his many problems. The wearing of a cold moist splint which cannot be covered when in bed, added to any pain he may have, plus the problems of learning how to negotiate the problem of turning or undressing must be experienced to be fully understood.

Facilities in most homes are not directed to patient care, particularly when an accident occurs; nothing will be ready, or the patient lives alone or with an aged frail partner. The parent managing a child with an above-knee plaster will have problems in negotiating stairs and doors while carrying the child. Using the toilet, wearing such a plaster, is also a problem.

A thoughtful nurse will always enquire about the facilities which exist at home and, if it is obvious that the patient cannot cope with the situation, arrange for admission to hospital for a period.

Child patients are especially vulnerable, particularly if they are small and do not understand. If a frog plaster (see Fig. 19.5 and 19.11) or jacket is applied to a child, careful supervision is required during the first few days; enclosure of the abdomen or thorax is a serious matter. Digestive and respiratory problems may occur and small babies in plaster may die from inhaling vomit. A small baby in a plaster cast immobilizing the body must not be put to sleep on its back. Before discharge from hospital the parents must be made aware of the dangers.

Lifting a patient in a cast. A large cast may crack or break if care is not taken in moving it, particularly while it is drying. During this phase the patient must be assisted by supporting limb plasters during turning; large casts such as spicas or jackets require three people to help during turning. Projecting portions of the cast must be supported separately.

Special coating for plaster casts. Casts which are liable to be heavily soiled with excreta may be waterproofed with fibreglass. When the plaster has completely dried out and the patient is well enough, an epoxy-resin covering may be applied according to the manufacturers' instructions. As chemicals which give off a strong smell must be used, a well-ventilated room away from the ward unit and other patients must be used.

Removal of plaster splints. Method. When a plaster splint is to be removed, the surgeon in charge of the patient will wish to examine the part supported by the splint before it is completely taken off the patient. He will examine the site of a fracture for clinical union, for example, by testing the efficiency of callous and will note if there is pain or not. This means that the splint must be cut into two sections; one section is lifted off, leaving the other to serve as a support. If it is decided that the limb should continue to be immobilized in the splint it can be replaced. Often the surgeon will indicate the lines along which the splint should be cut. For a leg splint it is divided behind the internal malleolus and in front of the external malleolus.

When the splint is well padded it may be cut along the lines indicated using an electric cutter. If the splint has no padding, slow, steady and careful cutting with shears or knives is required.

A plaster room will have a variety of sizes and shapes of plaster shears available. It does not follow that the largest are the best and small lightweight shears are suitable for thin casts. When shears are used they must be inserted slowly and gently to ensure that the patient's skin is not damaged.

Emergency situations

If swelling is likely to occur in a part enclosed in a cast, appliances for splitting the cast should be ready. An example of this would be when a plaster has been applied after surgery on a limb.

When a plaster is to be bivalved or split, it must be completely divided along the whole length of the splint and not just at the proximal end. Any bandages or wool rolls which encircle the limb under the cast must also be split longitudinally if there is any suggestion of circulatory impairment.

When swelling is likely to occur, two approaches in dealing with the situation are made:

(a) *Positional.* The limb is suspended or elevated so that gravity will help to assist venous return (see Fig. 8.10(b)).

(b) *Precautionary.* The limb is not completely enclosed in a splint. A shell or backslab is made to fit and is fastened on with cloth bandages which can easily be removed.

There are situations when a patient develops a secondary condition which requires urgent action and this becomes more important than the reason for applying the cast. An example here would be the patient wearing a plaster jacket or spica who develops an acute condition of his abdomen, such as appendicitis or a perforated gastric ulcer. In these circumstances the surgeon will require the jacket to be removed so that the abdomen can be examined. In such a condition the jacket or spica is divided into anterior and posterior sections. A new jacket or spica can be applied when the emergency is over or the old one is repaired.

The disadvantages of plaster fixation

1 The part is covered and cannot be observed.

2 The limb or part may be constricted either by the plaster being too tight a fit in the first instance, or the size of the part increasing in the second.

3 Encasement of the head, neck, thorax or abdomen causes secondary problems. Restriction of thoracic and abdominal movements with attendant respiratory and digestive distress to the patient are examples.

4 As with all forms of splintage, joints adjacent to the fracture and enclosed in the cast will become stiff and the muscles which move them will waste.

5 Localized pressure by the plaster on the heel or malleoli will cause ulceration. Complaints of pain at particular spots under the plaster must not be ignored. A window may be cut into the cast to examine the underlying skin. This must always be carefully repadded and replaced to avoid local swelling into it.

6 Crumbs, coins, beads or plastic toys, etc, may find their way inside the cast and cause sores.

7 When a limb is covered for a long time, the skin desquamates and forms large hard scales which are loose inside the splint. This can cause irritation of the skin.

8 A patient may develop a contact dermatitis from either the lining and padding, or from the plaster.

9 Pressure on peripheral nerves may be missed because a limb is covered up.

Instructions to patients

Some patients are extremely tolerant of pain and distress; others complain readily. There is no certain way by which the nurse or doctor can know which type of patient they are treating and there must be a standard set of instructions which are given to all patients who are going out of the hospital and away from observation.

These instructions must be given verbally to both the patient, if he is able to understand, and to his attendant relative or friend. The verbal instructions must be reinforced by giving the patient a printed document produced in the language he can read. These instructions may be pasted onto the cast in some hospitals.

If there is still doubt about the efficiency of communication, it is safest to admit the patient to hospital for observation or to communicate with the patient's general practitioner by telephone.

The instructions are:

1 To return to the hospital or seek other medical aid if there is any doubt.

There will be no resentment by either the hospital or the patient's own doctor.

2   To make use of the joints which can be moved and exercise them regularly.

3   The following are significant and must be immediately reported to the doctor or hospital:

(i)   severe discolouration,
(ii) tension and pain, even when the limb is elevated,
(iii) numbness,
(iv) unrelieved coldness.

4   If a leg plaster is fitted, the limb must be kept raised on a chair. If an arm plaster is fitted, the hand must be at the same height as the shoulder.

5   To report any localized pain under the plaster which may indicate the presence of a sore.

6   Avoid maltreatment of the plaster; particularly it must not be allowed to come into contact with water.

7   Not to interfere with the plaster.

8   To report to the relevant clinic on the given date.

The nursing management of a patient in a plaster splint

The drying of a plaster splint is described on p. 519.

Observations by nursing staff. The toes or fingers must be checked several times a day, particularly in the first few days after the application. The nails and skin of the patient on both limbs are compressed with the nurse's thumbs and comparison of the speed of clearance of the thumb-press is made. It should be equal on both the unsplinted and the splinted limb; the skin must appear healthy and adequately supplied with blood.

The skin at the edges of the plaster must be checked for soreness, particularly in a patient wearing a walking plaster. Rough edges on a cast can excoriate the skin.

Complaints of any form from the patient must never be ignored. There may be a sore under the plaster and unless the pressure here is relieved, extensive damage, requiring prolonged treatment may be caused.

A plaster sore will give off an offensive smell which must always be reported. If the sore is infected, as is probable if the odour exists, the patient will have all the signs and symptoms of infection, including a rise in temperature, restlessness and irritability, loss of appetite, thirst and an offensive breath odour.

Any staining of the plaster is significant and must be reported. A ballpoint pen mark around the edges of the stain will indicate where it is increasing in area or if it is static.

The management of plaster sores. A plaster sore is exposed by cutting a window in the plaster splint at the site of the pain. If the skin is unbroken, the padding is reapplied and the window closed off with new plaster bandage. Care is taken to ensure that the tissues do not bulge into the window area when it has been closed off.

If the skin is broken, the sore is treated in the same way as any surgical wound; when it is healed, the plaster window is sealed again.

Should the plaster sore be ulcerated and infected, then it must be dressed with a lotion such as Eusol and the doctor will order the relevant antibiotic after the organisms in the wound have been tested for sensitivity. Any anaemia or lowered haemaglobin level in the patient indicated by a blood test, must be treated so as to increase the rate of healing of the sore.

Care of the skin on removal of the plaster. Whilst the plaster has been in position the skin inside it has been undergoing the changes which occur over the whole surface of the skin of the body; this is replacement of the top layer with new layers from underneath. The top layer is normally rubbed away in friction from clothing and movement. Under the plaster the superficial layer remains in position to form thick scales usually held in position by hairs and some fibres.

Gentle washing of the skin with soap and water will take off many of the scales and any which remain should be left to fall away. It is unwise to pull them off as a sore may be caused in so doing. If urgent removal of the scales is required they may be softened with olive oil or arachis oil for easy removal.

Positive casts
To make splints, supports and appliances which fit accurately, an exact copy of the part is supplied to the splint manufacturer in the form of a positive cast. This cast can be used in the same way as the shoemaker uses a last to make an accurately fitting shoe.

Relevant points on the patient are first marked with indelible pencil. A negative cast is then made by making an unpadded plaster splint on the limb which has been coated with oil. This is removed with the minimal damage possible, while still wet, although it has set. The splint is then repaired down the line of the cut with an encircling plaster bandage and one end is sealed off with a layer of plaster bandage.

The whole negative cast is then smeared on the inside with a thin layer of petroleum jelly. A holder for the finished positive cast is placed down the centre of the negative cast; this may be a metal strut or wooden stick.

If possible, sufficient plaster cream is made to pour into the negative cast and fill it with one pouring. The cream is stirred as it is poured in to prevent air-bells in the plaster and to make a stronger positive cast. When set, the negative cast is removed and discarded, the positive cast is clearly marked with the name and reference number of the patient (Fig. 30.3). See also Chapter 29.

Wedging. This is a procedure used to correct a deformity in a joint or part. The cast to be wedged is cut with an electric saw. A piece of wood of required length is inserted into the gap that has been made. The cast is then re-closed, over the wooden wedge, with plaster bandages (Fig. 30.5).

When it is anticipated that a cast must be wedged, extra padding is applied beneath the cast.

Plaster of Paris jackets and posterior spinal supports
Plaster of Paris jackets and posterior spinal supports have the advantage that they can be made quickly and relatively cheaply on the hospital or clinic premises; they will last, with care, for up to one year and may be discarded and replaced as often as required. The method of application is related to the function they must serve.

1   *Immobilization of the sacral, lumbar and lower thoracic areas of the vertebral column.* This type of jacket is often applied following a period of complete bed rest, with or without traction, or immobilization on a plaster bed. The patient must therefore be carefully lifted by a team into position and the jacket must be applied with the patient horizontal, not standing (Fig. 30.6a). A stockinette vest is put on the patient while on his bed, or alternatively, a wool roll may be used. The patient is then arranged in the supine position on a plaster table with the following modifications:

(i)   A shoulder box is placed under the shoulders, and pillows of the appropriate height are placed under his head.

(ii)   A hip prop is used to elevate the pelvis to the same level at the shoulders.

(iii) A member of the team holds the legs in abduction and applies traction on the legs against the hip prop.

An alternative is to use an orthopaedic operating table with its various accessories to place the patient in the same position.

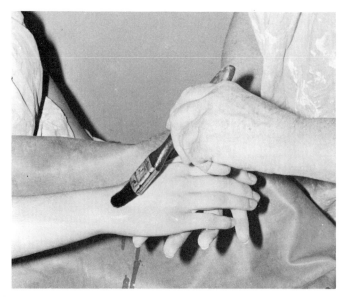

Fig. 30.3   (a) Painting the limb with oil to prevent the plaster sticking to the limb.

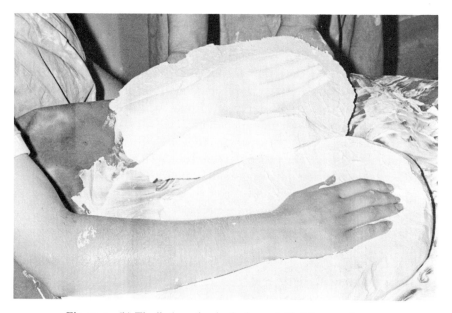

Fig. 30.3   (b) The limb resting in the lower half of the negative cast.

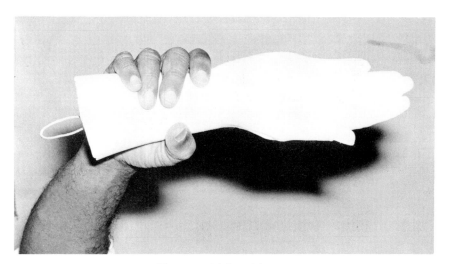

Fig. 30.3 (c) A positive cast.

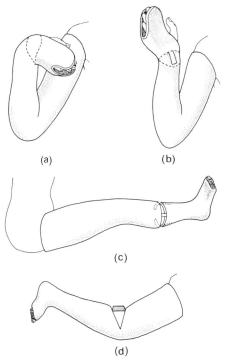

(a)

(b)

(c)

(d)

Fig. 30.4 (a) Plaster applied preparatory to wedging at wrist level to correct
flexion contractures of the fingers. A segment of plaster is removed from the
area marked. (b) Fully opened, cork in position over the front of the wrist.
(c) Wedging a long-leg plaster for re-alignment of the position of fracture.
(d) Correcting flexion contracture of the knee, by wedging.

Circles of orthopaedic felt are positioned over the stockinette to protect the anterior superior iliac spines. A wide strip of felt is also arranged along the spine and over the sacrum.

Wide plaster bandages (150 cm) are soaked and applied so as to encircle the trunk. The jacket extends from the top of the sternum at the front and the lower angles of the scapulae at the back, down to the level of the coccyx at its lower end. Extra slabs are incorporated in the area of the pelvis.

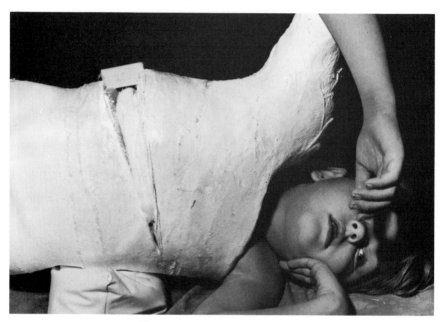

Fig. 30.5   Wedging a plaster jacket.

The jacket is completed by trimming sufficient off the front lower edge to allow the patient to flex the hips as in sitting. The upper and lower ends of the stockinette vest are then turned back over the jacket and fastened down with adhesive. It is important that the jacket should be firmly moulded over the pelvis. For comfort, a circle of plaster six inches in diameter may be removed over the patient's epigastrium.

2   *Immobilization of the spine in hyperextension.* The patient is placed prone and with the spine in hyperextension. This may be achieved either on an orthopaedic operating table or by using two separate tables, one nine inches higher than the other. The legs and pelvis of the patient are placed along the length of the lower table and the arms, shoulders, head and neck resting on

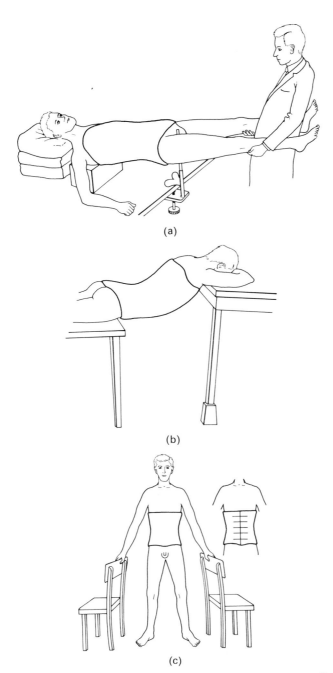

Fig. 30.6 (a) Patient in position on hip prop and shoulder box for application of a spica or jacket. (b) Hyperextension jacket applied between two tables. (c) A patient steadying himself, by grasping two chairs, for the application of a plaster corset or for taking a cast.

the higher table (Fig. 30.6b). Two assistants hold the patient in this position, one supporting the upper and one the lower portions of the body.

A similar jacket to that previously described is applied but a strengthening slab down the front is required.

This position is an uncomfortable one for the patient; it is difficult for him to sit, and lying down or standing is more tolerable.

3   *Immobilization of the cervical region.* After suitable modification, the plaster jacket described on p. 525 may have an additional section applied to include the head and neck. The jacket will be heavier and the weight will be received on the patient's pelvis, therefore the iliac crests are padded with crescents of felt and the jacket is carefully moulded in and on to the iliac crests.

When the jacket is completed the head and neck are enclosed in a thin layer of wool roll, leaving the face uncovered (Fig. 30.7). The axillae are also covered by wool roll.

Three helpers now maintain the correct position of the patient in either

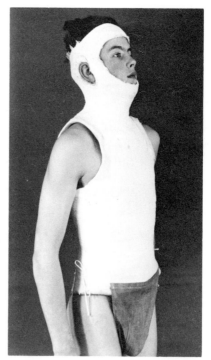

Fig. 30.7   A 'Minerva' jacket.

the sitting or lying position; the surgeon holds the head and the two others hold the shoulders. The plaster is continued upwards to envelope the head. Three 150 cm wide plaster slabs are used to reinforce the union between the jacket and the headpiece, one on either shoulder and one up the posterior surface. The forehead and chin are included in the headpiece. The plaster is cut away from the ears to free them. The top of the head is also left free. If the patient wears spectacles, gaps are left at each side of the face for the arms of the spectacle frames to enter. A convenient way of ensuring this is to insert a pencil over each ear during plastering. If dentures are normally worn by the patient they are fitted while the jacket is being applied. Pressure on the front of the larynx must be avoided. Alternatively, if the patient can tolerate sitting, the jacket may be applied with him sitting on a stool and his head suspended by a head halter attached to a rope and pulley.

4 *Making a model for the manufacture of a lumbo-sacral belt.* The patient stands with his legs astride (the feet are approximately one foot apart); a chair with the back towards the patient at either side serves to support the patient as he rests a hand on either chair and extends his spine upwards (Fig. 30.6c).

A thin plaster jacket is applied extending above and below the levels to which the belt is required to reach. The cutting line is marked and cross marks are made for rejoining. The jacket is cut off and converted into a positive cast as described in Chapter 30, p. 524.

5 *Posterior spinal support slab and tubular gripping bandage.* The advantage of this is that it can be worn or taken off by the patient as desired and necessary.

The unclothed patient lies prone as shown in Fig. 30.8a after a length of stockinette has been applied to the trunk. A slab of plaster, several layers thick, is made on the back extending from the level of the coccyx to the midthoracic region. This is carefully moulded to the curves of the patient's back. The slab is taken off after the stockinette vest has been slit down the anterior surface. The edges of the slab are neatly trimmed and the corners rounded. The stockinette is trimmed and stuck down on the posterior surface of the slab.

When dry the slab is re-applied to the patient's back and a length of strong tubular gripping bandage is rolled on to the patient's trunk to hold the slab in place (see Fig. 29.3a and b).

Plaster beds

A plaster bed is a shell made to fit accurately to the contours of the body of the patient. It usually serves to give complete support and rest to a lesion affecting the vertebral column; it may also be used, however, to assist the correction of a deformity (as in a divided bed for example, see in Fig. 30.8), or to apply traction to the hips when extensions bows, a pelvic band, and groin straps are used. The plaster bed may be modified by the addition of a headpiece and brow band for a cervical or high thoracic lesion.

Normally the plaster bed extends from the shoulder down the whole length of the body to the level of the malleoli of the ankles. At the sides of the trunk it extends up to a horizontal line drawn from the centre of the axilla downwards. The leg pieces should be as deep as is feasible for applying leg bandages to retain the patient's leg in the bed.

Preparation of the patient. The patient must be completely unclothed. It is therefore necessary to make the room warm (22°C), to adequately prepare before the arrival of the patient and to assemble a full team to reduce the time required for making the bed. The patient will be embarrassed and, because of his lesion, will probably tire easily.

Before going to the plaster room, an explanation to the patient of what is being done, and why, is necessary. The patient is bathed and given the opportunity to empty bowel and urinary bladder. A light meal prior to the event will ensure that he is not distended yet not hungry during the making of the bed.

Positioning the patient (Fig. 30.8a). The position of the patient is related to the shape of the finished bed. The patient is arranged comfortably in the prone position on a warm table or on his bed with the bedding adequately protected. The position of the patient can be adjusted to the requirements expressed by the surgeon by the use of small pillows. However, the standard position is with the patient prone with his feet extending over the edge of the bed or table. A pad is placed underneath each ankle to flex the knees to 5 degrees. The legs are abducted to give a distance of 33 cm between the internal malleoli. It is important to see that the vertebral column is straight and without lateral tilt. The arms of the patient may either be abducted and resting on the table or placed at the sides clear of the working area. The head may be positioned either with the face towards the table and the forehead resting on a small pillow; or with the head turned to one side. If a headpiece is to be added to the plaster bed, the former position is required.

Preparation of the skin. The highest point and the margins of the gluteal fold are marked with an indelible pencil. These marks will transfer onto the plaster shell to indicate lines for cutting a slot for bowel evacuation; this slot must not be wider than is necessary as the tissues of the buttocks may protrude through to cause cuts and sores as the edges of the bed dig into them.

Bony prominences on the body must be padded with strips and circles of 1 cm thick felt; the padding is retained in position with zinc oxide plaster (Fig. 30.8a). The number of points to be padded will depend upon the amount of subcutaneous fat on the patient; an emaciated patient will require padding along the whole length of the spine, across the sacrum and posterior spines of the iliac crests, the great trochanters of femur and the lateral and medial surfaces of the knees. When the bed is completed these will be represented as hollowed out areas in the plaster.

The skin not covered by padding is now painted with warmed arachis oil or olive oil. The perineum of the patient is covered with gauze soaked in petroleum jelly to prevent the plaster sticking to the hair.

Making the plaster shell. This may be made of:

(a) *Twenty-four 15 cm wide plaster bandages.* These are rolled out across the patient from one operator to another until sufficient area and thickness of plaster is built up on the trunk of the patient and then onto the thighs and legs (Fig. 30.8c). The bandages are constantly smoothed down on to the shell to avoid the occurrence of spaces in the layers; OR

(b) *Pieces of material soaked in a bowl of plaster cream.* Commonly plaster muslin is used for the material but other fabric will serve if it is porous and absorbent. Hessian may be used provided it has no oil in it.

Six pieces of material are needed, each greater than half the total required length of the plaster shell; three of the pieces form the upper half and three pieces the lower half and they must overlap where they meet. The three lower pieces are slotted for the length of the legs of the plaster shell; a neck slot is cut into the centre of the top edge of the upper pieces.

Careful timing is needed in using this method. The plaster cream is not mixed until the final moment when it is needed for use. A team of four, and preferably six, are needed, plus another operator for soaking the pieces. Half the team stand on either side of the table and, as the pieces are each soaked in the cream in turn, they are passed to the team who open them and position them.

It is necessary in this method to work quickly and to rub each piece on to the underlying piece to ensure that it is firmly laminated, particularly at the edges. Sufficient cream must be mixed at the start to last the whole procedure.

A bar, made either of wood or plaster of Paris, is used to connect the leg pieces at the level of the calf to give added strength.

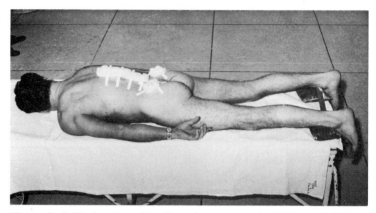

Fig. 30.8   (a) Patient in position for making a plaster bed. Bony prominences
have been padded to allow space in the finished bed.

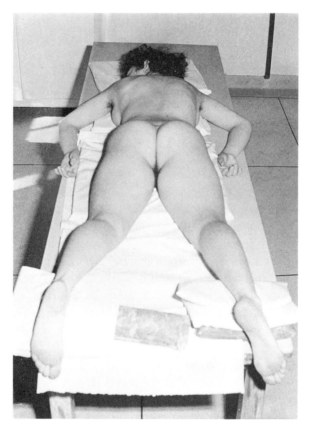

Fig. 30.8   (b) Patient in position (prone) for fitting of plaster bed.

Indelible pencil lines are now made on the exterior surface to indicate the lines for cutting the bed to shape (Fig. 30.8d and e). The plaster shell, when set, is carefully lifted off the patient (Fig. 30.8f), placed on a flat surface and the edges trimmed and rounded with sharp knives and files. At the same time the patient is cared for; the skin is cleaned of oil and debris and his body is covered with warmed blankets (Fig. 30.8g).

If it is intended to use the plaster bed to correct a kyphosis, two strips of a malleable metal such as aluminium are incorporated in the plaster bed which is then split transversely and the metal strips act as hinges. Alternatively, an adjustable metal stand can be used (Fig. 30.8h). The central support is adjustable by turning wing-nuts and if the plaster bed has been split and hinged, hyperextension can easily be obtained.

Finishing and lining the plaster bed. The shell is placed in the drying room until thoroughly dry. It is then passed to the carpenter who makes a base and

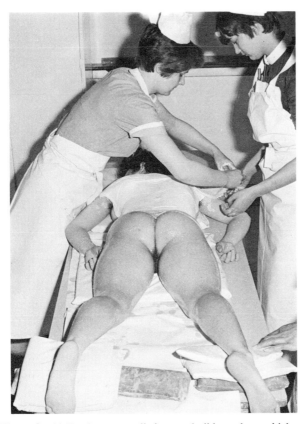

Fig. 30.8 (c) Bandages are rolled out to build up plaster thickness.

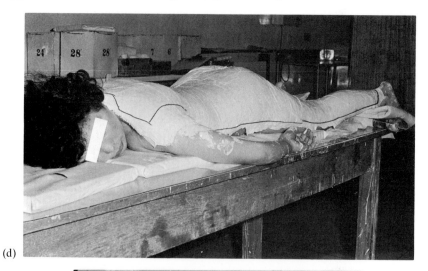

(d)

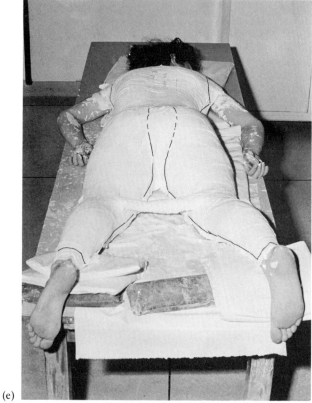

(e)

Fig. 30.8   (d) and (e) Lines on plaster for cutting bed to shape.

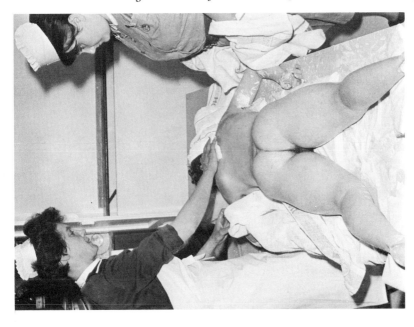

Fig. 30.8   (g) Cleaning skin after removal of shell.

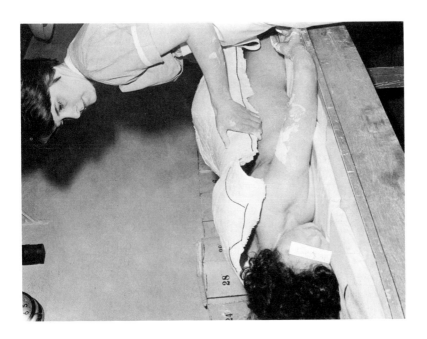

Fig. 30.8 (f) Removal of plaster shell.

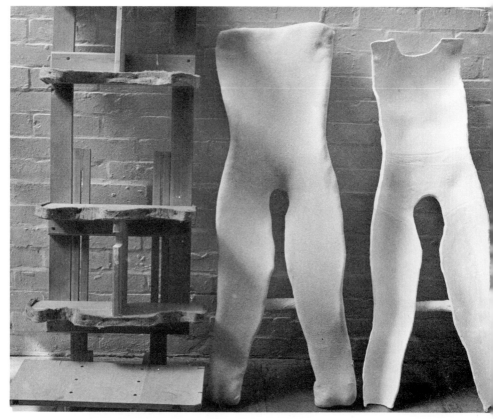

Fig. 30.8   (h) Stand for a plaster bed. (i) A lined plaster bed. (j) An anterior turning case.

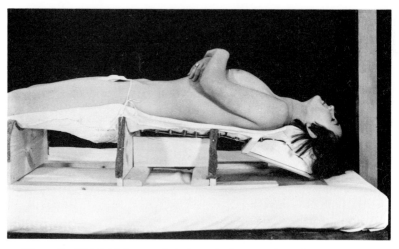

Fig. 30.8   (k) Divided (posterior) plaster bed. Correcting a flexion deformity of the spine.

stand for it (Fig. 30.8h). The stand is made from heavy deal 2·5 cm thick; it must support the bed at all points and leave sufficient space for the insertion of a bed-pan. The shell is *not* fastened to the stand.

If the shell is smoothed carefully during production by stroking the wet plaster with wet hands, the inside should be glossy and free from projections. It fits the patient so accurately that no lining to the bed should be necessary and the patient will not come to any harm if he lies on the bare plaster. It is, however, kinder and hygienic to fit a thin lining to the bed which can be replaced when necessary (Fig. 30.8i).

The lining is made of a thin layer of splint wool covered by stockinette. The stockinette is fastened to the exterior edges of the bed with either upholstery adhesive or a strong mucilage paste. Particular care is needed in the area of the genital and gluteal cleft of the bed to ensure that the lining is fixed down at all points. Particular care is needed to ensure that the lining is even and that there are no protuberances in the wool; that the stockinette is not so loose that it will ruck up and form a crease that will result in a sore on the patient's body; that the lining does not greatly reduce the volume of the interior of the shell.

Modifications for suspension of a plaster bed. The plaster bed described in this section may be modified either for suspension from a double balkan beam by weights, cords and pulleys (see Fig. 28.6) or for insertion in a turning bed. Instead of mounting on a wooden stand and base, transverse bars are fixed to the exterior of the bed.

Turning cases
A turning case is similar to the plaster shell used on a plaster bed but instead fits the anterior surface of the body of the patient; the plaster bed and turning case together are similar to an oyster shell. Its function is to enable a nursing team to change the patient from the supine to the prone position without affecting the alignment of the vertebrae and the lesion of the vertebral column.

Method of making the turning case. The turning case is made when the plaster bed has been completed and the patient is using it (see Fig. 30.8).

With the patient in his plaster bed, the skin is coated with warmed oil and the anterior-superior iliac spines of the patient are padded with circles of felt.

The anterior turning case is then made in the same way as the posterior plaster bed. If the lesion is in the upper thoracic or cervical regions and the

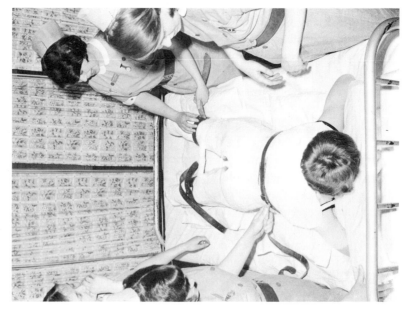

Fig. 30.9 (b) Turn completed; the straps are undone.

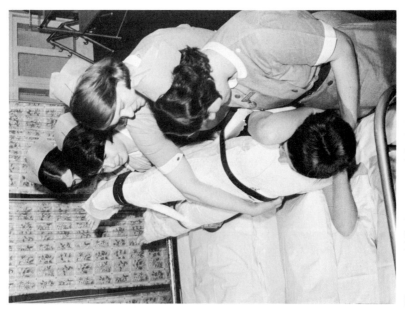

Fig. 30.9 (a) Patient strapped firmly into turning case.

plaster bed has a head piece, an anterior head and neck support is included in the turning case.

Turning the patient using a turning case and turning straps

A second bed is required. This is prepared with a number of pillows arranged on top of the mattress to receive the prone patient in the turning case.

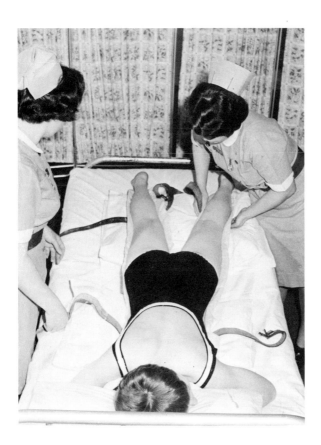

Fig. 30.9   (c) Patient rests on anterior turning case.

The turning case is placed on top of the patient in his plaster bed; this is strapped on to the patient with strong leather, buckled straps arranged around the trunk and both legs (Fig. 30.9a), so that the patient is firmly held between the plaster bed and the turning case.

A lifting team (at least four, depending upon the size of the patient) lifts the patient clear of the plaster bed stand, transfers him to the second bed (which is placed alongside), and turns the turning case, patient and plaster bed over on to the previously arranged pillows. When the turning straps and plaster bed are removed, the patient rests in the prone position on his anterior turning case.

31

The Paraplegic Patient

Definition

Paraplegia means paralysis of the lower limbs. The extent of paralysis in a patient is related to the level at which the spinal cord is cut, crushed or diseased. The nearer the lesion is to the brain on the spinal cord, the greater is the extent of the paralysis. If the spinal cord is affected in the neck, paralysis of all limbs and the trunk will result; this is known as tetraplegia. Most of the contents of this chapter apply equally to the tetraplegic patient and the paraplegic patient.

Relevant applied anatomy and physiology

The brain and spinal cord, with their coverings, constitute the main control centres of the body. They are composed of nervous tissue which is sensitive, soft and vulnerable to damage. Therefore they must be protected in a special bony and membranous covering.

The bony protection is provided by a cavity situated inside the skull and vertebral column which is entirely surrounded by hard bone which is sufficient protection from the normal stresses and trauma which will be applied to the body in everyday activities. Even a hard blow to the head or back will not usually affect the enclosed nervous tissue. Extreme force will, however, breach this defence.

The spinal cord is the trunk of nerve tissue which provides communication between the brain and the remainder of the body. It contains the pathways by which nerve impulses are conveyed from brain to muscles, blood vessels, viscera and skin; from muscles, tendons and joints to the brain in the reverse direction. Interruption of these pathways means that there is no communication between the structure at each end of each pathway.

As the peripheral pathways (peripheral nerves) leave the spinal cord at the first convenient point adjacent to the part they serve they will only be

543

involved in a lesion of the cord if that lesion occurs above the point where the relevant spinal nerve leaves the spinal cord. It follows therefore that the lower down the lesion in the cord, the less the disability which results, and the higher the lesion, the greater the disability will be. If the lesion is above the fourth cervical level the patient usually dies immediately. Thus, a patient with a sacral lesion will be less disabled than one with a lumbar lesion; a patient with a lumbar lesion will be less disabled than one with a thoracic lesion; a patient with a thoracic lesion less disabled than one with a cervical lesion. The level of the lesion in the particular region is also significant.

As each spinal nerve leaves the cord by two roots, one from the front and the other from the back of the spinal cord, it follows that some of the pathways from the anterior or posterior surface of the spinal cord may survive without interruption if the spinal cord is only partially transected. It is for this reason that some paraplegic patients may feel sensations in the skin and other tissues although their muscles are paralysed; the sensory pathways are intact but the motor pathways are interrupted.

Most paraplegic patients have paralysis of muscles and loss of sensation in skin, joints and bones below the level of transection of their spinal cord. They also have involvement of their urinary bladder, bowel and rectum, genital organs and abdominal wall with the problems attendant upon paralysis of these structures.

The causes of paraplegia

(a) *Traumatic*

1 *Road transport accidents.* Today road transport accidents are responsible for the greatest percentage of paralysed patients.

2 *Industrial accidents.* To miners, dockers and building workers, either by crushing injuries due to heavy weights falling on them, or by the worker falling from a height.

3 *Sporting accidents.* Such as a fall from a horse, or swimmers high diving into water too shallow to receive them.

4 *Accidents in the home.* Such as falling down a flight of stairs.

(b) *Non-traumatic.* Such cases are rare but may be classified as follows:

1 *Congenital.* Myelomeningocele and spina bifida. The infant is born with a defect both in the theca and the spinal cord.

2 *Deformities.* Severe scoliosis and kyphosis (see Chapter 18), caused either by congenital or acquired lesions which may progress to paraplegic unless effectively treated.

3   *Degenerative conditions.* Multiple sclerosis; scarring and fibrosis of various areas in the central nervous system.

Transverse myelitis; a section of the cord is destroyed and replaced by scar tissue probably because of a virus infection.

(c) *Infections.* Tuberculosis can affect the central nervous system. It may take the form either of tuberculous meningitis (inflammation of the meninges) or Pott's paraplegia (pressure on the spinal cord due to the presence of the products of a tuberculous abscess).

(d) *Vascular.* Arteriosclerosis may affect the spinal cord; it takes the form of progressive ischaemia until the spinal cord dies and its nerve fibres are replaced by a special type of fibrous scar tissue called gliosis.

Bleeding into the substance of the cord may also occur; this may be caused by trauma or disease.

(e) *Neoplasm.* Primary tumours may occur either in the membranes or the bone surrounding the brain and spinal cord, resulting in compression and constriction of the cord.

Secondary tumours from carcinoma elsewhere in the body may arise in the vertebrae and in other tissues adjacent to the spinal cord.

Relevant first aid. See Chapter 10.

Results of damage. Early: Spinal shock may be the immediate result of damage to the spinal cord. All the segments of the cord below the point of injury cease to function. The urinary bladder loses its power to contract and skin sensations cannot be felt. The muscles receiving a nerve supply from that segment cannot be moved and are flaccid and flabby without muscle tone. The rectum and sexual organs are also similarly affected but priapism may occur in the early stages after cord transection.

Spinal shock is often transient and a degree of recovery or sometimes even complete recovery may occur if there has not been significant permanent damage to nerve cells.

Later: After recovery from spinal shock, any paralysis remaining is permanent and residual. Although optimism is the keynote of paraplegic management, the attitudes of the patient and his relatives must be directed towards acceptance of the existing paralysis of the patient, and modification of his way of life to meet the new situation. Some recovery does occur much later in a few patients, but this is not a common occurrence.

Problems of paraplegia and tetraplegia

Classification
Pain.
Spasm.
Respiratory failure, acute or chronic.
Loss of urinary control.
Urinary infection.
Loss of bowel control.
Constipation.
Loss of sexual function.
Loss of sensation.
Vulnerability to burns and other injuries.
Pressure sores and decubitus ulcers.
Loss of movement in limbs.
Psychological distress.
Loss of occupation and earnings.

Pain. Pain will usually be the result of the initial injury. A later serious problem, however, is 'root pain' which is due to irritation of the affected nerve roots. This does not affect all patients but is a great trial to those it does affect. It presents serious problems for the doctor responsible for the patient, as the drugs provided must be carefully chosen in the light of the other problems of paraplegia. Pain is worse when the patient's mind is unoccupied. Games, handicrafts, interests and work all help to alleviate pain.

Spasms. Once the segment of the cord below the point of transection has recovered from spinal shock, it functions in a normal way but, being detached from the brain it can receive no instructions by the normal pathways and works independently. One pathway which is broken normally inhibits the reflex arc. This is a local phenomenon of muscle contraction dependent on a segment of the cord and a set of muscles. It uses the spinal nerve as a connecting link (see Chapter 16, p. 245, and Fig. 16.2). The absence of inhibition from the brain means that the reflex arc acts independently, erratically and with minimal stimulation. Thus, irritation of the skin, or a full bladder, constipation or emotion can cause the paralysed limbs of the patient to contract forcefully (Fig. 31.1). The contractions are usually accompanied by rhythmical shaking of the affected limbs.

Apart from the inconvenience for the patient and his attendants, such spasms may result in sores as the skin of the limbs is rubbed against the opposite limb and on other surfaces.

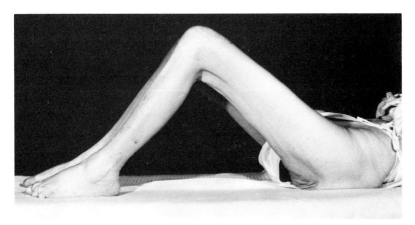

Fig. 31.1   Flexion contractures.

Because the reflex arc is intact, the muscles of the limbs do not waste so much as in paralysis due to peripheral nerve lesions; muscle tone is present and is usually excessive. Treatment of this problem may take the following forms:

1   Relieving the cause of the spasm if it can be found. Distension of bowel or bladder are obvious examples.

2   Nursing measures to hold the affected limbs and prevent them going into spasm.

3   Physiotherapy: Applications of heat and massage to the affected muscles; passive movements to prevent contractures of joint capsules and muscles.

4   Surgical means such as tenotomy, neurectomy or interruption of the reflex arc.

Respiratory failure—Acute. Soon after the injury, the patient may have difficulty in breathing if the level of his lesion is high enough up the spinal cord to involve the thorax. Later, an ascending paralysis may increasingly affect the chest and even the diaphragm. Regurgitation of stomach contents may also occur as part of the initial injury with inhalation of the vomit from the mouth.

Chronic. Efficient coughing requires the full use of the abdominal and thoracic muscles. If the abdominal walls are paralysed it is difficult for the patient to expel air from the thorax and secretions from the trachea and bronchi.

In patients with any paralysis of the abdomen, diaphragm or thorax, breathing is inefficient and mucous secretions gather in the bronchioles and obstruct respiratory efforts still further. Such patients are liable to chest infections.

Help may take the following forms:

1 Careful observation of patients with cervical lesions. They must not be left unattended, particularly during the acute stages.

2 The use of mechanical ventilators for patients with a cervical lesion.

3 Tracheostomy to assist the intermittent positive pressure ventilation provided by a mechanical ventilator, and to help evacuation of the respiratory passages by suction.

4 Assisted coughing; the nursing or physiotherapy staff apply pressure to the thorax and abdomen of the patient to help. Later, if possible, the patient compresses his own abdomen during coughing.

Urinary problems. During the phase of spinal shock, urine is at first retained in the urinary bladder which distends. When the limit of distension has been reached, the urine overflows, resulting in passive incontinence. This may last for a few hours or some days.

When the detached segment of the spinal cord recovers and is able to resume its activity, the bladder may return to the primitive ('reflex') function present in the young infant; in this state it contracts and empties as its walls are stretched. This creates an intermittent complete evacuation of urine. The management of the patient's condition may include training the patient to estimate the intervals between emptying so that he may arrange a toilet programme. Many patients learn to evacuate the bladder when they desire to do so by compressing the pubic area of the abdomen with the hand.

A major problem for every paraplegic or tetraplegic patient is the possibility of infection of the urinary tract with resultant serious illness. Until recently, urinary infection and resulting renal failure was the most common cause of death in paraplegics. Management of these urinary problems is discussed more fully later in this chapter.

Bowel problems. As a result of division of sensory tracts the patient is unaware of the contents of his rectum. Additionally, the absence of muscle tone in the bowel and rectum retards normal colonic actions and slows the normal forward movement of faeces and flatus.

Distension of the abdomen, digestive distress and constipation are paraplegic problems. These are discussed fully later in the chapter (p. 559 *et seq.*).

Loss of sexual function. Paralysis of the genital organs means that normal sexual function is not possible. The female paraplegic patient may become pregnant however. This inability to reproduce and the probability of remaining unmarried are causes of major psychological distress in many younger male paraplegic patients.

Intrathecal injection of pilocarpine can cause seminal emission in a paraplegic male. If he is married and his wife wants a child this is one way of achieving fertilization.

Loss of sensation and skin function. The paralysed patient with damage to the sensory nerves or tracts will have no sensation in the skin of the affected parts. This creates problems of temperature regulation for the patient as well as making him unaware of danger from burning or other hazards to his person. Such hazards as fires, radiators or exposure to severe cold with frostbite are to be avoided.

Related to this is the problem of poor muscle and skin tone. Prolonged unrelieved pressure on the tissues may not be felt and will result in the breakdown of the skin with necrotic ulceration, ultimately progressing to deep craters if untreated. Infection and anaemia may increase the problem.

The patient must be on his guard to prevent decubitus ulcers for the rest of his life.

Loss of normal mobility. This problem creates severe frustration for the patient who cannot now do the things he could before his accident. This is most serious in a person who was used to leading an active life in sports and other activities: it calls for major mental and physical readjustment in all patients. In addition, the loss of mobility causes osteoporosis and a high renal excretion of calcium with a tendency to form urinary stones.

Psychological distress. In the initial phase of paralysis the patient will not accept that he will never walk normally again; when he sees others who are paralysed, he thinks, 'I am different—it could not happen to me, *I* am going to recover.' Later, when his position becomes more obvious, he develops a severe mental depression. On recovery from this he may accept his lot and adapt to his new way of life.

The medical, nursing and physiotherapy staff must help him through the various stages of progression and create the optimism he requires for his rehabilitation. It is better if he is gently introduced to the inevitability of his state by graduated stages—a little information at a time.

Loss of occupation and earnings. A problem for any person who can no longer perform the work he has been trained to do is loss of earnings and thus dependence on welfare funds, compensation, or charity. A vigorous retraining and re-employment regime is undertaken for the paralysed person and many return to earning their living and paying income tax; but many do not.

The desire to earn and continue to support his family may provide the motivation to work for early rehabilitation.

Hospital management

The survival and rehabilitation of the paraplegic patient is more likely to occur in Spinal Injuries Units with teams of experienced specialist workers to care for him. The fastest possible means should be used to transfer the patient; the ideal is by helicopter or ambulance collection from the scene of the accident and direct admission to the spinal injuries centre. For relevant first-aid management see Chapter 10.

In the Spinal Injuries Unit the special equipment and accommodation required for spinal injuries patients is centralized.

Aims of management
The principal aim is to rehabilitate the patient in order that he may live in normal home surroundings and to take up an occupation with minimal dependence on others. These aims are ideals; many patients achieve them but others do not. There are many complications to be avoided. The end results of treatment depend upon the intelligence and motivation of the patient. To assist him in his rehabilitation the consistent efforts of skilled and conscientious members of the Spinal Injuries Unit are required.

Immediate treatment. In the period immediately following admission to the unit the patient will be ill—not only with his spinal injury but often with additional trauma to other parts of his body. Severe limb, abdominal, thoracic or cranial injuries may be present; there may be severe loss of blood; most certainly the patient will be shocked and bewildered. The injuries, other than the spinal injury, must be treated concurrently. The morale of the patient must be maintained and the attitude of his nursing team is related. There must be no disgust, revulsion or useless pity; the patient must be treated as a person—as should any patient. High standards of personal hygiene and grooming are important and must not be allowed to lapse, otherwise the patient will become dejected or ashamed. His mode of address by his proper name, Mr. —, is also essential.

The patient's bed. A conventional hospital bed is used with additional pillows or sorbo rubber pads. These pillows are used, (a) to roll the patient in turning; (b) to prevent pressure on bony prominences and (c) to adjust the patient in the desired position. A bed cradle, a bracket to support the urine receiving bag and a firm supporting pad for his feet which will maintain his ankles at a right angle are extra requirements. Electrically operated turning beds are also available (Fig. 31.2). A stryker bed is sometimes used.

The Egerton-Stoke Mandeville bed which turns the patient from side to side by an electric motor is an excellent way of treating any spinal patient (Fig. 31.2a). For tetraplegics or patients who already have sores, a similar bed with padded sides is useful (Fig. 31.2b).

The clothing. In the early management of the patient he is nursed without clothing. This is the most convenient way during the period of intensive care as otherwise bladder, bowel and thoracic management would require constant undressing and re-dressing of the patient if he was clothed.

The position of the patient. The patient's position is altered by a steady relentless routine of two-hourly turning. Each turn is charted and is carried out at exactly the time stated—that is every two hours, both night and day. A nursing team of sufficient numbers must be provided to maintain this routine in every spinal injuries unit. The method of turning is described in Chapter 10, p. 160. Once the turning routine is established the patient will wake automatically and, if he has the use of his arms, will eventually be able to turn himself as rehabilitation progresses.

In the interim period and whilst waiting transfer to a spinal injuries unit from the initial hospital, probably the greatest contribution the nursing staff can make is to commence and establish a turning routine for the patient. If turning is not carried out, or even if missed for one routine, pressure sores will occur.

The positions used are standard (see Figs. 31.3 and 31.4) and are considered the least likely to result in fixed deformity or pressure sores. The positions also contribute to the reduction of muscle spasm.

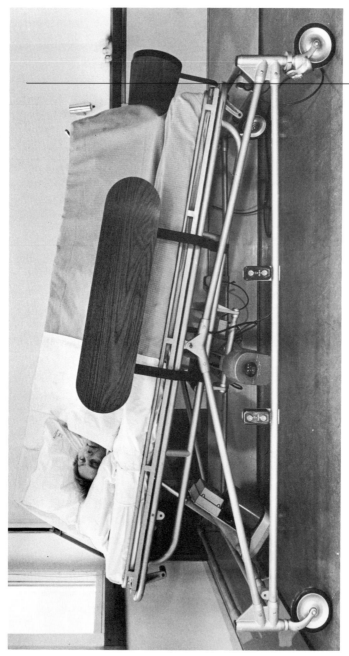

Fig. 31.2 (a) The Egerton-Stoke Mandeville Tilting and Turning bed shown in the turn position and in addition with the head tilting downwards. These beds will turn a patient on to either side to a maximum angle of 70 degrees and in addition will tilt the patient head or feet down by 15 degrees. The head and foot boards, supplied with each bed, may be arranged one at each end, one at each side, or both on the same side or in any combination of these arrangements.

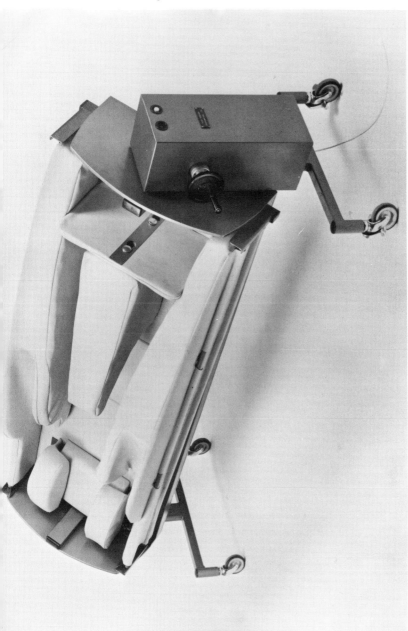

Fig. 31.2   (b) The Steeper Mini Co-Ro Bed. The bed is driven by electric motors which move the patient through an arc from one side to another in constant motion, the complete cycle of movement taking four minutes. Thus stasis cannot occur in any part of the patient. This contributes to the prevention of decubitus ulcers (pressure sores), renal calculi and pulmonary oedema. (By courtesy of Hugh Steeper (Roehampton) Ltd.)

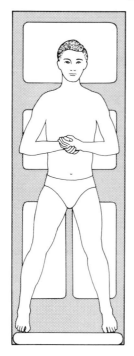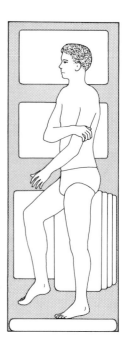

Fig. 31.3   Method of placing pillows around patient to prevent pressure sores
and deformities.

The management of the patient nursed on a
Steeper Mini Co-Ro bed (Fig. 31.2b)

The Steeper Co-Ro bed arranges a continuously changing attitude of the
patient's body to gravitational forces by a device which constantly moves
the patient and his mattress frame from one side to the other through an
arc moving 55 degrees each way. This means that a smaller nursing team can
manage the patient without the constant need for a manual turning routine.
It is particularly useful in managing heavy patients.

The patient is prevented from sliding off the bed by upholstered side
supports. The mattress and other supports are all covered by washable
p.v.c. cloth.

Preparing the bed and installing a new patient

1   With the bed level, remove all the upholstery with the exception of the
mattress, head pieces and bed pan cushion (check that hatch underneath is
closed and bolted.)

2 Loosen and slide inner thigh support tubes towards the foot end of their slots.

3 The bed can now be covered in one of three ways.

(a) Using disposable tissue sheets, lay some down the centre of the bed, wrap one around the bed pan cushion and some down each side for the legs if necessary, keeping clear of the slots in the mattress.

(b) Use draw sheets, folded so that one extends from the head and under the head pieces down to the beginning of the bed pan hatch. Wrap the bed pan cushion in a small piece of sheeting or disposable tissue, and another two sheets (one for each leg) folded and laid either side of the slots in the mattress.

(c) Fit suitably cut and tailored sheets as necessary.

N.B. Tuck in sheets and smooth out wrinkles and folds as much as possible.

4 Position pillow (wrapped in pillow case if desired) between head supports.

5 Adjust headpieces, side support brackets at head end and foot end outwards.

6 Lift the patient onto the bed. Position centrally and with the buttocks in the region of the bed pan hatch. Ensure that the shoulders are clear of the head support edges, i.e. a thickness of a hand should be sufficient. Put legs in the astride position and the arms across the body.

7 Fit foot board to inner thigh support by sliding the keyhole slots over the aluminium buttons. Position inner thigh support in tubes and slide thigh support up the bed until the feet are supported in a natural position. Tighten hand nuts under the bed.

IMPORTANT. Fit foam pads under lower leg to relieve pressure between heels and mattress.

8 Fit urine drainage tube, passing the tube through the slot nearest to the bed pan hatch and attaching tube and urine bag, to hooks provided underneath the bed.

9 Fitting *one side at a time* offer up the side supports to the side support brackets, sliding the tube ends down the channels provided. Push the side support in towards the patient until a firm but comfortable pressure is applied. Commencing at the head end, adjust the head support inwards to touch the ears and tighten nut with spanner provided and then lock foot end. Repeat the same procedure with the other side support.

If the patient is correctly placed in the centre of the bed, an equal amount of the support brackets will protrude either side of the bed.

Place the patient's arms in the side support channels if low sides are fitted. Cover the patient with a blanket.

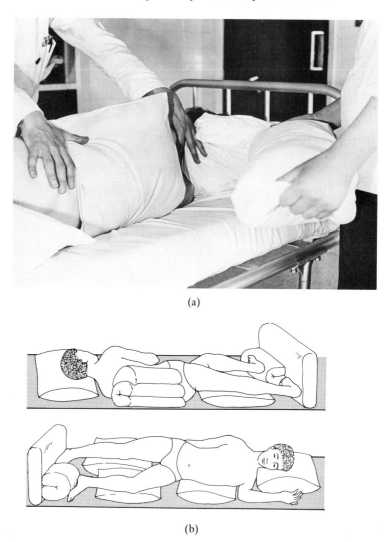

(a)

(b)

Fig. 31.4 (a) and (b) Method of placing the pillows when turning the patient to the lateral position.

Making sure that there are no obstructions in the way of the bed, i.e. chairs and bedside cabinet, the bed and patient are now ready and the bed can be switched on.

After a few rolls each side check whether any further adjustment is necessary.

Note. The correct supporting of the patient in the bed is the most important factor. If excessive side-play is allowed, i.e. slipping from side to side, a friction sore will be caused.

With certain patients, additional packing with pillows may be necessary, i.e. pillow between the legs instead of the inner thigh support, or the head pillow supplied may be too high or low. In this latter case the whole of the head support arrangement can be removed and replaced by pillows packed between the two side supports.

Note. The main side supports must always be used.

Once adjusted for a particular patient, the side support brackets and inner thigh support tubes locked, the removing and replacing of the upholstery to gain access to the patient can be achieved by anyone without altering the set-up. The main point to remember is that the patient should be adequately supported to avoid side-slip and yet not uncomfortably compressed.

Day to day use of the bed

The bed is powered by a small electric motor and therefore must be plugged into a 220–240 volt A.C. single phase supply.

The control panel is situated at the foot of the bed and consists of an ON/OFF switch, neon indicator light (to show when power is ON) and a fuse holder.

Assuming the patient is correctly installed in the bed and that there are no obstructions, switch on the bed and it will commence to roll slowly in one direction, when it reaches an angle of $55°$ it will automatically stop, reverse direction and roll to the same angle the other way, when it will reverse again. The complete cycle takes approximately 8 minutes.

The bed should be left running as long as possible, stopping of course for feeding, toilet care, visitors, T.V. viewing and general nursing.

A manual drive handle is situated at the side of the control box. To use, switch off the motor, push the handle in towards the box, keep turning and pushing inwards until it engages, turn the bed to the required position, keeping the inward pressure on the handle whilst turning. When it is required to switch on again, the handle will disengage itself.

For general examination of the patient and feeding, the patient can be rolled slightly to one side.

For toilet care roll the bed right over to one side, open the bedpan hatch, remove bedpan cushion, position bedpan, close hatch and roll to horizontal position. When the patient has completed his toilet, the reverse sequence is carried out.

To wash the patient in the bed. Remove one side support and the inner thigh support, the bed is then turned so that the patient rests up against the remaining side support and can be turned onto his face and chest on this side support. The whole of the patient's back can be examined, washed, and wiped dry, likewise the bed.

When putting the patient in or out of the bed, remove the side support completely. At other times the side support can be lifted and then swung down.

From time to time check that the patient has not slipped up the bed to such an extent that his shoulders are touching the head supports. If this persists use bed tilt adaptors.

Note. In the event of a power failure, the bed can be turned intermittently by winding the handle every 2 to 3 hours, or as necessary, with the advantage that only one person is required and causes less disturbance to the patient.

Toilet routine. As already stated, the morale of the patient will be improved by the maintenance of a high level of personal hygiene. He will perspire heavily; be either incontinent of urine and faeces, or require help to micturate and defaecate. A daily blanket bath is necessary and the genital and anal area must be kept clean by frequent washing. Shaving, hair washing and combing, oral hygiene and manicure for fingers and toes are all good points of patient care.

Diet. In the early stages a light nutritious diet is probably all that can be achieved. The most important diet content is that of fluid. Copious intake of all forms of fluid is a necessary part of the maintenance of kidney function and the prevention of renal failure.

As the patient progresses the diet content must be increased to about 2000 calories per day. If the patient has any pressure sores and is losing serum and protein, the intake of protein must be increased accordingly.

As soon as possible, the patient with full use of the upper limbs must be encouraged to feed himself; this may be difficult whilst lying supine but it is a skill which must be acquired.

The tetraplegic patient must be fed. To ensure an adequate intake, frequent small nutritious meals are more suitable than large quantities at longer intervals. The person feeding the patient must sit down and give an unhurried impression; he need not be a nurse—visitors, relatives, voluntary helpers and non-nursing staff can all help, particularly in a unit where there are several patients who are totally paralysed.

An important content of the patient's diet is roughage. The approach to establishing a pattern of regular defaecation with minimal assistance will require an adequate amount of cellulose and cereal in the diet.

Extra protein in the diet may be provided as meat or cheese, or other dairy produce, but powdered protein may be required for some patients to ensure a large enough intake.

When some paralysis of the upper limbs exists there will be difficulty in lifting food from the plate and transferring it to the mouth. The occupational therapist will contribute by providing devices such as those shown in Figs. 31.5a and b and training the patient in their method of use.

Management of defaecation

Because the patient is unaware of the contents of his colon he cannot know when defaecation is required. The abdominal muscles and colon walls contribute to the act of defaecation and as these are completely paralysed, they do not contribute much to the act of expelling either faeces or flatus. Pressure and massage by the hands on the abdomen may be necessary. The process of evacuation of the bowel therefore depends upon a regular timed routine each day.

In the early bed-management of the patient this habit must be established and a bowel action is caused at the same time each day. Ideally, before progression to a sitting or standing position, the patient's bowel routine should have become fixed at a definite time of day.

This bowel action should ideally be a natural process which can be achieved if all the factors related are considered:

1   *The diet content.* From the earliest days of management, roughage must be included in the food of the patient;

2   *The fluid intake.* This must be higher than was previously acceptable from both bowel and urinary considerations.

3   *Accurate timing.* A time schedule means that the patient will prepare for bowel evacuation even though the patient cannot feel the contents of his bowel.

4   *An awareness of distension.* Flatus in the bowel usually means that faeces is also present.

5   *The use of vegetable laxatives.* Peristalsis is increased if a suitable laxative is provided. If the patient is having difficulties, laxatives are supplied in the evening in preparation for bowel evacuation the next day.

6   *Suitable facilities and adequate time.* At first the patient will empty his bowel onto incontinence pads, but when he can be raised from his bed to a wheelchair the ward lavatory—with an inflatable ring cushion to cover the

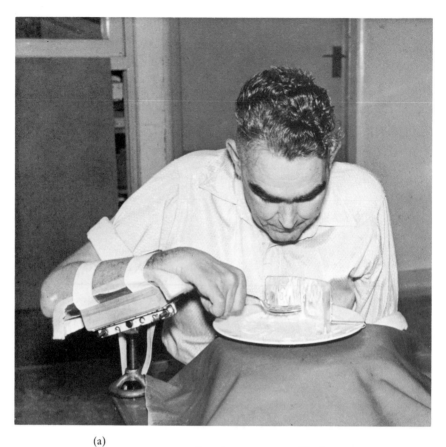

(a)

Fig. 31.5   Aids to independence
(a) Eating.
(b) Drinking.
(Hand paralysis patient managing a
drinking vessel: thumb passed
through handle of cup.)

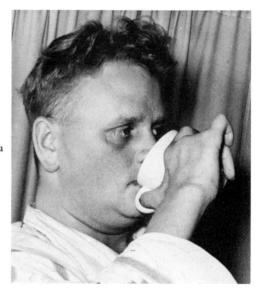

(b)

seat—must be available. This means that extra lavatories with adequate door width and cubicle width to accommodate the wheelchair must be part of the unit; suitable devices for the patient to use to transfer himself independently onto the lavatory from his wheelchair are supplied; a supporting rail attached to the wall near the washdown closet is helpful.

There must be no rush or hurry, although once the patient has established his own pattern he will require less time for the process.

7   *Suitable clothing.* Once the patient reaches independence in the lavatory, special clothing which can easily be removed is necessary.

The aim is that the patient will pass a soft malleable bowel content with minimal difficulty at a set time each day.

Constipation

Either constipation or diarrhoea are a problem for the patient. Constipation may be dealt with:

1   By the provision of a *laxative*.

2   By the use of a *laxative suppository* thirty minutes prior to the anticipated time of defaecation. In the early training the suppository must be used routinely.

3   *Enemata.* This is less desirable than the suppository because it may cause prolonged and repeated small bowel evacuation instead of a single movement. The small disposable enemata are preferable. When the faeces are hard and impacted three hundred ml of arachis oil or olive oil may be inserted thirty minutes prior to the purgative enema.

4   *Manual interference.* This is the least desirable method as it tends to dilate the anus and rectum so that any tonus in the muscle is lost. It must only be used as a last resort.

A lubricated rubber gloved finger is inserted into the bowel and any scybala are helped out with the crooked finger.

There is a danger that if constipation is not noted and reported and no action is taken, that the patient may become obstructed, requiring advanced surgical assistance to overcome the problem.

Charting of bowel action time and amount is necessary for the bed patient.

Urinary management

The excretion of urine from the body is necessary to maintain the normal chemical composition of the blood which is essential for health. Reduction of, or serious alteration in urine excretion results in a progressive increase in the blood stream of the organic wastes which should have been discarded from the body.

Management of the paralysed bladder and sphincters is essential for the patient's survival. When controlled and adequate excretion of urine has been established, the patient's general condition improves; he feels more socially acceptable and is capable of greater mobility.

The aims of urinary management

The patient should ideally be capable of expelling urine at a time and place which suit him. The next alternative is the wearing of a receptacle, hidden within his clothing, which is emptied when convenient (Fig. 31.6).

Early urinary management. During the phase of spinal shock, for the first forty-eight hours after the injury, there is no reflex activity of the bladder. The bladder neck is constricted; the walls lack tonus and the bladder becomes dilated by the increasing urine content. In a thin patient, the anterior abdominal wall is pushed outwards by the distended bladder and the swelling is visible as a protuberance. Such distension will take some hours to occur as the production of urine is inhibited by the spinal shock.

The bladder must be emptied by catheterization before becoming over-distended (see Fig. 31.6); otherwise the walls of the bladder will become over-dilated and back pressure along the ureters towards the kidneys will occur.

Later management of the urinary bladder. When spinal shock has passed, bladder retraining can begin. There are some conflicting views on the methods of achieving retraining and the wishes of the doctor in charge of the patient or the consulting urologist must be carried out.

Intermittent catheterization. The catheter is removed and re-inserted as the bladder fills, usually at approximately eight hourly intervals.

Intermittent catheterization requires a devoted nursing staff who will catheterize the patient regularly every eight hours with full surgical asepsis as in the operating theatre. If this high standard is not possible, continuous drainage through a thin plastic tube into a closed sterile container (Gibbon catheter) is an excellent method, but care must be taken that the tube is not blocked by mucus.

A large bore rubber catheter inevitably causes irritation of the urethra, infection, ulceration and stenosis.

It is necessary to regard the urinary bladder as a passive bag which requires the help of gravity for complete emptying. When the patient is supine there is often a quantity of stagnant urine remaining after emptying which may become infected. Turning the patient into the prone position will expel the residual urine.

Each patient presents different problems, but all require rigorous asepsis. When frequent insertion of a catheter must be carried out, there can be no lapse in the levels of asepsis by those responsible. Half measures will not do; the techniques used must be of the same aseptic standard as those used in the operating theatre; ideally the catheter should be inserted in an operating theatre reserved only for this purpose.

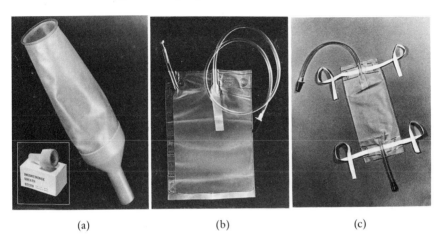

(a)   (b)   (c)

Fig. 31.6   (a) Incontinence sheath. (b) and (c) disposable urine bags.

Urinary infection

The patient with a urinary infection can be very ill. Apart from the local signs of an infected bladder and foul-smelling, turbid, flocculent urine, the patient will demonstrate all the symptoms of any generalized infection: he feels unwell, loses his appetite, has nausea and may vomit, looks feverish and has a raised temperature, pulse and respiratory rate, and may be irritable and confused. Irrational atypical behaviour is often the first sign that something is wrong.

If the patient's urinary tract becomes infected his progress towards rehabilitation will be seriously retarded; reflex automatic bladder control may not be possible. However, good nursing techniques can prevent infection.

The complications of urinary infection.
1   Pyelonephritis.
2   Urinary failure.

3 Inflammation of the ureters, urinary bladder and urethra with scar tissue formation and strictures.

4 Epididymo-orchitis occurs as the infection tracks along the vas deferens to the testicles of the male.

5 Generalized illness.

6 Secondary infection elsewhere in the body.

Catheters.

(a) *Red rubber catheters of the Jacques, Harris or Tiemann's type.* Such catheters are of value in intermittent catheterization—that is, the catheter is taken out of the urethra as soon as the procedure is completed. They are not suitable for fixing in the bladder as indwelling catheters, as they tend to irritate the lining of the urethra.

(b) *Latex rubber catheters of the balloon type.* These catheters offer a wide lumen for drainage when large amounts of debris are present. The balloon is inflated within the bladder with 5 mil saline and this protuberance serves to hold the catheter inside the urethra. The latex rubber is less irritating than red rubber.

(c) *Fine plastic catheters of the Gibbon type.* These are of much smaller external circumference than the lining of the urethra and are less likely to irritate or compress the lining. They are held onto the penis of the male or strapped to the medial side of the thigh of the female, using waterproof zinc-oxide plaster. They are ideal provided the urine does not contain debris as they can easily become blocked.

Hygiene of the patient with an indwelling catheter. The genitalia of either the male or female patient must be maintained scrupulously clean at all times. Thorough washing of these parts at least twice daily or when they become soiled is necessary. When an excessive amount of pubic hair is present this should be clipped.

Devices for collecting urine from the ambulant patient. There are several excellent devices for collection of urine into a portable receptacle available for the male patient (Fig. 31.6) but the female genital organs are not suitably shaped for the attachment of devices to facilitate urinary drainage. It may be necessary to help the incontinent female paraplegic patient by surgical means as described in the next paragraph, although some female patients manage with an indwelling catheter.

Ileal loop bladder for the female paraplegic patient. The female patient is provided by surgical means with an artificial bladder formed from a detached segment of the small intestine. The two ureters are detached from their lower insertion into the bladder and re-attached to the loop of intestine; this loop opens onto the anterior abdominal wall in a similar fashion to a colostomy or ileostomy opening. Thus the urinary bladder is by-passed and no urine passes through the urethra. A device can now be attached to the anterior abdominal wall to receive urine and keep the patient dry. This operation is specially useful if there is chronic incurable bladder infection.

Hygiene of the receptacles. As these receive urine they soon become fetid and smell badly unless properly cleaned. The patient must have at least two and preferably three. The reserve urinal is cleaned carefully with detergent and antiseptic, dried, and hung up to allow air to reach the inside.

An essential factor for the self esteem of the patient is the knowledge that the receptacle is reliable and will not let him down.

Surgical resection of bladder-neck. At a later stage if good emptying of the bladder is not achieved per urethra, resection of the bladder neck may be necessary. Long continued urinary obstruction is inevitably fatal. In the male, incontinence is better than obstruction.

Rehabilitation

The rehabilitation of the patient is the function of a large team who are specialized in the care of paralysed patients.

The medical staff

In addition to the medical officer directly in charge of the unit in which the patient is nursed, help may be required from consultants who have other special skills: neurology, radiology, orthopaedics, urology, gynaecology, general medicine, general surgery and psychiatry are some of the specialist fields which may be needed for the paralysed patient.

Physiotherapy

Efficient rehabilitation of paralysed patients is unlikely without the help of skilled and conscientious physiotherapy staff. They are part of the team who are essential for the intensive care of the patient on his admission and they must work for him right through to his return to his home.

There are so many aspects of physiotherapy care of the paralysed patient that they are best classified in list form:

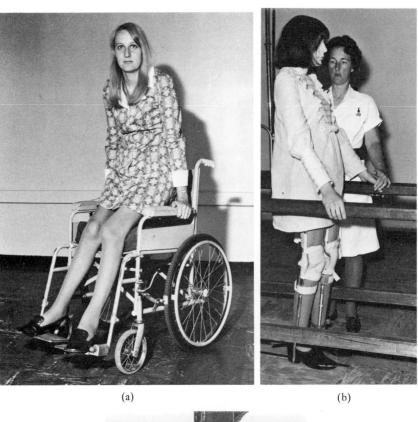

(a)   (b)

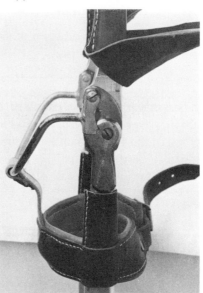

(c)

Fig. 31.7 Exercises for the paraplegic patient. (a) Patient demonstrating
'press-ups'. (b) Patient walking with calipers. (c) Locking device on knee-
hinge of calipers.

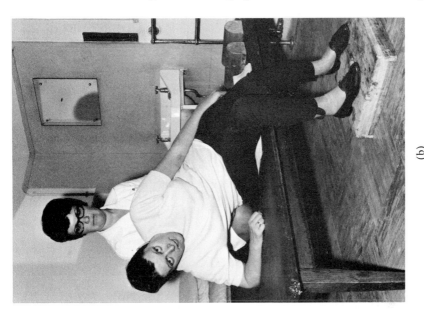

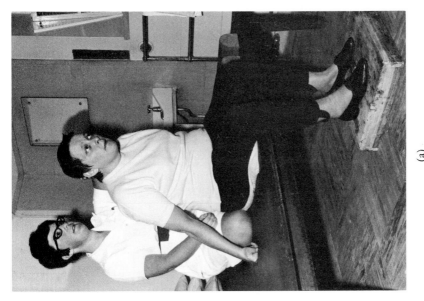

(a)

(b)

Fig. 31.8   Exercises for the paraplegic patient. (a) and (b) Regaining balance.

Early

1 Improving breathing methods of both tetraplegic and paraplegic patients.
2 Helping the patient to cough and clear the bronchioles of mucus.
3 Maintaining musculature of unparalysed muscles so as to prevent wasting.
4 Preventing contractures of muscles.
5 Preventing stiffness of joints.
6 Inhibiting excessive reflex action.

Later

Teaching methods of:

1 Transferring from bed to chair and chair to bed.
2 Transferring to and from the toilet.
3 Transferring to and from bath or shower.
4 'Press ups'; developing automatic habits in the patient who must elevate his buttocks and sacrum from his wheelchair at frequent intervals by using his arms (Fig. 31.7a).
5 Standing in calipers or a special walking frame.
6 Mobility—i.e. walking in calipers (only useful for patients with low lesions). (See Fig. 31.7b.)
7 Picking up items from the ground.
8 Wheelchair management.
9 Sports activities—netball, swimming, etc.
10 Strengthening the musculature of the pectoral girdle.
11 Regaining balance (Fig. 31.8).

All these activities are related to the patient's ability to balance himself without the use of the lower limbs. This is a difficult task and one of the prime functions of the physiotherapist is to establish new patterns of balancing so that the patient does not fall over.

The occupational therapist

The duties of the occupational therapist in relation to the rehabilitation of the patient frequently overlap those of the physiotherapist. They must work as a team towards the improvement of the patient. The functions of the occupational therapist may be classified as:

1 Developing the ability of the patient to use any function of the limbs and body that are not lost. Thus the patient with limited use of his hands is taught methods of grasping the knife, fork and spoon, the razor, pencil, etc. Often the equipment must be adapted to suit the patient (see Fig. 31.5), or new trick methods of using the equipment devised.
2 Retraining the patient in techniques of everyday habits. Thus methods

of fastening buttons and shoes, or putting on and taking off clothes must be taught.

3   Developing alternative hobbies and diversions for the patient. The accident may have altered everything the patient had done formerly so that previous interests can no longer be followed and others must be developed.

4   Retraining for existence outside the hospital precincts. Entering public transport or places is an ordeal which the patient must overcome both physically and psychologically.

5   Retraining for re-employment.

The social caseworker

The length of stay of a patient in a spinal injuries unit often depends on the efforts of the social caseworker. She works towards the discharge of the patient to his home and family. In the simplest terms this may mean only orientating the family to accepting a chair-bound invalid among them. In more complex terms it involves complete rehousing of the patient in a bungalow with ramps instead of stairs or steps, doors wide enough to receive a wheelchair, modified bathroom and toilet facilities, with light switches, door handles and other devices at wheelchair height.

Financially and legally there is much to be done. Money must be found for the patient's family during his hospital stay. He must not become distressed through worrying about their welfare or about debts which are mounting because of his unemployment through hospitalization. Legal advice may be needed to gain the compensation which is due to the patient from the accident and the social caseworker may help in arranging this.

A paraplegic's happiness in life depends upon his character and material circumstances. If he has enough money to build a bungalow with the special adaptations which are needed he can live a reasonable life. But if he has no money he may have to spend most of his time in a hospital or other institution. If he has the motivation and some financial help he can achieve much. If he is likely to obtain some financial compensation it is important that this should be settled as soon as possible.

The disablement resettlement officer

This worker is the liaison between the hospital, the patient's employer, government retraining centres and a new employer if one must be found. There are many situations in employment which can be found for a chair-bound person of reasonable intelligence.

Transport

A vital factor in helping the paralysed patient to enjoy a full life after re-habilitation is his transport. There are many forms of vehicle available, from conventional cars specially adapted for the disabled to simple electrically-propelled vehicles.

An adequate number of hand-propelled wheelchairs is also necessary, e.g. one light, folding transit chair; one for use at home and one for use at work.

Mobility

The ability to drive and possess a car makes a vast difference to a disabled person's happiness. In England patients who 'cannot walk or are virtually unable to walk' are entitled to a mobility allowance. Unfortunately the interpretation of 'virtually unable to walk' is variable and ambiguous and some patients who previously had invalid cars now have no help.

32

Amputations and Prostheses

Amputations of the leg

Indications for amputation
An amputation may be indicated for a number of different reasons:
1 To improve the patient's general health.
2 To improve function.
3 To improve appearance.
4 To free the patient from pain.
5 To prolong his life.

Amputation is a drastic and irrevocable step; nevertheless, a well-judged amputation can make a big contribution to a patient's life and although a limb should never be amputated lightly, it is probable that there is still a tendency for amputation to be delayed too long. If one considers the above reasons in more detail, the conditions for which the surgeon advises amputation will become clearer.

1 *Health.* If there is chronic infection of a limb, and especially of the bones, then in time this infection will have adverse effect on the kidneys and liver and may even lead to amyloid disease. Therefore, if the chronic infection cannot be eradicated by widespread local excision of bone, or if such an extensive local excision of bone would impair the use of the limb till it was inferior to an artificial limb, amputation should be advised. This, of course, does not mean that every patient with chronic osteomyelitis which cannot be cured should have an amputation; there are many patients with a small persisting sinus or with occasional recurrences of infection who remain in good health for many years with a reasonably efficient limb, but it does mean that, at the first sign of impairment of general health, for example, chronic anaemia or evidence of chronic nephritis as manifested by the appearance of casts in the urine or a high blood urea, amputation should be seriously considered. Usually the improvement in general health is very striking.

Naturally, conservation of an arm is more important than conservation of a leg.

2   *Function.* In the case of the lower limb, an efficient prosthesis can be provided for almost any level of amputation, and indeed, with a below-knee prosthesis, the patient can take part in many varied activities, including sports. In any limb which has been severely damaged either by injury or disease, or if there is a severe persisting limitation of function, the question whether or not the patient would be better off with an amputation and a prosthesis must be considered. For instance, for certain occupations the combination of a stiff knee and a stiff foot may be extremely disabling, and under such circumstances it might be wise to advise an amputation.

Clearly, very considerable experience is needed to know exactly what a given patient is likely to be able to do if he has an amputation and compare it with what he can do at the moment, and what the ultimate function of his limb may be. For instance, in certain crush injuries of the foot or lower part of the tibia, even though the extremity may be technically viable, we may know that the ultimate function will be inferior to that which the patient would have with a prosthesis. Therefore, it may be advisable to perform an early amputation, especially if the patient is unlikely to tolerate a prolonged stay in hospital and multiple operations.

Naturally, each case must be considered on its merits, but the important principle in treating any lower limb injury is to assess the likely result against the functional efficiency of a similar patient with an amputation and prosthesis. The better the prosthesis, the stronger the indication for amputation.

3   *Appearance.* Especially in girls, the appearance of a limb is very important, and whereas a man may hide a thin, short or deformed limb by trousers, a girl cannot always do so. In many cases a very short or a very thin limb may be so ugly that the girl would prefer to have an amputation and wear a prosthesis. This applies, for instance, to the deformed limbs of poliomyelitis or certain severe congenital deformities. As a general rule, it is a mistake to amputate for the sake of appearance until the girl is at least fourteen, and only then if she wants it herself. Most children, even with grotesquely deformed limbs, will tolerate the wearing of an appliance and get about quite well until they reach the age of puberty. It is important that before an amputation is performed the girl should visit an amputation centre to see what an artificial limb looks like and what she will be able to do if she has one. The success of an amputation for cosmetic purposes depends very largely on

the patient wishing to have it done and knowing what she will look like afterwards. As with function, the quality of the prosthesis is very important.

4   *Freeing from pain.* At first sight the problem of performing an amputation for intractable pain would appear to be simple, but experience shows that actually it is a very complicated question. The patient's reaction to and tolerance of pain depends on his psychological and physical constitution, and a patient who has a low tolerance to pain is more likely to develop a painful stump and to suffer from a painful phantom limb than would a more robust individual. If there is a well-defined and purely localized cause for the pain—for example, a tumour or gangrene—and the patient is mentally stable, amputation is frequently a great relief, but experience has shown that amputations for conditions such as peripheral nerve lesions or causalgia or for the painful sequelae of industrial injuries are often unsuccessful. It is as though, when such a patient has experienced pain for a number of months, certain nervous pathways become permanently sensitized and the patient continues to experience pain even after amputation and removal of the original source of the pain. In this connexion it is possible for a patient suffering from a complete traumatic paraplegia to experience unpleasant phantom limb sensations after one of his legs has been amputated.

The problem of when it is wise to advise amputation for the relief of pain is a complicated one and requires an assessment of the whole patient; a careful estimation of his personality and his usual tolerance for pain, and the relative importance of purely local and peripheral factors and central factors in the genesis of pain.

5   *Prolonging life.* At first sight it must seem surprising that this indication has been placed last, and there must be many people who would consider that the only real indication for amputation of a leg nowadays is to save life. It is true that the first indication given—namely, amputation for the sake of the patient's general health—is, in the long-term, life saving, but if we restrict the indication of amputating to save life to pathological conditions, we have to consider malignant tumours, gangrene and uncontrollable sepsis. Amputation for malignant tumours will not save life, if, as is often the case, tumour cells have already spread to other sites in the body. The optimal level of amputation for gangrene is highly debated and depends on the exact degree of circulatory impairment and the collateral circulation.

As the intention when amputating is to fit an artificial limb to practically all lower limb stumps, the exact length of the stump should be designed in close co-operation with the limb maker. Amputations through joints, e.g. the knee or ankle joint, may present problems to the limb maker because he will either have to provide a very bulky prosthesis or the artificial joints of the prosthesis will not be in the correct anatomical position. Such amputations, e.g. through-knee and the Symes' amputation, have their place; in general, the cosmetic appearance of the limb is less satisfactory than with the tibial or mid-thigh amputation and therefore these are more applicable to men than to women. In many cases the level of amputation is determined by the pathological condition, and it is true that the majority of leg amputations are either mid-thigh or upper tibial. A Symes' amputation, however, has certain advantages, especially in boys or young men, and provided the patient's circulation is adequate and the patient does not object to the rather thick ankle which the prosthesis produces, most patients with a Symes' amputation can perform rather more efficiently than with the conventional below-knee amputation.

Similarly, through-knee amputation has certain advantages, particularly in the bilateral amputee, but healing is less certain, and in peripheral vascular disease in the elderly it is not generally recommended. Nevertheless, in younger people, where there is extensive scarring of the skin in the upper tibial region which precludes the conventional below-knee amputation, it may give a more efficient stump than the mid-thigh amputation.

Figure 32.1 shows the percentage disability for amputations at different levels.

After-treatment
Although there are exceptions, it is probably safer to drain most amputation stumps for 36–48 hours because the accumulation of a haematoma at the tip of the stump may delay healing and cause breakdown of the wound. If a simple rubber drain is inserted, it is removed 36–48 hours later and it is unlikely that a haematoma will form. A more efficient and refined way of achieving the same object is to apply continual suction into a vacuum bottle to the stump for the first 48 hours through a fine polythene tube in which side holes have been cut.

In the first fortnight after amputation the most important thing is to keep the tissues at rest so that sound healing occurs as soon as possible. It is also important during this period to avoid the development of deformities such as flexion deformity of the knee, or flexion and abduction deformity of the hip. The application of a simple back splint to a below-knee amputation, with the end of the splint protruding beyond the stump, will both protect the stump from injury and prevent a flexion deformity of the knee occurring. For an above-knee amputation it may be wise to prevent a flexion deformity of the

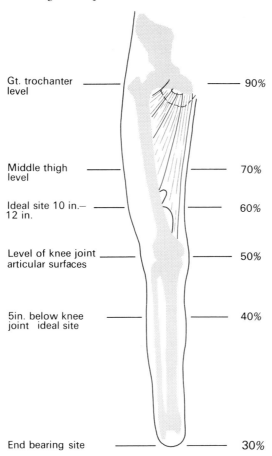

Fig. 32.1   The percentage of disability for amputations at different levels.

hip by placing a firm bandage or towel over the limb, the towel held down on each side by sandbags so that the hip is held in the extended position.

In the case of Symes' amputation, it is essential that the skin of the heel and the fibro-fatty tissues of the heel should be held in place directly under the end of the tibia. That is, it is extremely important to transfix the skin and sub-cutaneous tissue with a small Kirschner wire or a long, straight needle which goes through skin and subcutaneous tissue into the end of the bone. Recently, immediate post-operative limb fitting and early weight-bearing on a plaster of Paris pylon have been advocated. The scope and indications for this technique are still uncertain.

Once the skin is soundly healed it is time for the patient to start stump exercises and, in particular, to cultivate the movements which will be necessary in walking, and to prevent a fixed deformity occurring. At one time great stress was laid on firm bandaging in order to produce a conical stump; it is true that the stump should be adequately bandaged and that oedema of the tip of the stump should be avoided; nevertheless, tight bandaging which might interfere with the blood supply and delay healing or cause breakdown of the wound should be avoided, and a simple tubular cap of the tubigrip type, combined with proper stump exercises, will usually produce a well-shaped stump more efficiently than any other method.

The object now is to achieve a firm stump over which the patient has good control and to which a suitable prosthesis can be applied. Change in the shape of the stump continues for some three or four months after amputation and it is seldom possible to fit an adequate final prosthesis before this time. Nevertheless, it is often important for the patient that he should get up and walk about, and the fitting of a temporary prosthesis or skeletal pylon is often a great advantage, and the socket can help in moulding the stump.

Patients vary very much in their ability to learn to use an artificial limb; a child with a below-knee prosthesis requires hardly any training, but at the opposite end, the elderly person with bilateral above-knee amputations will require a prolonged period of training and will have to start to use short prostheses such as 'penguins' before graduating to full-size ones. Indeed, some elderly patients with bilateral amputations for peripheral vascular disease may never learn to use full length prostheses.

Complications

There are three main complications of amputations:

1   There may be failure of healing due either to wrong shaping of the flaps or inadequate blood supply due to the surgeon failing to assess the viability of the tissues correctly.

2   There may be recurrence of the disease, infection or neoplasm for which the amputation was performed, due to the amputation being too close to the diseased area.

3   The patient may develop a painful stump. This is a complicated problem. All patients after an amputation experience the phenomenon of phantom limb—that is, they feel as if the limb was still there. These sensations are always unpleasant, and if there is any emotional disturbance they will be interpreted as pain. To a large extent the degree of which the painful phantom upsets the patient will depend on the patient's psychological outlook, the development of outside interests, whether his attention is directed in more useful directions, and the advice he receives from his medical and nursing attendants. Occasionally, a true painful neuroma develops which

requires local treatment. In any amputation nerves must be divided, and these will form neuromata; usually, if the nerve is cut cleanly across and allowed to retract into muscles, the neuroma will not be subject to pressure and will not be a source of trouble, but if the neuroma is superficial and a source of trouble, painful impulses can often be deadened by continuous repeated percussion of the neuromatous area. If this fails it is occasionally necessary to divide the nerve at a higher level; but it should be pointed out that even this measure often fails, and repeated operations on amputation stumps are usually an indication of the patient's psychological inadequacy, and are seldom indicated.

There are a number of more infrequent complications of amputations such as persistent spasm of the limb and, in children, continued growth of bone may create a problem—for example, in below-knee amputations in children, the fibula may grow through the scar and may require resection later for this reason.

Other complications of amputation are really complications caused by wearing artificial limbs. An artificial limb subjects areas of skin to pressure which are not adapted for it. This may lead to changes such as pathological thickening of the skin, furunculosis and excessive sweating but, if the amputation has been well designed and if the artificial limb is a good fit, such complications can be avoided provided the patient gives his stump and his prosthesis reasonable care and attention.

Gait after amputation

This has been the subject of extensive study in many centres. In general, the patient expends considerably more energy in walking and has to lift the pelvis excessively in the swing phase and dips unduly in the stance phase. Above-knee amputees often need to use a stick. The aim in artificial limb making is to smooth out the gait and reduce the strain on the patient.

The Blatchford modular assembly prosthesis

This is, as the name implies, a system enabling a complete range of lower extremity prostheses to be assembled from interchangeable stock components, thereby ensuring rapid fitting and delivery. Above-knee and patella tendon bearing type below-knee limbs may be built from these interchangeable units and components to suit a full range of prescriptions. A permanent built-in alignment device, readily adjustable at the fitting stage, is incorporated in the system to eliminate the necessity for duplication of alignment when finishing the limb. This type of limb also offers the facility for changing

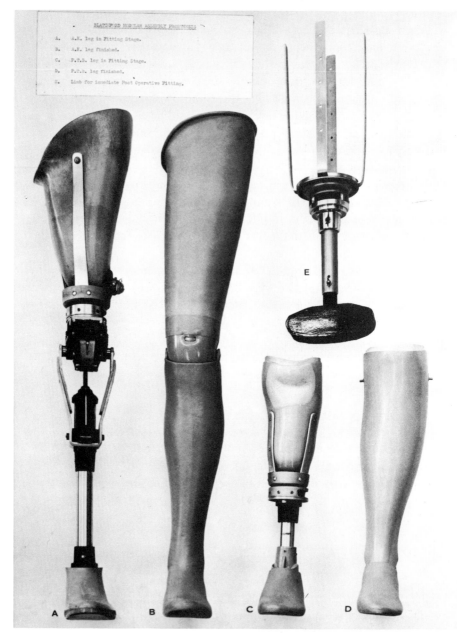

Fig. 32.2   Blatchford modular assembly prosthesis. (a) Above-knee (AK) leg
in the fitting stage, (b) AK leg finished, (c) patella tendon-bearing leg in fitting
stage, (d) patella tendon-bearing leg finished, (e) limb for immediate post-
operative fitting.

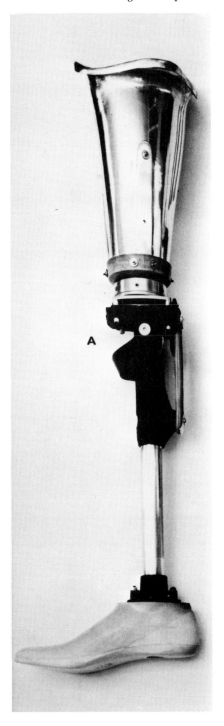

A

Fig. 32.3 Blatchford modular assembly prosthesis.
(a) Assembled limb with uniaxial knee.
(b) Socket attachment struts.
(c) Alignment device.
(d) Stabilized knee unit.
(e) Shin stirrup casting.
(f) Shin tube.
(g) S.A.C.H. foot ankle adaptor.
(h) Back check casting.
(i) Back check ligament.
(j) Internal calf spring.
(k) Wood socket attachment item.
(l) Knee mechanism with wheel type control.
(m) Pneumatic swing phase control.
(n) Uniaxial ankle.
(o) Geriatric type socket attachment.
(p) Knee mechanism with semi-autolock.
(q) Cosmetic cover for shin.
(r) Latex shin cover.

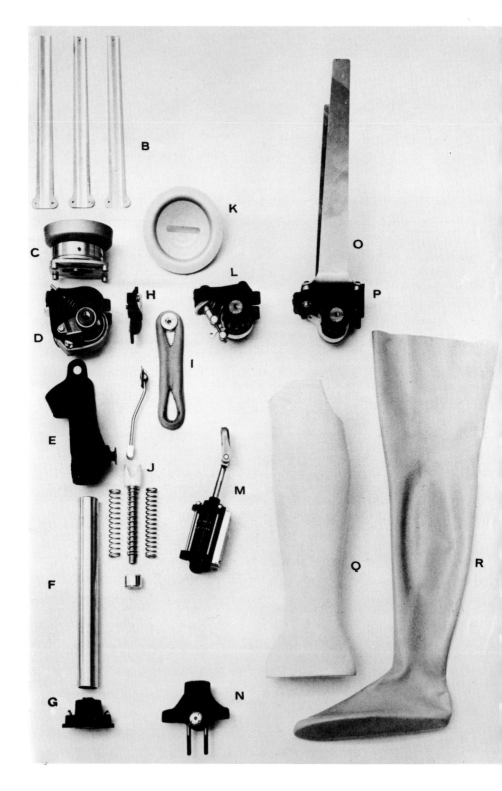

or adding to the prescribed type of control at the fitting stage by simple substitution or addition, to the benefit of the patient.

The following notes show the versatility of the system.

Socket. Any type of socket can be accommodated, i.e. total bearing, suction, or open ended sockets in plastic, wood or metal. The socket being attached by means of high strength aluminium alloy members to the 'built-in' alignment device.

Alignment device. This 'built-in' adjustment feature enables the fitter to make adjustments in the Anterior/Posterior, and Medial/Lateral plane. The device also enables independent angular adjustments of flexion, abduction/ adduction and rotation (Fig. 32.4).

Knee mechanisms. There is a large range of controls available that may be used either independently or in suitable combinations:

(a) Uniaxial knee with a *wheel type knee control,* a mechanism giving the familiar constant friction control.

(b) *Internal calf spring* (kicker spring) which when coupled with the wheel type knee control gives a simple unsophisticated control of the swing phase.

(c) Uniaxial knee with a *manual knee lock* suitable for the more active type of patient, who may require a knee lock due to the nature of his work, etc.

(d) *The Blatchford stabilized knee,* a mechanism giving full stabilizing control of the knee during the stance phase, and, also, when used on its own, providing a constant friction type of control of swing phase.

(e) *The Blatchford swing phase control,* a pneumatic device giving full control of gait at all speeds of walking, with valves controlling the overall level of activity of the unit and giving independent control of flexion and extension.

(f) *Uniaxial knee with a semi-automatic knee lock* (suitable for the geriatric patient) allowing the patient to walk with a locked knee, the lock being released to allow the patient to be seated.

Shin assembly. A structure using lightweight castings and a load-bearing aluminium alloy tube. The tube length may be adjusted to give an accurate centre of knee to ground dimension.

Foot and ankle. The system can accommodate either the standard wooden foot with uniaxial ankle joint or the *S.A.C.H.* type foot. A Metalistic foot and ankle may be substituted if required.

Cosmetic covering. The definitive limb would normally be finished with a soft foam fairing both above and below the knee. This foam fairing is in turn protected by a thin washable latex cover. This combination gives a pleasing appearance and feel to the limb. An alternative type of covering consisting of a laminated rigid foam is also available.

If it is preferred not to build the alignment device into the finished limb, adaptors are available for use with the Staros-Gardner type of alignment coupling. When these are used the limb is finished by removing the alignment coupling and duplicating the alignment.

Patella tendon bearing. This is of a similar type of construction to the above-knee limb. A conventional plastic P.T.B. socket is attached to the alignment device now located in the shin. This permanent built-in alignment device offers the fitter the same range of adjustments as in the above-knee limb. The shin, ankle and foot, and cosmetic covering are again similar to those fitted in an above-knee limb.

This type of below-knee modular prosthesis may also be used as a re-usable temporary limb for immediate post-operative fitting.

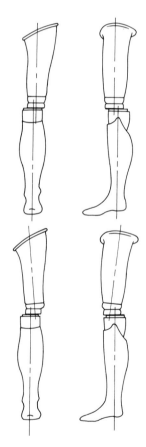

Fig. 32.4   The range of adjustments in limb with built in alignment coupling.

Included in the modular assembly range is a below-knee *immediate post-operative pylon* that has a built-in alignment coupling and adjustable length shank.

The system has been developed since 1965, when the specification was laid down by the Research Department of the Ministry of Health at Roehampton for immediate post-operative fitting techniques. One exception being the Blatchford Stabilized Knee which has been in regular supply to the Ministry of Health since January 1963. The system is currently being developed with the co-operation of the Bio-Mechanical Research and Development Unit of the Ministry of Health at Roehampton where it has undergone full structure, static and dynamic tests, as well as the normal clinical trials.

Summary

Amputation of the lower limb is, of course, an irrevocable procedure; it should never be undertaken lightly and, if possible, two experienced surgeons consult together before advising a patient to have an amputation. But, if the indications have been assessed correctly, amputation of the lower limb can lead to improvement in the patient's health, function and appearance, and amputation is still one of the most successful operations in the surgeons' repertoire.

Amputations of the arm, and artificial arms

Compared with leg amputations, arm amputations are relatively infrequent and, in particular, peripheral vascular disease, which is the most common reason for a leg amputation in this country, rarely affects the arm sufficiently severely to require amputation (in some countries, e.g. Burma, peripheral vascular disease affecting the arms is relatively common and does necessitate a considerable number of arm amputations).

The most common reasons for amputation of the arm are, therefore, for malignant tumours and crushing injuries. Again it should be noted that clean-cut injuries, e.g. the clean-cut division of arteries and veins, can usually be repaired successfully in the arm, and indeed there have been instances of restoring a completely severed hand after a clean-cut injury. This, of course, is not possible if the tissues have been damaged by crushing. In addition to surgical amputations, the whole or part of an arm may be absent due to a congenital anomaly, and these are often referred to as congenital amputations.

The problem of rehabilitating such patients is in many ways different from that of rehabilitating an adult patient who has lost an arm following surgical intervention or injury.

In addition there are instances, e.g. after an injury to the brachial plexus, where an arm is paralysed and anaesthetic, when it is advisable to amputate the arm if it has become a useless, swollen, ulcerated appendage.

Artificial arms

The arm, including the hand, is basically a sensory organ and we derive much of our knowledge of our environment through the skin of our fingers, hand and arm. In addition, the movements of our arms are very varied, unlike the somewhat automatic, repetitive and stereotyped movements of the legs, e.g. in standing, walking or running. For these two reasons the problem of providing a substitute for an arm is quite different from providing an artificial leg.

In the first instance, certainly after injury, it is wise to preserve every possible shred of tissue, and even stumps of fingers, as their sensitivity may prove of great use to the patient at a later date—indeed, many patients develop remarkable skills using even portions of their arm; for instance, they learn to hold a needle in the crook of their elbow, or to hold things between two forearm stumps, and especially when they have skin sensation such stumps, although comparatively inefficient mechanically, may be of more use to them than the best of artificial arms. In addition, the function of the two arms is rather different—the dominant arm (usually the right one) is used for movement, the other arm for holding and fixing; therefore, if the patient loses part of one arm it may still be useful for holding objects while the other arm is still able to act as the dominant one. Nevertheless, there are certain circumstances under which artificial arms are extremely useful. These may be divided into two types:

1 The conventional arm. In this the artificial arm is activated by a system of wires and pulleys attached to some other part of the body—e.g. the opposite shoulder, and by this means the patient can learn to bend the elbow of his artificial arm and grip or release objects with his artificial hand. In particular, artificial arms are invaluable for certain sports, golf or cricket, or certain hobbies such as carpentry or metal work, or for driving a car; an artificial hand for driving purposes is also often very desirable.

2 In the last few years a number of mechanized arms have been devised. These are basically of two types—firstly, those in which the power is provided by compressed carbon dioxide cylinders, and secondly, those in which the power is supplied by light electric batteries (Fig. 32.5).

The power-operated arms can be controlled either by the patient activating

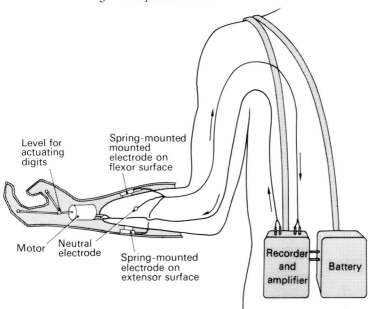

Level for
actuating
digits

Spring-mounted
mounted
electrode on
flexor surface

Motor

Neutral
electrode

Spring-mounted
electrode on
extensor surface

Recorder
and
amplifier

Battery

Fig. 32.5   A power-operated hand. This power-operated hand developed in Moscow makes use of the electric currents which are generated when a muscle contracts. These are picked up by electrodes placed on the surface of the skin, amplified, linked with the battery and converted into mechanical power by the electric motor. The motor is powerful enough to lift weights of from 4 to 5 pounds.

a switch from another part of his body, or by the stumps of fingers, or the stump of his leg; or secondly, by electric currents from the muscles of the amputated arm which can be amplified and used to activate an electric motor.

Some patients develop great skill in using such power-operated arms, but the question of control, lightness and replenishing the power source still presents certain difficulties, and, in general, one could say that for the loss of one arm, the conventional—that is, the fully operated arm, is still most useful for ordinary purposes. Nevertheless, it is likely that future development will lead to greater improvements and that power-operated arms will become of increasing importance in the future.

Figure 32.6 shows a patient with phocomelia fitted with a prosthesis which provides control of: (1) hook/shoulder distance; (2) elevation of the arm with respect to the shoulder; (3) inward and outward rotation; (4) hook rotation; and (5) prehension. Throughout all movements his hook is kept at a fixed angle to the horizontal.

In addition he is provided with separate prehension on the left side. The left arm is passive except for prehension and is used to carry the gas tank to power the right arm.

The control of the four movements are taken: two functions from each shoulder, prehension of the powered arm is from the digit, and chest expansion controls the occasional operation of the passive arm. The four principal movements of the arm are controlled on a system which ensures that the amount of movement of the arm is proportional to the amount of movement of the shoulder and because of this relationship there is an apparent extension of proprioception of the clavicles into the limb and this

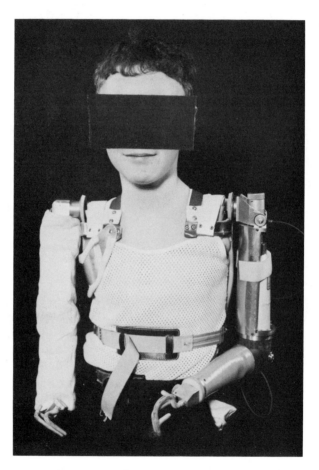

Fig. 32.6 Motivated prostheses on a patient with phocomelia. This photograph is of a boy with a single small functional digit on his right side, on his left side he does have a digit-like appendage but this is simply soft tissue and has no function whatsoever.

(a)

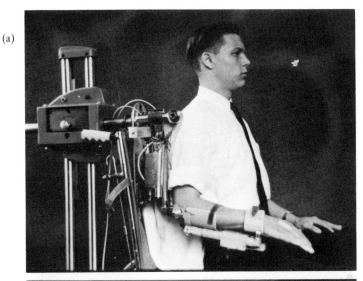

(b)

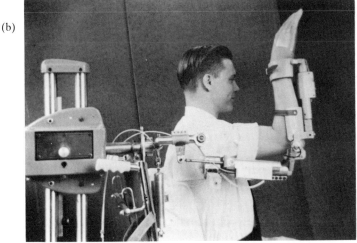

Fig. 32.7 (a) and (b) Experimental motivated limb.

system is therefore known as e.p.p. (extended physiological proprioception).

This extension of proprioception means that the use of the arm can be learnt in a matter of one or two hours and thereafter it is simply a matter of gaining experience. This is in marked contrast to other systems which rely on visual feedback for monitoring the arm's operation.

Artificial muscles

A further development is the substitution of springs for paralysed or absent muscles. There the problems are:

(a) Fixation to bone;

(b) Choosing the right alloy so that the spring does not corrode or break but still retains its elasticity, and

(c) Preventing connective tissue ingrowth which can stop movement between the coils of the spring.

Nursing management of the amputee

Pre-operative preparation

The thought and anticipation of losing a limb or part of one, excites considerable emotion in the patient and his relatives. Much help is required for them to accept the idea and both the medical and nursing staff must work to prepare the patient, his relatives and friends as gently as possible.

Amputation is often done as a secondary procedure in disease such as diabetic or vascular impairment of blood supply to the limbs; the patient is often ill as a result of the primary condition and may also be aged and frail. Careful physical assessment is therefore usually carried out before operation as special consideration must be given to the anaesthetic and drug regime of the patient.

Preparation of the skin (see also Chapter 27, p. 435). For most amputations the preparation of the patient's skin is no different to that at any other orthopaedic operation. When an ischaemic state exists, however, extra care must be taken. Clostridium welchii is the organism of gas gangrene. The ideal culture medium for clostridium welchii, in the animal body, is necrotic tissue in which the flow of blood is reduced or absent.

Careful skin preparation and bathing with thorough cleansing of skin creases in the groins, perineum and anal cleft are necessary.

A special skin preparation with povidone-iodine is recommended; this is commercially produced and is applied as follows:

Iodophor-povidone-iodine skin preparation
In the ward

1   The skin is thoroughly washed with detergent and water and then dried.

2   A compress made of several layers of surgical gauze soaked in Iodophor-Povidone-Iodine is applied to the skin and left in position for thirty minutes.

It should cover the skin over a wide area beyond the anticipated point of the incision. (See also p. 438.)

3   The skin is washed with sterile water; dried with a sterile towel and then covered with sterile cloth coverings which are fixed in position. The patient's skin is then considered to be pre-operatively prepared.

In the operating theatre

4   In the operating theatre the skin is painted with a lotion of Chlorhexidine 0·5 per cent in Alcohol 70 per cent.

Other recommendations

1   A prophylactic course of Penicillin G from the day before operation, at least 500 000 International Units intramuscularly six hourly for seven days. For patients who are sensitive to penicillin, Erythromycin is used instead; 100 mg six hourly intramuscularly, or 2 grams daily by mouth.

Post-operative care of the patient

Most amputation operations are basically similar to other forms of operation as far as wound healing is concerned. The surgeon ligates the blood vessels, drains the subcutaneous tissues and sutures the wound in a way that will provide a stump that is firm and well muscled.

Traditionally it has been considered necessary for patients with amputation stumps to be very carefully observed for haemorrhage but this is mainly a relic of the days when limbs were removed hurriedly, without aseptic technique and minimal or no anaesthesia. The modern surgeon has time and facilities to ensure that the blood vessels were efficiently tied off and only in very exceptional circumstances will bleeding from the stump occur. However, it is the usual practice in nursing to return the patient to a special amputation bed, with the bandaged stump visible on the surface of the bed, and with a tourniquet on the foot-end of the bed. Both of these may be demoralizing for the patient and consideration must be made after discussion with the surgeon, to decide if they are necessary.

Haemorrhage from the stump

Bleeding may be classified as:

(i)   *Primary*. That which occurs at the time of surgery or trauma.

(ii)   *Reactionary*. That which occurs as the blood pressure rises as the patient recovers from the anaesthetic.

(iii)   *Secondary*. That which occurs some days after operation because infection erosion through blood vessels has caused a portal of exit for the blood. This is nearly always caused by infection or gangrene of the stump.

It is for this last form of haemorrhage that the stump must be under observation so that rapid action can be taken to control the loss of blood. Therefore, patients who show the general signs of infection or have a condition that may result in gangrene on the stump are those who should be nursed with the stump exposed.

A tourniquet is a difficult implement to use in an emergency and it is not really of value in dealing with haemorrhage from a stump wound. The same principles apply as in other forms of harmorrhage and direct manual pressure on the site of bleeding over the dressings, is more effective. It should be maintained by the nurse until other help is available.

Post-operative problems

1   *Control of stump movements.* In the days following amputation the patient will not be used to the absence of the limb from the stump. He will apply the same muscle power to move the stump as he would to move a full limb. This results in sudden unpleasant jerking of the stump which may distress him. It is necessary to restrain the jerking until the patient has accepted that the limb is no longer attached to the stump. The usual method is to place a roller-towel crosswise over the stump and roll long, slim sand-bags in either end until they lie alongside the stump; thus the stump is held down by the weighted towel. As soon as possible, however, this restriction must be removed and the patient encouraged to move the joints, controlling the stump in every direction. It is unwise to permit the patient to hold the limb in one set position as the tissues may shorten and hold the limb in a flexion contracture or some other unhappy fixed position.

The physiotherapist takes an active part in teaching the patient to use the stump and make it firm in preparation for the fitting of the prosthesis.

2   *Shaping the stump.* During the operation the surgeon will devise a stump which is suitably shaped, with ample muscle tissue over the bone-end, and with the wound in a position which will avoid compression of the wound by the weight of the body against the socket of the prosthesis.

After this the nurses contribute by dressing the wound until it is healed and firm. They will apply bandages in a way that will form the stump into a shape as near to that of a cone as is possible. The cone shape is not essential, however, and the limb maker can provide a socket on a prosthesis which will accept most shapes. The bandages are replaced and made taut on the stump as often as necessary.

When ready, the physiotherapist will teach exercises to the patient which will make him use his stump and the adjacent joints in a sufficiently vigorous manner to make it a useful appendage.

3 *Gait.* Loss of a limb, particularly of a leg, produces imbalance of posture. The patient must re-learn the use of his muscles so that he can disguise his loss.

As soon as possible after the operation, the patient is provided with a pylon and encouraged to leave his bed and move about. A pylon is an appendage which is fitted with a socket for the stump at one end and a footpiece at the other; it is as long as is required to correspond to the length of the opposite limb; it has no joint at knee level. The important purpose of the pylon is to help the patient to realize that mobility is possible. When the more refined and finished artificial limb is made and ready to wear, walking with a balanced even gait is possible, particularly if the stump is long enough.

4 *Care of the stump.* The remains of the limb to which the prosthesis is fitted, must be healthy and free from tenderness or soreness. The patient is instructed either to bath or wash and powder the stump every day. A stump sock is worn over the stump and this must be changed for a clean one each day. Any sore or tenderness should be reported by the patient to his doctor; it may be necessary to leave the artificial limb off until the sore has healed.

5 *Fitting the prosthesis.* There are several ways to attach the prosthesis to the stump. The most common way is with a harness or shoulder strap passing from the prosthesis to the shoulder on the opposite side.

It is possible to attach an artificial limb by a suction device which grips the stump because of the vacuum created between stump and socket. A bung is removed from the base of the socket first; the stump is inserted into the socket so that there is a close fit between the skin and the walls of the socket; the bung is re-inserted. The stump will not leave the socket unless the bung is removed from its base. A complication of this method is that air may rush in and out at the edge of the socket and excoriate the skin of the stump, as well as causing embarrassing noises.

6 *The care of the prosthesis.* The prosthesis is precision made for the individual patient. It must be maintained in a good condition. A patient will usually have a spare artificial limb available so that one can be rested whilst

the other is worn; the second limb can also be sent away to the maker periodically for overhaul.

A child will need frequent replacement of the prosthesis to correspond to his increase in height.

7   *The general health of the patient.* The general health of a patient who is an amputee and must wear an artificial limb must be maintained at a high level. Advice must be given as follows:

(a) To avoid obesity. An increase in weight will create many problems of mobility and balance.

(b) To report to the doctor pain or stiffness in the joints of muscles of the opposite limb.

(c) To report pain or stiffness in the spine or pelvic region; this may be caused by imbalance between the length of the artificial limb and the good limb.

(d) To strive to achieve as full and normal a life as possible in spite of his disability; there are far worse disasters than loss of a limb.

Hints on the use of an artificial limb

This section has been prepared from a Ministry of Health booklet* intended for those who are being issued with an artificial limb for the first time. It does not aim at recapitulating the advice that will have been given, but rather at emphasizing certain points regarding care of the stump and of the artificial limb. It also attempts to give a general idea of how some of the common daily activities may be tackled, as well as of some of the further possibilities which lie ahead.

In the early stages in hospital the future may seem to some to be rather an uncertain quantity. Moreover, it is unlikely that the average man or woman who loses a limb will have concerned himself with the subject of artificial limbs, or know the things which those who have been fitted with limbs are capable of doing.

Reassurance comes quickly from surgeons and nurses, and the patient hears, with something like incredulity, for example, how even those with an amputation of the thigh can be taught to walk—and walk well—with a special type of limb.

* Available from the Secretary, The Research Department, Artificial Limbs & Appliances Med. 5.P.L., Roehampton House, London S.W.15.

A close accord springs up almost spontaneously in the ward and heads are put together from an early stage on how this or that problem of locomotion or adjustment can best be tackled. This grows later into a strong bond of fellow feeling among all users of artificial limbs, wherever they may meet, and contributes very largely to the ease with which the various difficulties, both physical and mental, are overcome.

There is also this further point, and it is one which concerns the inner feelings of the patient. Many experienced limb-wearers will agree—although they may not admit it openly—that they gain a certain feeling of satisfaction in learning to do things which they once may have thought they would never do again. Sometimes, too, certain faculties appear to be sharpened, perceptions and insight become keener and ambitions stronger. Indeed many have found that from what at one time may have threatened to be a calamity there grows, in some mysterious way, an actual strengthening of character. This is not to say that there are no limits to the activities that can be indulged in with an artificial limb, in a strictly literal sense, but rather that these limitations have their compensations, and further, that these compensations are of a kind of which the patient, with his growing insight into the problem, may make the greatest use.

Those who help themselves deserve the help of others, and sound advice throughout the hospital and limb-fitting periods is given on many aspects of limb-wearing. It is clear, however, that the individual problems of different limbless patients will vary considerably. Moreover, it is not until the wearer of a new limb goes out into the world that he becomes faced with many of the small difficulties of accommodating himself to the demands of everyday life. The necessity for these adjustments remains throughout life, but experience has shown that the reaction to them of the great majority of the limbless is very good. Whilst most British people are strong individualists who like to work out their own methods of doing things, the information which follows may be helpful for those who have not yet adopted or evolved their own ideas.

Instruction

Legs. Special instruction in walking is given in all limb-fitting centres and in some hospitals. The properly fitted modern leg, in the case of a below-knee amputation, will enable a person to walk so that the disability should hardly be noticed. Above-knee amputees will need to continue to bear in mind the instruction that has been given to correct the more common faults, such as allowing the leg to swing out, rising on the ball of the good foot and taking too long a step with the artificial foot. By adjusting the knee brake and elastic pick-up (if used) according to the strength of the muscles, the weight of the shoe and the speed of walking, the properly fitted limb, in the case of a mid-thigh amputation, will enable a man with practice to walk very nearly naturally. On boarding buses, or going upstairs, the sound foot goes first: on stepping off a bus or going down stairs, the artificial precedes the sound foot. When using escalators it is best to step both on and off with the sound foot first. For men non-skid crampons to prevent slipping on ice or snow are available for issue.

Arms. Owing to the numerous functions which the natural arm and hand are called upon to perform, it has always been more difficult to supply an artificial arm which will meet with as much general satisfaction as an artificial leg. Consequently, those who have lost arms are sometimes too ready to regard an artificial arm merely as something 'to fill the sleeve', and tend to concentrate on doing everything with their 'good' arm. Many appliances designed for use with an artificial arm are available to enable the artificial arm wearer to be efficient at work, to be independent in the home, and to enjoy sporting and other activities.

Some of the appliances are designed for use in a variety of ways, whilst others have been specially designed for one particular purpose. If a particular tool is habitually used in an occupation or trade, it is often possible to adapt it to be used with an artificial arm. Patients with both below- and above-elbow amputations can be taught to write well with the modern writing hand. All are advised to accept arm training.

Medical officers experienced in solving the problems met by arm amputees are at all Limb Centres, ready to advise on the appliances most suitable for individual needs. If a special appliance is required and is not already available, the possibility of designing one will be considered. Suggestions for new appliances are always welcome.

A list of the main appliances is given below. Arm amputees who would like to know more about these appliances, or who would like advice whether any particular appliance would meet their individual needs, should ask about them at the Limb Fitting Centre.

General appliances
    Split hook for left or right hand.
    Split hook (small) for children.
    Split hook push rod type.
    Variable spring operated split hook.
    'C' hook plain.
    'C' hook, 'Williams' type with link spring action.
    Plain hook, long, medium, or short for men, women or children.

Spade grip (Steeper type) adjustable for 'T', 'D', or other shaped handles, (suitable for pick-axe, sledge-hammer, hoe, rake and other agricultural tools).

Universal tool holder (functions similar to spade grip).

Ring appliance for garden or farm workers.

'A and W' type tool holder.

Saw appliance; also holds plane.

Hammer holder (with various types of adaptor).

Finger appliance (small or large).

Rubber hand (for cycling, etc.).

Other appliances for workshop, home and office use

Double or Sack hook.

Hammer, claw or ball pen type.

Quick grip pliers (Steeper types).

Pliers, long or square-nosed.

Welding rod holder.

File holder.

Knife, hooked, for pruning, lino-cutting or leather work.

Tweezer appliance, thong control or push rod type.

Nailbrush holder.

Table knife, fork or spoon.

Office appliance (prong, flat or adjustable type).

Typing appliance.

Pencil holder.

Potato holder: also useful for holding meat or bread whilst cutting.

Rubber sleeve, to fit over end of forearm to protect mechanism when washing dishes, etc.

Knitting appliance.

Darning appliance.

Postman's sorting hand.

Motoring appliance with cup in palm of hand or as a rod and ball fixed to steering wheel.

Special appliances

Picknell push rod operated split hook.

Painter's hook.

Laxton split hook (for use with McKay arms).

Golfing appliance, wrist type or clamped to club handle.

Fishing appliance and rod holder.

Dressmaker's appliance.

Telephone appliance, plain or desk type telescopic.
Radio pliers with insulated link.
Sailing appliance.
Blow-lamp holder.
Scissors appliance.
Spray-gun holder (with foot pedal if necessary for double amputees).
Axe-swinging appliance.
Heavy-duty welding appliance.
Sanding appliance.
Rifle shooting appliance.
Trumpet holder.
Violin bow holder.
Test-tube holder.
Special typing finger (to fit over index finger of hand with rigid fingers).
Glazier's appliance.
Plumber's appliance.
Book holding appliance.
Piano playing device.
Paintbrush holder.
Milking appliance.
Electric razor holder.
Baker's appliance.
Appliance for holding crutch hand grip.
Camera holding appliance.
Billiard cue holding appliance.
Bowling hand.

Appliances for double arm amputees
Toothbrush holder.
Shaving brush holder.
Hairbrush holder.
Hair comb holder.
Safety razor holder.
Drinking glass grip.
Food pusher.
Toilet appliance.
Plate clamp.

When preliminary instruction in general uses and possibilities has been given at Ministry of Health arm training schools, there are more specialized courses at Ministry of Labour and National Service training centres where particular trades may be learned. In fact, thanks to the greatly increased interest which the public and employers of labour are showing in the capabilities of wearers of artificial limbs, there is no need today for those who have been so fitted to fear that they will not be able to play an effective part in the modern world.

Dressing and clothing

Dressing. The first difficulties are soon overcome where there is an amputation of only one limb. Patients suffering from double amputations have more difficulty and although they are in most cases able to dress and undress, the time taken to do so is necessarily longer. Those who have lost both arms usually require assistance.

Where a single artificial arm is used, it should be passed through the sleeve of the jacket or other garment before the other arm.

Many wearers of one artificial leg find it easiest to dress the limb with pants, trousers and shoe before fitting it on the stump and before dressing the sound leg. Others, in order not to pass a dirty shoe through the clothes, put the shoe on last, i.e. after the leg has been passed through the clothing. Others again may find it possible to clothe the limb after it has been fitted to the stump.

In double leg amputations, both legs are usually dressed completely before fitting them on to the stumps.

Clothing. This should tend to be light in weight and loose fitting. However light the artificial limb, and however good the fit, there will always be more exertion expended in using it than there is with the natural limb, and loose-fitting clothes will give more ventilation and comfort, besides lasting longer. At the same time, flimsy material for underwear should be avoided, as this is liable to be damaged by the harness and suspenders, which are usually worn over the vest and under the shirt. Where possible, a hard-wearing material should be selected which, even though it may be more expensive to buy, will prove to be more economical in the end owing to its much longer life. For women, dresses or frocks which button or zip-fasten up the front are preferable to blouses and skirts. Extra slotting guards may be fitted if necessary and ladies' stockings can be protected by stocking guards. Ladies may also prefer to have a flock or matt finish to their limbs instead of a polished finish.

Socks. The sock on the artificial foot will wear out quickly if the shoe is a loose fit on the foot. Less damage is done to the sock if a thick sock is used underneath the outer sock. If the under sock makes the leg too bulky, the leg and ankle part of the sock may be cut off.

When buying socks it is advisable to buy more than one pair of exactly the same pattern, since if the sock on the artificial foot wears out, there are then a number of serviceable socks remaining. If a single pair of pattern socks is bought, and one sock is worn out, then the remaining sock is wasted. It is better to change the socks over from one foot to the other as often as possible to get the maximum amount of wear out of each.

Some people give up the battle of mending holes in socks altogether, and cut the feet off all the socks that they use on their artificial foot. Instead, the tops of these socks are fixed to the artificial foot with adhesive tape, just below the level of the shoe. This can be regarded as an extreme measure, however.

Sock suspenders. It may be difficult to keep these from slipping down on the artificial leg. One or two metal studs can be riveted or screwed on to the shin by the limb-makers to hold the suspender in the proper place.

Boots and shoes. Light shoes have the advantage over heavy boots or shoes. The light shoe does not add appreciably to the weight of the leg, and it gives a greater sense of security and balance in walking : also, the sole is more flexible in walking and so bends more easily with the joint movement of the artificial foot. It will be found that the shoe on the good foot will wear out far more quickly than that on the artificial foot: it will pay to have two shoes, if possible, for the good foot, to one for the other. It will also add to comfort if the shoe of the artificial leg is kept in good repair and not allowed to get worn down at the heel. Women with amputations above the knee should decide the height of heel of shoe they intend to wear in future, and this should not be varied without reference to the Limb Fitting Centre, because the alignment and stability of the limb may be affected by the change, and the risk of a fall increased. There is not as much risk for the below-knee wearer in such circumstances, but any gross change of height of heel should be reported to the Limb Fitting Centre. A device for varying the height of the heels of certain types of legs for ladies can be supplied if thought desirable by the limb surgeon.

Long pants present a difficulty when used with artificial legs. Some patients have the leg of the pants cut off near to the top of the artificial leg. Short pants or trunks, although not so warm in winter, are more convenient.

Trousers may need to be protected from damage by a clothing pad of leather fixed to the back of the thigh piece by the limb-maker or by a lining inserted into the back of the trouser leg to prevent wear by the artificial limb. Joints on artificial limbs are now provided with leather or plastic protective covers, and protruberances are either cut down to a minimum or rounded off. Nylon braces may be supplied if preferred in place of webbing ones and a spring clip for shoulder harness in place of a fixed tab is also available. If it is found that the protection is unsatisfactory, the fact should be reported to the Limb Fitting Centre.

Gloves are issued singly to the wearers of artificial hands to meet their special needs, as it may be that the glove on one hand will wear out more quickly than that on the other, or it may be necessary for a different size or even a different type of glove to be worn on each hand.

Care of the stump

It is necessary not only to develop the stump muscles, but also to remember the correct method of bandaging. It is as well to put a bandage on if more than a day has to be spent in bed without using the leg, otherwise the stump may swell, and it may be impossible to get a comfortable fit for a day or two after getting up, until exercise has reduced it again. Some people find that a bandage every night is necessary in order to reduce this tendency of the stump to swell while at rest.

The most important treatment for the skin of the stump is to wash it every day with soap and water. After washing, remove all traces of the soap and then dry the stump thoroughly, taking especial care to dry all scars. Talcum powder may be applied afterwards if considered necessary or desirable. Spirit lotions may dry the skin too much and make it liable to crack.

Washing is necessary to remove salt deposited from perspiration. Salt retains moisture and keeps the skin damp and sticky, causing friction between the skin, stump-sock and socket, with consequent irritation.

Stump-socks. A healthy condition of the stump is maintained by the right size of stump-sock and care should be taken in putting it on, to avoid forming creases or folds in it: it should not be pulled too tightly over the end of the stump. Some amputees attach a piece of tape to the tip of the stump-sock so that, when the sock is put on, the tape can be threaded out through the ventilation hole of the container, enabling the wearer not only to pull the stump into the socket but to pull the tip of the sock away from the end of the stump and by so doing to eliminate creases.

Stump-socks are supplied by the Ministry and should never be washed in hot water or rubbed. The best method of washing is to dissolve soap flakes in lukewarm water: then squeeze the sock in this water by hand only, and never by wringing. To keep the stump in a healthy condition, the stump-socks should be changed as frequently as possible, especially in hot weather. A shrinkage of the stump may cause discomfort. If the shrinkage is slight, comfort may be restored by wearing an extra stump-sock.

In some cases, shrinkage continues to such an extent that several stump-socks have to be worn. Too many stump-socks should not be worn for any length of time, and if it is necessary to wear more than two stump-socks, the Limb Fitting Centre should be told. When the stump increases in size the limb feels too long, and also uncomfortable: in such a case, the Limb Fitting Centre should be informed immediately. Stump-socks which are no longer serviceable will be replaced on application to the Limb Fitting Centre.

Care of the limb

The Ministry of Health is responsible for the maintenance of both the original and duplicate limbs. At the same time every reasonable care should be taken to prevent loss or damage. Remember that these limbs are valuable articles which have been fitted to individual requirements.

Repairs and adjustments. To ensure that a patient is never without one serviceable artificial limb, it is essential that immediately a limb requires repair or alteration of any kind, the patient should at once report the fact on the stamped form provided for the purposes (MHM 169) to the appropriate Limb Fitting Centre. If the form is not available, full particulars as to the repair or adjustment required should be sent by letter to the Limb Fitting Centre.

If the information given on the form or the letter indicates that only a mechanical repair is needed, a box (with a carriage free label) will be sent to the patient (if one is not already in his possession) in which to forward the limb to the Centre for the necessary repair.

If, on the other hand, the information given indicates the need for a refit, the patient will be called to attend the Centre, in which case the limb should be brought or sent in advance. Arrangements can be made for the limb to be conveyed to the Centre in a box with a carriage free label in advance of attendance, if it cannot be brought by the patient. The patient should not in any circumstances continue to wear the limb after a defect has been noticed or a repair become necessary, as by so doing a minor repair or adjustment may become a major repair. Special tools are necessary for the assembly or dismantling of any part of the artificial limb and no attempt, therefore, should be made to take it apart in any particular.

Cleaning the limb. A limb that is kept clean and free from dust and fluff will last longer and will give less trouble than one which is neglected in this respect, and when sent in for repair or examination it should be in a clean condition. Detergents should not be used in washing suspenders and appendages which have leather tabs as they will damage the leather. Leather may be washed in good quality soap and water and the leather tabs, metal buckles and slides should be well dried after washing to prevent deterioration.

Lubrication. The use of lubricating oil is unnecessary as all bearing parts are packed with grease when the limb is delivered, and the grease will last a long time without any attention. The lubrication will automatically receive attention whenever the limb is returned to the Limb Fitting Centre for repair or adjustment.

Try to avoid getting the artificial foot wet, as this may cause deterioration of the foot and ankle joint. For those whose occupation demands it, rubber foot socks can be supplied by the Limb Fitting Centre.

Sport and recreations

Besides the normal everyday activities, there are many sports and hobbies open to those who wear artificial limbs. A great deal will depend on the energy, the inventiveness and the tastes of the individual, as well as on the nature and condition of the stump. Generally speaking, anything which results in the over-straining or chafing of the limb should be avoided, and in cases of doubt the advice of the limb surgeon should be sought. It would be beyond the scope of this booklet to detail the many pastimes which are possible, but swimming, billiards, dancing and bowls are obvious examples of the less strenuous activities. Swimming is regarded as beneficial to the stump. Many persons, both leg and arm amputees, are able to indulge in golf, tennis, badminton, squash, cricket, fishing and shooting. Provided these games are tackled in the right way, they will add greatly to one's confidence and will help to dispel, as nothing else will, any lurking impression that one is a cripple. The Limb Fitting Centre will be ready to advise those interested in any of these sports.

Motoring. The loss of one limb, or even two, does not necessarily prevent a man from driving a motor vehicle, and there are many double leg amputees who have passed the driving test. Any amputee who wishes to know more about motoring for the disabled should ask at the local Limb and Appliance Centre.

Advice to leg amputees who may accidentally be thrown into deep water

These notes have been prepared by the Standing Advisory Committee on Artificial Limbs following swimming experiments by male leg amputees wearing artificial limbs. It is thought that they may prove helpful to leg amputees who are unexpectedly thrown into deep water and they should be memorized.

General. Your clothes can be helpful in keeping you afloat because of the air trapped in them; on the other hand, they are an encumbrance if you want to swim any distance. In addition, the action of swimming will tend to force out the air sooner than if you just float.

The recommendations given here are based on these facts, and in any case should be regarded as a guide only, since what you decide to do will depend on how powerful a swimmer you are as well as on the other factors mentioned.

The guidance given is for the benefit of both above-knee and below-knee amputees; the periods and distances shown in brackets ( ) refer to below-knee amputees only.

If rescue is expected within three minutes (twenty minutes) or thereabouts:
(a) Float on back holding head well back. Do not undress or remove artificial limb.
(b) Gentle paddling motion with the hands may prove helpful in keeping you warm and afloat.
(c) Remove shoe from natural foot if easy to accomplish. If land is within swimmer's range up to a distance of 100 yards (150 yards) or thereabouts:
Remove coat, but nothing else, and swim to land.

If rescue is not expected within three minutes (twenty minutes) or land is beyond swimmer's range:
(a) Remove clothes and artificial limb immediately on entering the water, as suggested below.
(b) Float on back with head held well back until rescue arrives. Alternatively, swim towards land.

N.B. It is recommended that clothes be removed in the following order:
(i)   Coat and waistcoat. If harness permits, these may be retained until last in order to provide extra bouyancy.
(ii) Remove shoe from natural foot.
(iii) Undo braces and lower trousers sufficiently to enable shoulder strap and pelvic band or belt to be undone.
(iv) Remove trousers and pants from the sound leg, allowing these, together with the artificial limb, to fall away—helping with the hands if possible.

Conclusion

As has been pointed out, different individuals will have varying needs, as well as different methods of approach, and it is not claimed that these notes include all that can be said.

If there are any further suggestions which it is felt would help those who wear artificial limbs, they should be sent to the address shown at the foot of p. 592.

33

The Future of Orthopaedics

The pioneers of orthopaedic surgery were mainly occupied in treating the deformities arising from tuberculosis, poliomyelitis and malunited fractures.

They were handicapped by the then limitations of surgery—poor anaesthesia, poor resuscitation facilities, no antibiotics, inadequate knowledge of the body's reactions to metals, etc. Conservative treatment was safer than operation; small operations were much safer than big ones. In chronic infections the surgeon relied chiefly on time and fresh air. For this reason the early orthopaedic hospitals were usually situated in remote country districts.

Today the position is different. Tuberculosis and poliomyelitis have almost disappeared in the United Kingdom and malunion of fractures is rare. With modern anaesthesia and resuscitatory techniques operations are often safer than conservative measures. Antibiotics are more important than fresh air. A general hospital with good supporting ancillary services provides more efficient treatment than a country hospital with an inadequate laboratory. The orthopaedic surgeon mainly treats fresh injuries, congenital deformities, degenerative and other joint diseases and the orthopaedic consequences of neurological disorders. What will be the scope of orthopaedics in the future? Certainly the orthopaedic surgeon will depend even more on scientific and technological knowledge from other sources. Genetics, immunology, endocrinology, metallurgy, virology and psychology are a few of the subjects, a knowledge of which will be increasingly necessary for the future orthopaedic surgeon. Here are a few illustrations of the way orthopaedics is likely to develop.

Congenital conditions

Prevention is now more of a practical proposition in this field because of a better understanding of the development of the embryo and fetus. Thus, toxins from infectious diseases, such as rubella, and the effects of drugs used during pregnancy and their effects on the delicate embryo or fetus in the uterus are understood. Such afflictions as hare-lip and cleft palate, congenital club foot, spina bifida and absence of bones or limbs may be prevented by improved knowledge of fetal development.

Prevention may be demonstrated in the concept of careful examination of infants at birth in diagnosing and treating congenital dislocations of the hip before the condition becomes firmly established.

Recent advances enable the doctor to detect certain types of severe fetal anomaly such as anencephaly and myelomeningocele at an early stage of pregnancy. Detection of an unusual protein in the mother's blood is the first screening test. If this is positive the amniotic fluid is examined: if this is again positive the probabilities can be explained to the parents who can then choose to have the pregnancy terminated or not.

The very early diagnosis of gross fetal abnormalities is obviously of great importance.

Progress in methods of treatment are also seen in children born with defects in the neural canal of the vertebral column. In the past such patients died in early infancy as the result of infections affecting the central nervous system through the opening. In recent years repair of the spina bifida or meningocele has meant the survival of these patients. Similarly, children with hydrocephalus can be helped by the use of the Spitz-Holter valve.

Congenital conditions

During the last few years it has become increasingly apparent that seemingly identical clinical syndromes can be caused by different agents. For instance spinal dysraphism may be of genetic origin, i.e. inherited due to an unfortunate union of adverse genes or it may be due to toxic or other adverse agencies acting on the developing fetus at an early vulnerable stage. An important recent development in this regard is the diagnosis of gross fetal abnormalities at an early stage by aspirating and examining cells in the amniotic fluid. This enables the doctor to present the facts to the parents and discuss with them the best course of action.

Growth conditions

Much research and new principles are applied in the treatment of young people with osteochondritis (softening and deformity of the growth centres of bones). Investigation into the causes of these conditions has moved orthopaedic scientists towards the field of endocrinology.

Biological principles are applied in the treatment of idiopathic scoliosis of the spine by growth arrest of the epiphyseal cartilages of the vertebrae (epiphyseodesis). Similar principles are applied in the attempts to increase the blood supply of the epiphyses of long bones to stimulate the growth of a short limb by the surgical induction of an arteriovenous fistula.

Engineering principles are applied in the lengthening of short limbs by osteotomy and bone grafting, and the use of metal staples in growth centres to retard the growth of a bone. Engineering principles are also applied in the correction of spinal curvature by the use of metal rods and jacks.

Infections

Most of the orthopaedic centres in the United Kingdom owe their origins to skeletal tuberculosis. Although this is rare in the more fortunate countries of the world, it is still a major problem in others. Such countries still await the progress in the public health fields that has overcome the tuberculosis scourge in the wealthier countries. The tuberculostatic drugs (Streptomycin, Para-aminosalicylic acid and Isonicotinic acid hydrazid) used in concert have reduced the length of stay in hospital for sufferers from tuberculous infections and completely altered orthopaedic attitudes. After a relatively short course of treatment spinal tuberculosis is approached surgically, the abscess cleared away and bone grafting performed; previously the treatment of this condition kept the patient on a plaster bed, at complete rest, for some years.

Acute osteomyelitis, an unhappy disease which often became chronic, can be cured by the prompt administration of antibiotics.

Spinal surgery

The surgeon may now perform many operations on the vertebral column and spinal cord which could not have been attempted in the recent past. This has been made possible by the new directions of approach to a spinal lesion which could not have been previously considered when only the posterior approach was known. Thus the front, sides and posterior surfaces of the spine are accessible and osteotomies, fusions, growth arrests and intervertebral disc surgery are now all possible. Much if not most of the advances in spinal surgery are due to a combination of better pre-operative diagnosis by improved radiological techniques and improved anaesthesia, e.g. controlled hypertension to diminish bleeding.

Blood supply of the spine

In all operations, injuries and disorders of the spine the integrity of the blood supply of the spinal cord is of paramount importance. In the thoracic region the blood supply to the spinal cord is often precarious. It is easily impaired by operative interference and even by conservative treatment such as forced correction, corrective plaster jackets or halo-pelvic traction if great care is not taken.

One promising line of investigation to diminish this risk is to take direct electrical records of the action potentials of the spinal cord during treatment. Another is to investigate the blood supply of the spine by vertebral angiography before starting treatment.

Congenital dislocation of the hip

Early diagnosis and treatment of hip laxity in the neonate has diminished but not eliminated the incidence of dislocation of the hip. It seems probable that in addition to the common capsular laxity type there is a rarer type in which there is an intrinsic failure of acetabular development. In this type the hip does not appear to be lax at birth but slowly subluxates as the child grows and starts to walk. Operative interference to deepen the acetabulam is often needed.

Accident surgery

The twentieth century has seen the transference of interest away from poliomyelitis and chronic infection towards the problems created by the increased speed of travel throughout the world. The automobile, aircraft, new fast rail vehicle, and the space vehicle all now move at speeds which result in new dimensions of injury should an accident occur. The numbers of people involved and the multiplicity of their injuries means that there must be new concepts of administration of accident services, better communications, superb accident centres at optimum points, better training for ambulance personnel and the creation of a new person—that is, the mutation of the orthopaedic surgeon and general surgeon, who may be called an accident-surgeon.

In recent years there has been considerable research into the causes of accidents both at home, at work, on roads and in factories.

The causes are complex and include faults in the environment, emotional instability, lack of elementary protective devices, fatigue, drugs, alcohol and lack of training.

On roads, better protective devices, e.g. crash helmets and safety belts in cars, the elimination of blind areas, better warning signs, attention to tyres and good mechanical upkeep of the car are all important. But most accidents involve at least an element of human failure and irritability, bad temper, fatigue, alcohol and undue haste can all be important contributory factors.

Safety guards on machines, protection, particularly for head and feet, are obviously important in factories, mines or building sites.

Injuries to bones and other tissues

The pioneer orthopaedic surgeon used a conservation attitude to the repair of bone and joint lesions out of necessity. 'Rest, prolonged, enforced, and uninterrupted', was found to be the best method in the light of the knowledge and facilities that then existed.

The modern surgeon can reduce the length of the patient's stay in hospital and hence, speed his recovery by surgical intervention at the correct moment in the internal fixation of broken bones and the repair of damaged joints. The pressure of work and the need for the more efficient use of hospital beds has, of course, contributed to this climate of opinion.

Intramedullary nails, the use of plates and screws and bone grafting, using stored, frozen bone are now frequent practice. Other tissues such as skin, fascia, cartilage, tendons and blood vessels may also be replaced by stored, frozen replacement grafts.

The degenerative diseases

The conditions affecting the patient in the 'senior citizen' category have come into the range of progress also. In the treatment of arthritis of the hip, replacement of the joint with metal implants has now progressed to commonplace. Displacement osteotomy of the upper end of the femur to relieve pain, is applicable to a wider range of patients since compression devices for reuniting the bone have been used.

When such procedures are not feasible, synovectomy—the removal of the synovial membrane of a joint—is carried out in concert with the use of the many new drugs now available.

Chronic diseases

Chronic diseases of joints continue to make increasing demands on the orthopaedic surgeon's time.

There is still considerable uncertainty about the relative importance of on the one hand purely mechanical factors such as articular surface incongruity and on the other hand intrinsic deficiencies of cartilage metabolism. It also appears likely that weakness of the subarticular bone with microfractures and areas of collapse plays an important part in degeneration of the joint. Treatment is ideally directed to the most important aetiological factor. If there is mechanical incongruity this should be corrected, if a hypertrophic synovial membrane is having an adverse effect on the joint surfaces (directly or indirectly) it can be removed. If, however, the joint surfaces have been destroyed or there is extensive collapse of the adjacent bone joint replacement should be undertaken.

It is possible in young people to transplant a joint from either another part of their own body (e.g. toe to finger) or from another individual (cadaveric joint complex transplant) but such operations are only indicated in carefully selected young people.

In the majority of patients with rheumatoid or degenerative joint disease, if the joint is badly destroyed they can be helped by implanting an artificial prosthetic joint. These can be classified under four main headings.

1   Interposition arthroplasty, e.g. cup arthroplasty for the hip.

2   Replacement of one joint surface, e.g. Moore prosthesis for the head of the femur; McIntosh prosthesis for the superior surface of the tibia. A sophisticated development of these is the Monk prosthesis for hip replacement. This consists of a metallic femoral head replacement surrounded by a plastic cup manufactured as an integral whole so that movement occurs within the prosthesis, i.e. between the metal and the plastic so that a complete joint replacement is effected although only one of the joint components is replaced.

3   Replacement of bone joint components, e.g. in the case of the hip both femoral and acetabular surfaces are removed and replaced. There are many successful examples of this both in the hip and the knee. The problems are firstly the choice of materials and secondly fixation of the prosthesis to the adjacent bone. At the moment a combination of stainless steel and high density polyethylene appears to be the best combination of materials.

4   Finally the joint may be replaced by a hinged prosthesis as in the knee or finger or by a flexible silastic prosthesis as used in the finger.

Replacement of severed limbs
Recently there has been some success in the suturing and replacement of arms, or hands, legs or feet torn off in accidents. Such success is usually related to rapid action by the surgical team in replacing the part and to the full use of all the facilities that a modern hospital offers.

Prostheses
Engineering progress in providing useful, functional and cosmetically acceptable false limbs has meant much to the amputee or patient born without a limb. Motivated limbs are operated electrically, using transistorized circuits, or with gaseous compression and micro-switches to control them.

Metabolic disorders
Much progress has been made in the control of diseases such as osteoporosis, osteomalacia, and others affecting the composition, structure and thus the

efficiency of bones. This work has mainly been done in specialist metabolic and endocrinal units.

Organ transplantations

Definitions. (i) An *auto* transplant is a transplant of a tissue or organ from one part of the body to another part of the same individual's body.

(ii) A *homo* transplant is a transplant of tissue or organ from one individual to another of the same species.

(iii) A *hetero* transplant is a transplant of a tissue or organ from one animal to another animal of a different species.

Tissue rejections. Normally the body reacts to a foreign protein by what is known as an immunity reaction, which makes it reject the tissue or organ containing the foreign protein—this is analogous to the body's defence mechanism to bacteria which, of course, contain foreign protein.

Until recently, although it was possible to transplant tissue from one part of a patient's body to another, e.g. skin, bone and cartilage grafts, the only tissue which could be successfully transplanted from one individual to another was the cornea. During the last few years, however, there has been great progress in the knowledge of the reasons why tissues from other individuals are rejected by the body, and it is now possible to transplant whole organs from one individual to another. For example, the kidney, the heart and the liver have all been successfully transplanted. Previous to this, transplantation of organs, e.g. the kidney, from one part of an animal's body to another part had been done.

In order to achieve the homotransplantation successfully, it is first of all necessary to suppress the lymphoid tissue responses of the recipient by immunosuppression agents such as azathioprine, corticosteroids and anti-lymphocytic serum.

The donor. The problem of a suitable donor is, of course, a far more complicated one, and either a live donor who is willing to give one of his kidneys has been used or, in the case of unilateral organs such as the heart and liver, these have been taken from patients whose cerebrum is dead although their heart and lung actions have been artificially maintained sufficiently long enough to keep the cells of the donor organ alive.

The recipient. Hitherto, most agents which have been used to suppress the body's immunity reactions—that is, those which enable it to accept a tissue or organ containing foreign protein—also suppress the body's normal defence mechanism for combating infection; therefore, after an organ transplant operation the patient must be nursed in a sterile environment.

In addition, tissue typing—a means of detecting whether the donor's and recipient's lymphocytes are compatible—holds out future promise for advances in this field. Following operation, the recipient must be maintained on continuous immunosuppressive therapy and must be isolated from all infection, being nursed in sterile surroundings. Needless to say, such operations at the moment should only be performed by specialized units with adequate equipment, organization and a specially trained team. In addition to the great technical skill required to join the transplanted organ's blood vessels to the recipient's arteries and veins, an extensive knowledge of immunity is required.

Bone grafting is a well established orthopaedic procedure, more recently surgeons have been performing cartilage grafting to 'reline' joints in which the articular cartilage has been damaged. The cartilage is usually transplanted with a thin slice of underlying bone. Total joint transplants have also been done, using joints from cadavers and some success has been claimed for this method which has been extensively used in Moscow.

Conclusion
This picture is a very favourable one for those of us who acquire orthopaedic conditions in the future. There is still much to be done however. We are still very ignorant about many conditions, such as neoplasms of bone, joint, and cartilage and osteochondritic diseases such as Perthes' disease and the muscular dystrophies.

Appendix

The following sections are reprinted from memoranda issued jointly by The Medical Defence Union and The Royal College of Nursing of the United Kingdom (revised versions 1978).

Safeguards against wrong operations

This Memorandum sets out recommendations based on consultations between the Medical Defence and the Royal College of Nursing, and suggests precautions to avoid the risk of an operation being performed on:
(A) The wrong patient; or
(B) The wrong side, limb or digit.

There may be occasions when the recommendations are not followed, but it must be stressed that standardization of routine procedures will minimize errors, particularly as medical and nursing staff move from one theatre or department to another.

Efforts should be made in all hospitals and by all health authorities to agree on a routine procedure, incorporating the safeguards recommended in this memorandum. Joint committees of medical and nursing staffs should be set up locally for the purpose.

(A) Operating on the wrong patient

Potential causes of error

(i) Patients are not always labelled immediately on admission to hospital.

(ii) In hospitals which undertake a substantial amount of casualty work, and where emergency patients are admitted in quick succession, some of them unconscious, the clinical notes may become attached to the wrong patient. An identity label is sometimes attached to the patient's clothing immediately on his arrival in the casualty department but mistakes may occur if the labelled clothing is taken off the patient when he is admitted to the ward.

(iii) Mistakes may arise if on the day of the operation the beds are changed round. This risk is increased if the day of operation coincides with a change in the nursing staff.

(iv) Mistakes may occur when changes are made in theatre lists after the start of the operating session, particularly if such changes have not been notified to all concerned immediately they have been made. Operation lists should be altered as little as possible and never by telephone.

(v) The absence of a reliable and routine procedure for identifying patients when they are taken to the anaesthetic room or brought into the theatre carries considerable risk. *There may be other patients of the same or similar name in the ward.*

Recommended safeguards

(a) All patients should be labelled immediately on admission to hospital.

(b) The identity bracelet should be of a reliable pattern and bear the patient's name, including the forenames in full, hospital number and if possible address and age. Departmental numbers should never be used in place of the hospital number.

(c) The labelling of an unconscious patient admitted through the casualty department should be the responsibility of the casualty sister or her deputy, or at night the nurse in charge or her deputy. The identity bracelet is the most reliable means of labelling an unconscious patient.

(d) The ward sister or her deputy should be responsible for checking that all patients who are to undergo an operation have been properly labelled.

(e) Day patients who are to undergo any operative procedure should be labelled in the same way as in-patients.

(f) As the case history of a child must be taken from the patient's relatives (who may not be present immediately before the operation), care must be taken to ensure that in the notes no error occurs in reference to the side, limb or digit on which the operation is to be performed. In a children's ward the identity bracelets should be of a type which can be removed only by an adult.

(g) The ward sister or her deputy should be responsible for seeing that:

    (i)   the correct patient is sent to the operating theatre;

    (ii) the appropriate form of consent to anaesthetic/operation has been completed and signed;

    (iii) the patient has received the prescribed pre-operative preparation, including premedication;

    (iv) where appropriate, the side of the operation has been marked;

    (v) the correct case papers, radiographs, etc. accompany the patient to the theatre.

(h) The operation list should be typed and photo-copied and should show the nature of the operation and the patient's full name and hospital number.

A copy of the operation list should be displayed in the anaesthetic room, the operating theatre and the post-operative recovery room. The list should also be sent to all wards in which patients are awaiting operation and displayed in all places where the patient is to undergo operation.

(i)   Any alteration in the operation list must be made on every relevant copy by a designated person.

(j)   In the operating theatre one person should be responsible for sending for patients. This should normally be the senior nurse in charge of the theatres but in large operating suites it may be necessary for her to delegate this responsibility to some other person, such as the nurse in charge of a particular theatre, the nurse taking the list in a particular theatre or another designated person.

(k) Patients should be sent for from the operating theatre by name and number and never as 'the patient from such and such a ward'. Where it is the practice for a porter from the theatre to collect the patient from the ward he should bring with him a slip bearing the full name and hospital number of the patient.

(l)   When the patient is to be given a general anaesthetic the anaesthetist has a responsibility for ensuring that the right patient has been brought to the anaesthetic room or to the operating theatre. Before induction of anaesthesia he should check the consent form and examine the other records accompanying the patient to make sure that they relate to that particular patient. If the patient is not to be given a general anaesthetic the practitioner who is to perform the operation or carry out the examination should be responsible for ensuring that the correct patient has been brought to the anaesthetic room or operating theatre and that the correct side, limb or digit is identified.

(m) The surgeon has a responsibility to see the patient before he is anaesthetized. He should make sure that the accompanying documents relate to that particular patient. If the surgeon cannot examine the patient's clinical records before the start of the anaesthetic he may delegate this responsibility to his assistant. Before beginning the operation the surgeon or his assistant should check that the patient's full name and hospital number, and the nature of the operation, as set out on the operation list, correspond with the entries in the patient's notes.

(n) *If for any reason the identity bracelet is removed from an unconscious patient special care must be taken to ensure that no mistake is made about his identification. The bracelet should be replaced as soon as practicable.*

(B) Operating on the wrong side, limb or digit

Potential causes of error

(i) Wrong information on the case papers of the patients—'right' instead of 'left'.

(ii) Failure to examine the patient clinically in the immediate pre-operative period.

(iii) Abbreviation of the words 'right' and 'left'.

(iv) Illegible writing on the case papers.

(v) Fingers referred to by number instead of by name.

(vi) Failure to check immediately before the administration of the anaesthetic that the entry on the operation list agrees with the notes taken to the operating theatre.

(vii) Wrong case papers accompanying the patient.

(viii) Preparation of the wrong side, limb or digit.

(ix) Absence of routine procedure for marking the operation site.

(x) Radiograph being incorrectly and inadequately labelled.

Recommended safeguards

(a) The side on which the operation is to be performed should be marked before the patient reaches the operating theatre suite and the mark should be made with an indelible skin pencil which may be seen clearly by the surgeon before starting the operation. The mark may be made on or near the operation site and this is particularly important in the case of digits. A possible exception would be the accident case with obvious wounds needing attention. The side and site of operation in a small child should be marked on the child in the presence of the parent or guardian while the consent form is being completed.

(b) Marking should normally be the responsibility of the surgeon or house surgeon. If there is no resident staff the surgeon should himself accept this responsibility.

(c) If the ward sister or her deputy finds that the site of the operation has not been marked when the patient is due to be sent to the operating theatre, she should ensure that the surgeon who is to operate is informed but *she should not herself undertake the marking*.

(d) If a patient is taken direct from the casualty department to the operating theatre the practitioner who decides upon an immediate operation should be responsible for marking the operation side.

(e) The words 'right' and 'left' should be printed in full on the patient's notes and on the operation list.

(f) In order to avoid ambiguity concerning the digit(s) on which the operation is to be performed, the following nomenclatures should always be used. The fingers should be described as thumb, index, middle, ring and little fingers and not as 1st, 2nd, 3rd, 4th and 5th, and the toes as hallux (or big), 2nd, 3rd, 4th and 5th (or little).

(g) All reference to the operation type or site should be written in full.

Year	Total	Wrong patient or operation	Wrong side	Wrong digit
		Wrong operations		
1960	9	1	6	2
1961	23	3	12	8
1962	16	5	11	—
1963	13	3	5	5
1964	29	2	11	10
1965	16	4	11	1
1966	11	6	3	2
1967	26	5	16	5
1968	13	4	7	2
1969	16	3	10	3
1970	23	6	13	4
1971	17	5	8	4
1972	22	7	8	7
1973	16	8	7	1
1974	16	5	9	2
1975	22	12	7	3
1976	20	5	8	7

Safeguards against failure to remove swabs and instruments from patients

This Memorandum sets out recommendations after consultations between the Medical Defence Union and the Royal College of Nursing. While it may not always be possible to follow all the recommendations, it is stressed that standardization of routine procedures will minimize errors, particularly when medical and nursing staff move from one theatre to another during an operating session.

Unintentional failure to remove a swab or instrument from a patient's body is negligence on someone's part and provides grounds for an action against the surgeon, the health authority or both; if the patient suffers ill effects he will be entitled to damages.

The surgeon has a duty to take resonable precautions to ensure that all swabs and instruments used during the operations are removed. The extent of his personal obligation will vary from case to case. Sometimes he may be compelled to discharge his duty in part or in whole by relying on the nurses, for example if the patient's condition becomes so grave during the operation that it is necessary to finish as speedily as possible. In such a situation the surgeon may have to cut short or even dispense with his own check and rely on the nurse's swab and instrument counts. The health authority also has a duty in this matter as the employer of the nursing staff and as the supplier of the swabs and instruments. There are steps which the health authority, as well as the surgeon, must take to avoid such a mishap. Every hospital should have an operating department committee composed of representatives of the surgical, anaesthetic and nursing staffs to keep theatre procedure under review.

Retained foreign bodies
(swabs, instruments, needles, drains and tubes)

cases reported to The Medical Defence Union

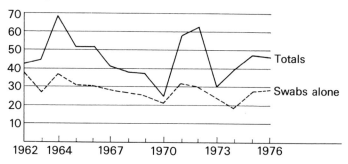

(A) Swabs and packs
Potential causes of inaccurate counts and failure to remove swabs and packs

   (i)   Emphasis on speed either for its own sake or because the patient is critically ill at the start of the operation or becomes so during the procedure.

   (ii) Working under pressure.

   (iii) The above may result in there being insufficient time for a careful first count or in the next patient being brought into theatre before it has been ascertained that no swabs have been left from the previous operation.

(iv) A scrub nurse who is insufficiently experienced or who has insufficient authority to insist on the surgeon following an effective procedure for the care of swabs; a dangerous situation is created if the operating surgeon is new to the hospital or inexperienced.

(v) Failure to make an efficient check that all packs have been removed, especially when packs without clips attached have been used.

(vi) Attaching a swab or instrument to a specimen which is removed from the operating theatre during the operation.

(vii) A change in membership of the operating team during the operation.

(viii) Multiple operative procedures on the same patient.

Recommended safeguards—Accounting

(a) A count should always be made by the scrub and circulating nurse of the swabs and packs used by the surgeon and his assistants during any operation, however minor or superficial. Whatever holds them together should be counted and checked, including rubber bands.

(b) All swabs and packs to be used should be in bundles of FIVE and should be counted again before the start of the operation and the number recorded in accordance with the practice of the particular theatre. Each bundle should be opened and the contents counted to ensure that it contains five swabs or packs and that each has a radio-opaque marker. It should not be assumed that packs from manufacturers contain five; more or less than five have sometimes been discovered.

(c) Before the operation wound is closed both the scrub and circulating nurses should count the swabs and packs used and satisfy themselves that the count is correct. *The surgeon must allow sufficient time for the check to be made.* Before the completion of the operation the surgeon should ascertain by direct inquiry whether all the swabs and packs have been accounted for.

(d) A count of all swabs and packs should be made before closing any internal cavity or organ.

(e) If the surgeon decides to close the wound before the nurse is satisfied about the accuracy of the count or if there is an unsatisfactory count, the nurse should inform the senior nurse in charge of the theatre immediately.

(f) After the first count has been taken and found to be correct the scrub nurse and the surgeon should keep a careful check on any swabs or packs still in use, as mistakes may occur at this time. On completion of closure and before the patient leaves the theatre a final count should be made.

(g) Tapes and other materials used for retracting ureters or blood vessels should also be checked.

(h) Swabs, packs and instruments should not be removed from the theatre until all incisions are closed and final checks are completed and found to be correct.

(i) If the swab count remains unsatisfactory after all steps have been taken the relevant part of the body should be X-rayed before the anaesthetic is discontinued to ensure that a missing swab is not in the patient.

(j) When a count shows a discrepancy the head of the nursing services should be informed by the nurse in charge of the theatre and the surgeon should inform his chief. A record of the discrepancy should be made in the patient's notes and be recorded in the theatre register.

(k) If a mistake in the swab or instrument count is discovered after the operating session is concluded, it should be reported at once, through the appropriate channels, to the surgeon.

Types of swab

(1) All swabs and packs used by the surgeon should be white and should contain radio-opaque material.

(2) All swabs, including throat packs, used by the anaesthetist and his assistants should be coloured and contain radio-opaque material. The anaesthetist should personally be responsible for the removal of any swabs that he inserts into the patient's mouth or throat.

(3) Variation in the size of packs and swabs should be avoided so far as possible. The use of small swabs should, in general, be avoided, or they should be clamped in swab holders. It is appreciated that in certain types of surgery small swabs and strips of gauze have to be used.

(4) All swabs and packs, both white and coloured, should conform to the British Pharmaceutical Codex standard.

During operation

(1) Swabs used for swabbing the skin before the incision is made should contain a radio-opaque marker and be included in the count.

(2) Packs or swabs should not be cut or divided.

(3) In general packs should have tapes attached to which clips or forceps should be fixed by the nurse or surgeon, but it is recognized that on occasion a surgeon may have a good reason for not attaching a clip or for using packs without tapes.

(4) The scrub nurse should control the number of swabs and packs on the table at every stage of the operation.

(5) As an additional safeguard the surgeon should tell the other members of the team whenever he introduces a swab or a pack into a particular area of

the operation field. Theatre practice should allow for this information to be recorded.

Post-operative procedure
(1) Gauze containing radio-opaque material should never be used for skin dressings, as it may be misleading in subsequent X-rays.
(2) When a patient is returned to the ward after an operation with a swab, pack or tube deliberately left in the vagina or other cavity or in a wound, this should be recorded in the notes.
(3) All tubes and drains should have a retaining device to prevent retraction into the wound. Clear written instructions should be given about removal.

(B) Instruments
(1) The scrub nurse should count all the instruments on her table before the start of the operation.
(2) The scrub nurse should check that the instruments and parts of instruments are correct before the operation wound is closed. This particularly applies to haemostats. *The surgeon must allow sufficient time for the check to be made.* He must inquire whether all the instruments, as well as the swabs and packs, have been accounted for.

(C) Needles
(1) The scrub nurse should count all the needles on the table before the start of the operation.
(2) The scrub nurse, after handing a needle to the surgeon, should not part with another needle until the used one has been returned to her.
(3) No needle should be removed from the theatre until the final count has been made and the operation completed.
(4) If more than one needle is in use at the same time, the scrub nurse should ensure that all the needles are returned to her. The number of atraumatic needles must correspond with the number of packets opened: the empty packets should be kept and counted.
(5) Needles should be counted before closure of the wound and the scrub nurse should inform the surgeon at once if the count is wrong.
(6) *The co-operation of the surgeon is essential in carrying out this count and in allowing time for it to be completed.*

Special situations
(a) When the surgeon is working alone without the assistance of a scrub nurse, whether in an operating theatre, in the casualty or out-patient theatre

or in the labour ward, it is more than ever necessary to ensure that no swab, instrument or needle is left in the patient's body.

(b) Swabs are easily left in body cavities. The risk in operations through the mouth, such as adenoidectomy, is especially great.

(c) In obstetric operations, where there may be considerable bleeding, it is a good rule never to put loose swabs into the vagina; a tampon with an attached tape which can be left outside is safer.

(D) Training and instruction

Nursing staff

(i) All nurses who work in the operating theatre must be made fully aware of their responsibilities.

(ii) A detailed routine procedure for the care of swabs and instruments should be set out in writing. Each nurse whose duties necessitate her entry into the operating theatre, whether trained or in training, should be handed a copy of the instructions and have them explained to her. The nurse should sign a statement that she has read and understood this procedure.

(ii) After each operation a record should be kept indicating that the checks were satisfactory at the conclusion of the operation. This should be signed by the nurse who has scrubbed for the case and by the circulating nurse who checked the swabs and instruments with her. This should be kept in a special column in the operation register. This is important because litigation concerning the leaving of a foreign body in a patient during an operation may not be started for months or years after the date of the operation. The names of those involved should be recorded.

Surgical and radiological staff

(a) Where this has not already been done a theatre procedure should be agreed by the committee referred to on page 2 and be set out in writing.

(b) All medical officers, in particular surgical registrars and house surgeons new to the hospital, should be given copies of the procedure.

(c) The surgeon must satisfy himself that the system for counting swabs and instruments is efficient and that the persons responsible are familiar with the system and competent to carry it out. This is particularly important when the surgeon is working with a nurse who does not routinely scrub for him, and applies especially in nursing homes and private wings of hospitals where visiting surgeons operate.

(d) *The surgeon himself must take all reasonable precautions to minimize his dependence on the nurse's swab and instrument counts and at the appropriate stage in the operation must search the operation field as far as is possible and compatible with the safety of the patient.*

(e) All members of the surgical and radiological staff should be aware of the type of swabs and packs in use in the hospital and be familiar with their radiological appearance.

(f) Any change in the type of radio-opaque material in the swabs and packs supplied to the hospital should be notified to the surgical and radiological staff. There is a wide variety of opaque markers. A radiograph of all the types of radio-opaque swab markers should be available and continually updated.

An Orthopaedic Glossary

Abduction   To move the arm, leg or thumb away from the median line of the body. The reverse of *adduction*.

Acetabulum   The socket of the hip joint situated in the pelvis.

Achondroplasia   Absence of growth at the epiphyseal cartilages.

Acromioclavicular   The region of the shoulder where the clavicle and scapula meet.

Adduction   Movement of the arm, leg or thumb towards the median line. The reverse of *abduction*.

Amputation   Severance of all or part of an extremity.

Analgesia   Reduced sensitivity to pain but not unconsciousness.

Ankylosis   Stiffening or fusion of a joint as the result of disease.

Anterior   The front or foremost surface or area of the body, or organ, or part, when in the anatomical position.

Approximate   To bring together as in manipulating bone fragments, the ends of ruptured tendons, or the edges of the wounds.

Arthritis   Inflammation within a joint.

Arthrodesis   An operation performed to stabilize or fuse a joint so that no further movement will occur in that joint.

Arthroplasty   Reconstruction of a joint by a surgical procedure.

Arthrotomy   To surgically enter, or open, a joint.

Articular cartilage   The tissue covering the ends of the bones involved in the formation of a joint.

Arthrogryposis   Congenital stiffness of many joints of the arms and legs.

Articulation   Point of union of two or more bones. A joint.

Aseptic necrosis   Death of bone cells without infection or inflammation.

Aspiration (of a joint or cavity)   To drain pus or fluid via a hollow-needle.

Ataxia   Loss of co-ordination. Disorganization of voluntary movements.

Athetosis   A pathological state in which there are useless, uncontrolled, involuntary movements.

Atrophy   Wasting. Cessation of growth.

Avascular necrosis   Death of bone cells (and thus bone) due to cessation of a blood supply.

Avulsion   Separation, by force, of two connected parts.

Axillary   Pertaining to the armpit.

Bilateral   On both sides.

Bloodless field   An operation performed after the blood has been removed and prevented from returning to the site.

Bursa   Sac made of synovial membrane containing synovial fluid. It serves as a cushioning device.

Cartilage   Hard yet flexible material which serves as a shock-absorbing cushion.

Cancellous bone   Tissue in bone which is light in weight and has many spaces in it, containing marrow.

Cavus   Hollowed.   The foot deformity in which the longitudinal arch becomes abnormally high.

Cervical   Pertaining to the neck.

Chisel   An instrument with one sharp bevelled edge used to cut bone.

Chondromalacia   Erosion of the articular cartilage.

Closed reduction   To re-align a broken bone without making an incision into the skin.

Compact bone   Tissue in bone which is dense and devoid of spaces in it.

Complicated fracture   An injury which combines a fracture with involvement of a nerve, blood-vessel or organ.

Compound fracture   An injury which combines an open wound and a broken bone.

Cortex   The peripheral portion of a bone. Usually made of compact bone.

Coxa   The hip-joint.

Crepitus   To rub against or grind. Usually at a site of fracture.

Cubitus   Pertaining to the elbow-joint.

Cyst   A cavity or space.

Debridement   Surgical removal of dead and foreign tissue from a wound.

Defect   Absence of continuity.

Degenerative bone disease   Any condition which results in a progressive deterioration of bone.

Devitalised   Deprived of a blood-supply.

Diaphysis   The shaft of a long bone.

Disarticulate   Amputation or separation through a joint.

Dislocation   Displacement from an original position. Usually applied to joints.

Distal   End of an extremity or bone furthest from the trunk.

Donor   Source of bone or other material to be used at another site or another person.

Dyschondroplasia   Abnormality of growth or development of the epiphyseal cartilages.

Dyscrasia   An abnormal state of the body.

Dysplasia   Abnormality of development or formation.

Dystrophy   Abnormal growth.

Elective surgery   A surgical procedure performed at the convenience of the patient and surgeon.

Electrolytic reaction   A phenomenon which occurs when two dissimilar metals are in contact in a salty medium.

Epiphyseodesis   Retardation, by surgical means, of development at a growth centre.

Epiphysis   The two ends of the long bone before ossification is complete.

Equinus   A deformity in which the foot points downwards (plantar flexion) and the patient walks on the heads of the metatarsal bones.

Erosion   Degenerative destruction.

Exostosis   A bony outgrowth.

Extracapsular   Exterior to the capsule of a synovial joint.

Fibrous-union   Broken bone which has united with soft, not bony, tissue.

Fissure   Groove or crack in a tissue.

Fracture   Any break in the continuity of a bone.

Geriatrics   The medical management of the elderly patient.

Gouge   An orthopaedic instrument with a curved sharp cutting edge for cutting a furrow or channel.

Graft   Transfer of tissue from one site to another, possibly to a different person.

Immobilisation   Fixation so that no movement can occur.

Implants   Plates, screws, nails or other devices used, in a surgical wound.

Inert   Produces no reaction in the tissues.

Intertrochanteric   Between the two bony processes (trochanters) on the femur.

Intramedullary   Within the medullary canal of a long bone.

Intrathecal   Within the cavity containing the spinal cord.

Involucrum   The excessive growth of new bone underneath the periosteum at the site of a lesion in the bone.

Ischaemia   An inadequate or deficient blood supply because of obstruction of blood-vessels to a part.

Kyphosis   A deformity of the spine which causes a hump on the back.

Ligament   Band of strong fibrous tissue which joins bones at a joint.

Lordosis   A deformity which occurs when the spine is bent backwards.

Loxotomy   An oblique amputation.

Lumbar   Pertaining to the lumbar region of the vertebral column.

Myelitis   Inflammation of the spinal cord.

Malignant   Grows worse and resists treatment.

Mal-union   Broken bone which has united but in an incorrect position.

Manipulation   The use of the hands as in reducing a fracture or dislocation.

Marrow   Soft material found in the spaces of bone. It is mainly concerned with the reproduction of blood.

Median line   An imaginary line at the exact centre of the body.

Metaphysis   The portion of a child's bone between the epiphysis and diaphysis where growth activity occurs.

Metatarsalgia   Pain in the part of the foot in the metatarsal region.

Mobilization   Allowing mobility after treatment by immobilization.

Muscle atrophy   Wasting away of muscle tissue because of disuse of paralysis.

Necrosis   Death of bone cells.

Neuritis   Inflammation of nervous tissue.

Neuroglioma   A tumour of the special connective tissue of the nervous system.

Neuroma   A tumour of a nerve.

Non-union   Failure of broken bone fragments to heal and unite.

Nutrient vessel   A blood vessel which serves a bone.

Open reduction   Re-aligning the broken fragments of a bone, and securing them, through a surgical wound.

Orthopaedic appliance   Traction apparatus, splints, calipers, supports and any similar equipment used in orthopaedic management.

Osseous tissue   Bone tissue.

Osteochondritis   An inflammatory reaction affecting bone and cartilage.

Osteoid   Immature bone tissue.

Osteomalacia   Failure of calcification of osteoid tissue with resultant bending of the soft bones.

Osteomyelitis   Infection of bone.

Osteoporosis   Condition in which bones become demineralized and soft and spongy.

Osteotome   A sharp bone-cutting implement similar to a chisel but bevelled on both surfaces.

Osteotomy   A surgical operation in which bone is cut.

Periphery   The outermost boundary or limit.

Pes   Pertaining to the foot.

Posterior   The hindmost surface or area of an organ, or part of the body.

Prosthesis   Metal or other device used to replace a bone, part of a bone, a joint, or a complete limb.

Proximal   The end of a bone or limb nearest to the trunk.

Pseudoarthrosis   A false joint.

Sacral   Pertaining to the sacral area of the spine.

Scoliosis   The deformity of the spine which exists when the spine is curved to the side.

Sequestrum   A necrotic fragment of bone which has become detached and protrudes from a wound.

Spasticity   Imperfect voluntary control of muscles with stiff jerking movements.

Spondylitis   Arthritis of the vertebral column.

Spondylosis   Non-infective disease of the spine in which there is ankylosis.

Stability   Steadiness, firmness.

Stress   Abnormal strain such as that to which a metal implant might be subjected.

Subluxation   Displacement of two articular surfaces short of a dislocation.

Suppurative arthritis   Inflammation within a joint including the presence of pus and related debris.

Synovial membrane   The secretory membrane which lines joints and covers structures within them.

Talipes   Deformities in which the tarsal joints are involved.

Tendon   Fibrous tissue connecting muscle tissue to bone and other parts.

Tendonitis   Inflammation of a tendon.

Tendosynovitis   Inflammation of the lining of a tendon sheath.

Tendovaginitis   Mild chronic inflammation of the wall of a tendon sheath. This prevents the free movement of the tendon within the sheath.

Thoracic   Pertaining to the chest or thorax.

Thoracotomy   Opening the chest cavity by surgical incision.

Tourniquet   A device used in the operating theatre to obstruct the blood supply to a part.

Traction   Pulling along the length of a limb or part.

Transient paralysis   Temporary loss of sensation and ability to move a part.

Trauma   Injury or damage to the body.

Unilateral   One side only.

Valgus   Initially this meant bow-legged, but has since become the opposite, i.e. knock-kneed. When applied to the hip, as in coxa valga, it refers to the fact that the angle between the shaft and neck of the femur usually 120° is increased. When applied to the foot, as in talipes valgus, it means eversion of the foot. In hallux valgus the great toe is angulated towards the other. It means, therefore, a divergence of the part indicated away from the mid-line. Cubitus valgus is an angulation of the elbow.

Varus   This denotes that the part named is angulated towards the mid-line of the body, e.g. talipes varus, inversion of the foot. In coxa vara, the angle between the shaft and neck of the femur is decreased. Genu vara now means bow-legged and cubitus vara means a similar angulation at the elbow.

Z-plasty   Repair of skin defect by the transposition of two triangular flaps.

Index